Fast Facts for the **NURSE PSYCHOTHERAPIST**: The Process of Becoming *(Jones, Tusaie)*

Fast Facts About **NURSING AND THE LAW**: Law for Nurses *(Grant, Ballard)*

Fast Facts About the **NURSING PROFESSION**: Historical Perspectives *(Hunt)*

Fast Facts for the **OPERATING ROOM NURSE**: An Orientation and Care Guide, Second Edition *(Criscitelli)*

Fast Facts for the **PEDIATRIC NURSE**: An Orientation Guide *(Rupert, Young)*

Fast Facts Handbook for **PEDIATRIC PRIMARY CARE:** A Guide for Nurse Practitioners and Physician Assistants *(Ruggiero, Ruggiero)*

Fast Facts About **PRESSURE ULCER CARE FOR NURSES**: How to Prevent, Detect, and Resolve Them *(Dziedzic)*

Fast Facts About **PTSD**: A Guide for Nurses and Other Health Care Professionals *(Adams)*

Fast Facts for the **RADIOLOGY NURSE**: An Orientation and Nursing Care Guide, Second Edition *(Grossman)*

Fast Facts About **RELIGION FOR NURSES**: Implications for Patient Care *(Taylor)*

Fast Facts for the **SCHOOL NURSE**: What You Need to Know, Third Edition *(Loschiavo)*

Fast Facts About **SEXUALLY TRANSMITTED INFECTIONS**: A Nurse's Guide to Expert Patient Care *(Scannell)*

Fast Facts for **STROKE CARE NURSING**: An Expert Care Guide, Second Edition *(Morrison)*

Fast Facts for the **STUDENT NURSE**: Nursing Student Success *(Stabler-Haas)*

Fast Facts About **SUBSTANCE USE DISORDERS**: What Every Nurse, APRN, and PA Needs to Know *(Marshall, Spencer)*

Fast Facts for the **TRAVEL NURSE**: Travel Nursing *(Landrum)*

Fast Facts for the **TRIAGE NURSE**: An Orientation and Care Guide, Second Edition *(Visser, Montejano)*

Fast Facts for the **WOUND CARE NURSE**: Practical Wound Management *(Kifer)*

Fast Facts for **WRITING THE DNP PROJECT**: Effective Structure, Content, and Presentation *(Christenbery)*

Forthcoming FAST FACTS Books

Fast Facts for the **ADULT-GERONTOLOGY ACUTE CARE NURSE PRACTITIONER** *(Carpenter)*

Fast Facts About **COMPETENCY-BASED EDUCATION IN NURSING**: How to Teach Competency Mastery *(Wittmann-Price, Gittings)*

Fast Facts for **CREATING A SUCCESSFUL TELEHEALTH SERVICE**: A How-to Guide for Nurse Practitioners *(Heidesch)*

Fast Facts About **DIVERSITY, EQUITY, AND INCLUSION** *(Davis)*

Fast Facts for the **ER NURSE**: Guide to a Successful Emergency Department Orientation, Fourth Edition *(Buettner)*

Fast Facts for the **L&D NURSE**: Labor & Delivery Orientation, Third Edition *(Groll)*

Fast Facts About **LGBTQ CARE FOR NURSES** *(Traister)*

Fast Facts for the **NEONATAL NURSE**: Care Essentials for Normal and High-Risk Neonates, Second Edition *(Davidson)*

Fast Facts for the **NURSE PRECEPTOR**: Keys to Providing a Successful Preceptorship, Second Edition *(Ciocco)*

Fast Facts for **PATIENT SAFETY IN NURSING** *(Hunt)*

Visit www.springerpub.com to order.

FAST FACTS HANDBOOK for
PEDIATRIC PRIMARY CARE

Kristine M. Ruggiero, PhD, MSN, RN, CPNP-BC, began her career in nursing after graduating from Yale University as a pediatric nurse practitioner in the primary care track, with a special concentration in pediatric chronic illness management. After her son was diagnosed with a congenital heart defect (CHD), Dr. Ruggiero obtained her doctorate and focused her research on the care coordination of children with chronic illnesses. Her research validated that understanding a parent's perceptions of their child's health status is important, as parents drive healthcare utilization in the pediatric setting.

Dr. Ruggiero has extensive clinical experience as both a pediatric nurse and pediatric nurse practitioner in various inpatient and outpatient acute care and primary care settings. Currently, Dr. Ruggiero practices clinically at Boston Children's Hospital.

Dr. Ruggiero is also actively involved in research and presents her research nationally and internationally. She is a nurse scientist at Boston Children's Hospital in the Department of Medicine. Dr. Ruggiero has held academic appointments for the past 15 years and serves currently as an assistant professor of nursing at MGH Institute of Health Professions, teaching in both the pediatric nurse practitioner and accelerated BSN programs. Dr. Ruggiero is also co-founder of the Boston Nursing Institute (BNI), an educational and consulting platform for nurses.

Michael S. Ruggiero, MHS, BS, PA-C, graduated from Quinnipiac University with a master's degree in health science and physician assistant studies. Studying sports medicine and athletic training in his undergraduate studies, Michael built on his interest in orthopedics by starting out his career as a physician assistant (PA) in orthopedic surgery. Since then, Michael has practiced and served for the past 17 years in the fields of orthopedic medicine, pediatric and adult urgent care, and physician assistant education.

Michael has been an assistant professor of physician assistant studies at the University of New England, and he currently teaches at MGH Institute of Health Professions. In addition to teaching, Michael has held many leadership roles in PA education, including as the director of clinical education and remediation coordinator, working with at-risk PA students. Michael's leadership at the institute has been recognized with the Partners in Excellence (PIE) award thrice, honoring him for outstanding work in the areas of leadership and innovation in PA education.

FAST FACTS HANDBOOK for PEDIATRIC PRIMARY CARE

A Guide for Nurse Practitioners and Physician Assistants

Kristine M. Ruggiero, PhD, MSN, RN, CPNP-BC

Michael S. Ruggiero, MHS, BS, PA-C

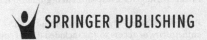

Springer Publishing Company, LLC
11 West 42nd Street, New York, NY 10036
www.springerpub.com
connect.springerpub.com/

Acquisitions Editor: Elizabeth Nieginski
Compositor: Amnet Systems

ISBN: 978-0-8261-5183-4
e-book ISBN: 978-0-8261-5184-1
DOI: 10.1891/9780826151841

20 21 22 23 24 / 5 4 3 2 1

The author and the publisher of this Work have made every effort to use sources believed to be reliable to provide information that is accurate and compatible with the standards generally accepted at the time of publication. Because medical science is continually advancing, our knowledge base continues to expand. Therefore, as new information becomes available, changes in procedures become necessary. We recommend that the reader always consult current research and specific institutional policies before performing any clinical procedure or delivering any medication. The author and publisher shall not be liable for any special, consequential, or exemplary damages resulting, in whole or in part, from the readers' use of, or reliance on, the information contained in this book. The publisher has no responsibility for the persistence or accuracy of URLs for external or third-party Internet websites referred to in this publication and does not guarantee that any content on such websites is, or will remain, accurate or appropriate.

Library of Congress Cataloging-in-Publication Data

Names: Ruggiero, Kristine M., author. | Ruggiero, Michael S., author.
Title: Fast facts handbook for pediatric primary care : a guide for nurse
    practitioners and physician assistants / Kristine M. Ruggiero, Michael S.
    Ruggiero.
Other titles: Fast facts (Springer Publishing Company)
Description: New York, NY : Springer Publishing Company, LLC, [2021] |
    Series: Fast facts | Includes bibliographical references and index.
Identifiers: LCCN 2020019769 (print) | LCCN 2020019770 (ebook) | ISBN
    9780826151834 (paperback) | ISBN 9780826151841 (ebook)
Subjects: MESH: Primary Health Care | Pediatrics—methods | Infant | Child |
    Handbook
Classification: LCC RJ61 (print) | LCC RJ61 (ebook) | NLM WS 39 | DDC
    618.92—dc23
LC record available at https://lccn.loc.gov/2020019769
LC ebook record available at https://lccn.loc.gov/2020019770

Contact us to receive discount rates on bulk purchases.
We can also customize our books to meet your needs.
For more information please contact: sales@springerpub.com

Kristine M. Ruggiero: https://orcid.org/0000-0001-5602-2637
Michael S. Ruggiero: https://orcid.org/0000-0002-1268-0520

"While we try to teach our children all about life, our children teach us what life is all about."
—Angela Schwindt

This book is dedicated to all the pediatric patients and families who we have cared for in our practices over the years and who we have learned so much from. To our own four beautiful children, Jagger, Brody, Cruz, and Lola Mae, who are our greatest gifts in life and remind us every day to be thankful for our blessings and to keep laughing and loving life. We love you more than words.

Thank you to the MGH Institute of Health Professions PA program for their kindness and support in writing this book. Thank you to my co-author on this book and in life—I have learned so much from you on how to love, live, and learn. If life is like a box of chocolates, you have made mine full of sea-salted caramel! (Mike)

To my collaborator in life and on this book, thank you for your unrelenting love for me and our family. I am lucky to be on this journey with you. (Kristine) And lastly, I would like to dedicate this book to the memory of my late grandparents, Mary E. McCue and James P. McCue III (Bunka), who were endless believers in all of their children and grandchildren. I carry their memory and inspiration with me every day. (Kristine)

Contents

Part III   POINT-OF-CARE TESTING

Contributors

Laura Cline, MSN, RN, CPNP, FNP
Pediatric and Family Nurse Practitioner
Department of Medicine
Boston Children's Hospital
Boston, Massachusetts

Leah Hecht, MSN, RN, CPNP
Pediatric Nurse Practitioner
Division of Genetics & Genomics
Boston Children's Hospital
Boston, Massachusetts

Sharon Lincoln, MS, CGC
Senior Genetic Counselor
Division of Genetics & Genomics
Boston Children's Hospital
Boston, Massachusetts

Elizabeth Maloney, MSN, RN, CPNP
Pediatric Nurse Practitioner
Department of Neurology
Boston Children's Hospital
Boston, Massachusetts

Josh Merson, MPAS, MS-HPEd, PA-C, EM-CAQ
Associate Director and Assistant Professor
MGH Institute of Health Professions
Boston, Massachusetts

M. T. Parsons, MSN, RN, CPNP
Pediatric Nurse Practitioner
Department of Cardiology
Boston Children's Hospital
Boston, Massachusetts

Kristine M. Ruggiero, PhD, MSN, RN, CPNP-BC
Pediatric Nurse Practitioner and Nurse Scientist
Department of Medicine
Boston Children's Hospital
Assistant Professor of Nursing
MGH Institute of Health Professions
Boston, Massachusetts

Michael S. Ruggiero, MHS, BS, PA-C
Assistant Professor
MGH Institute of Health Professions
Physician Assistant
Partners Urgent Care
Boston, Massachusetts

Rebecca Sarvendram, MSN, RN, CPNP
Pediatric Nurse Practitioner
Department of Neurology
Boston Children's Hospital
Boston, Massachusetts

Meredith Scannell, PhD, MSN, MPH, CNM, CEN, SANE-A
Clinical Research Nurse
Center for Clinical Investigation
Brigham and Women's Hospital
Boston, Massachusetts

Allea Scifo, MSN, RN, CPNP
Pediatric Nurse Practitioner
Department of Cardiology
Boston Children's Hospital
Boston, Massachusetts

Casey Sweeney, PhD, MSN, RN, FNP
Family Nurse Practitioner
Partner's Urgent Care
Boston, Massachusetts

Preface

This book was written for the busy clinician working in pediatric primary care, family medicine, and urgent care. It was developed to be a quick reference to help providers navigate through some of the most common presenting complaints and symptoms encountered during the pediatric office visit. It is not a "textbook" to help write a dissertation. It is a book designed for, and by, busy clinicians in the trenches of ambulatory practice. In developing this book, we spoke with many advanced practicing clinicians and asked them what they wanted in a book. Not surprisingly, they all want the same thing—a book that is easy to use and gives quick practical guidance. Whether you are an experienced clinician, a newbie nurse practitioner (NP), or a physician assistant (PA) student going into your peds rotation, this book will serve you well. This book is unique in that it has been written by both NPs and PAs who work in and teach pediatrics to advanced practicing clinicians. This book has been organized as a concise and focused review of the most common presenting symptoms within a system.

Kristine M. Ruggiero
Michael S. Ruggiero

Acknowledgments

I (K.R.) would like to thank and acknowledge the vice president of nursing at Springer Publishing Company, Elizabeth Nieginski, for her creative vision for this project, but more so for her sincerity, kindness, and ongoing encouragement, and endless assistance and feedback at every turn of the way. She is an incredible leader and supporter of advanced practicing clinicians. And I would like to also thank Hannah Hicks, assistant editor at Springer, who has been an invaluable resource, from whom I have learned so much.

I also would like to acknowledge my dearest friend Meredith Scannell for all her support, who is in her own right an amazing nurse author, speaker, researcher, clinician, and professor.

On a personal note, I want to acknowledge my love and gratitude for my family and coworkers for their love and support. And a special thank you to Dr. Jennifer Irani, Dr. Andrea Enzinger, Giuliana DeMarchi (nurse practitioner), Kathleen (my amazing infusion nurse), and Suzanne. Thank you for the brilliant care and support you have shown me during my very recent battle with cancer.

These wonderful people have helped me in some way to write this book. I want to share my passion, knowledge, and expertise in caring for children, and I hope this book is a great resource for others who are (or students who will soon be) providing care to pediatric patients.

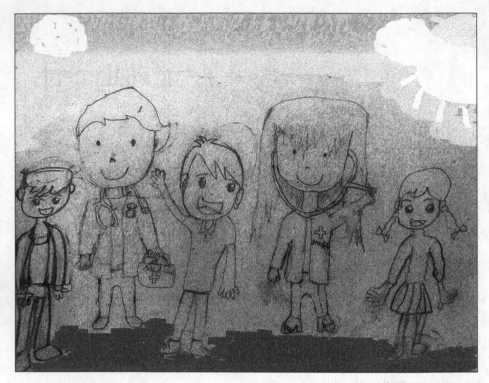

Art by Brody Ruggiero.

I

Essentials of Pediatric Primary Care

1

Assessment of a Pediatric Patient

Kristine M. Ruggiero

INTRODUCTION

The history and physical exam (PE) remain a clinician's most important tools. Many times a complete history and PE reveal findings unrelated to and unexpected from the patient's chief complaint and major concerns (Boxes 1.1 and 1.2).

An age-specific approach to the pediatric PE is another important consideration when caring for children. Remember historical information depends almost completely upon the caregiver for the patient, especially in infants and very young children.

OBJECTIVES

1. To understand the differences in the approach to care of a pediatric patient based on the child's age and developmental level:
   a. Prenatal and birth history
   b. Developmental history
   c. Social history of family
   d. Immunization history
2. Overview of how to approach the history and PE of a pediatric patient based on their age and in the context of the parent/caregiver–child relationship during the pediatric healthcare encounter.

KEY POINTS IN OBTAINING THE HISTORY

Key elements of the history-taking process (Box 1.1) are to establish a warm, caring atmosphere and be nonconfrontational. It is important to greet everyone in the room in a polite manner, with a friendly demeanor. Remember to wash your hands before and after your exam while in the patient's exam room. Getting down to the child's eye level upon entering the room (and not towering over them) is also important, especially when examining toddlers and preschoolers. Distraction is a valuable tool. Be honest. If something is going to hurt, tell the child that in a calm, age-appropriate fashion. Do not lie, or else you will lose credibility. Remember that the birth history and the impact that this has on the child's growth and development are key differences between a pediatric and adult patient (Hagan, Shaw, & Duncan, 2020).

- Infants under 6 months of age who tend to not have stranger anxiety are best examined on the exam table.
- For infants older than 6 months and anxious toddlers who are leery of strangers, the exam may be more comfortable if sitting on their parent/caregiver's lap.
- While children over 3 years of age tend to be generally more cooperative during the exam without being held, they may like to play with the equipment beforehand (i.e., allowing patients to hold the stethoscope or otoscope before using it on them).
- The PE of children aged 5 to 12 years old and adolescents are easier to perform because they also tend to cooperate more.

OUTLINE FOR PEDIATRIC HISTORY AND PHYSICAL EXAM

BOX 1.1   OUTLINE FOR PEDIATRIC HISTORY AND REVIEW OF SYSTEMS

I.   **Presenting Complaint (Informant/Reliability of Informant):** Document the chief complaint and its duration in the patient's or parent's own words whenever possible.

II.   **Present Illness:** Begin with statements that include age, sex, color, and duration of illness (note source of information and relationship to the patient, i.e., mother, father, grandparent, caregiver).
History of the present illness (HPI): "OLDCART" (acronym for onset, location, duration, character/quality, aggravating/alleviating, relieving factors, timing).

How and when did the illness start?

Health immediately before the illness.

Progress of disease; order and date of onset of new symptoms.

Specific symptoms and physical signs that may have developed.

Any pertinent negative data (i.e., no fever, denies sore throat, etc.).

Aggravating and alleviating factors.

Significant medical attention and medications given, dosages, and over what period and when the last dose was given.

In acute infections, ask about the type and degree of exposure. For the well children, ask how they have been since their last visit. Any concerns?

III.   **Birth History/Neonatal History**
   A.   **Birth History:**
      1.   **Prenatal:** Did the mother receive prenatal care? Use of prenatal vitamins? Health of mother during pregnancy. Medical supervision, drugs, diet, infections such as rubella, other illnesses, vomiting, toxemia, other complications.
      2.   **Antenatal:** Rh typing and serology, maternal bleeding, mother's previous pregnancy history.
      3.   **Natal:** Duration of pregnancy, birth weight, kind and duration of labor, type of delivery, presentation, sedation and anesthesia (if known), state of infant at birth, resuscitation required, onset of respiration, first cry.

BOX 1.1 OUTLINE FOR PEDIATRIC HISTORY AND REVIEW OF SYSTEMS (*continued*)

    B. Neonatal:

        1. Ask what the Apgar scores were. Sometimes parents/caregivers do not know this information. Another way to ask if there were complications after the baby was born is to ask if the baby went home from the hospital with the mother/parents or stayed in the hospital longer. Also ask if the baby went to the NICU.

        2. Ask about any congenital anomalies or birth injuries.

        3. Ask about any jaundice, transfusion, sepsis, or other neonatal problems.

        4. Ask if the baby had any difficulty in sucking, any rashes, excessive weight loss, or feeding difficulties.

IV. Previous History (Including Past Medical History [PMH], Past Surgical History [PSH], Past Illnesses)

    A. Past Illnesses:

        1. First document the child's previous general health (i.e., "Previously healthy 1-year-old male"), and then the specific areas listed below should be explored.

    B. PMH (Including all diagnoses, infections, accidents, and injuries [including ingestions]): age, type/nature, severity, sequelae.

    C. Past Hospitalizations: Including place of hospitalization, for what reason, and duration of hospitalization. And/or past ED visits, including what hospital, for what reason, and when.

    D. Past Surgeries: Where and by whom for what diagnosis.

V. Vaccination History/Immunizations

    A. List date and type of immunization, facility providing immunization, and any complications or reactions.

    B. Do not list: "Up to date per parent report." If no immunization record is available, then note this in the problem section of the plan so this can be followed up on.

VI. Developmental History (Growth and Development)

    A. Development: Remember to ask about motor (gross and fine) and social (interaction with others) as well as some major milestones achieved (i.e., age smiled, sat, crawled, walked, first words). Can ask about school performance or comparison with siblings in the older child.

    B. Gross motor (e.g., head control, sitting, pulling to stand, walking).

    C. Fine motor (e.g., raking, pincer grasp, refined pincer grasp).

    D. Social (e.g., social smile, smiling, interaction with toys).

    E. Cognitive (e.g., object permanence, school performance).

Note major growth and development milestones for age and if parent/caregiver has any concerns about infant's development (i.e., first raised head, rolled over, sat alone, pulled up, walked; Feigelman, 2018).

Note any formal developmental screening when appropriate and also if infant/child is receiving services for any delay.

(See Chapter 2, Pediatric Growth and Development.)

VII. Nutrition History

    A. Breast or formula: Type, duration, major formula changes, time of weaning, difficulties.

    B. Be specific about how much milk or formula the baby receives. How does caretaker mix the formula?

    C. Vitamin supplements: Type, when started, amount, duration.

    D. "Solid" foods: When introduced, how taken, types.

    E. For older child, ask about diet, meals/snacks per day, and types of foods consumed.

    F. Appetite: Food likes and dislikes, idiosyncrasies or allergies, reaction of child to eating. An idea of child's usual daily intake is important.

(*continued*)

BOX 1.1 OUTLINE FOR PEDIATRIC HISTORY AND REVIEW OF SYSTEMS (*continued*)

VIII. **Medications and Allergies**
- A. Allergies, with specific attention to drug allergies: Detail type of reaction. Results of allergy testing if performed.
- B. Medications that patient is currently taking: Prescribed, over the counter (OTC), homeopathic, including dose, formulation, route, and frequency.

IX. **Family History (Use Family Tree Whenever Possible)**
- A. Age and health of family members (parents, grandparents, siblings).
- B. Stillbirths, miscarriages, abortions; age at death and cause of death of immediate members of family.
- C. Known genetic diseases.
- D. Conditions with a genetic contribution: Allergy, blood dyscrasias, mental or nervous diseases, diabetes, cardiovascular diseases, kidney disease, rheumatic fever, neoplastic diseases, congenital abnormalities, cancer, convulsive disorders, and others.
- E. **Health of contacts: Any recent ill exposures** (i.e., TB).

X. **Social History**
- A. Type of habitat, age of habitat, number of people in home and relationship(s) to patient
- B. Marital status of parents and involvement with child
- C. Parents' employment
- D. Child care or school

XI. **Environmental History**
- A. Environmental tobacco smoke
- B. Water source to home
- C. Pets
- D. Smoke and carbon monoxide (CO) detectors
- E. Firearms

REVIEW OF SYSTEMS (ROS)

A system review will serve several purposes:
- A. It will often bring out symptoms or signs missed in collection of data about the present illness.
- B. It might direct the interviewer into questioning about other systems that have some indirect bearing on the present illness (e.g., eczema in a child with asthma).
- C. It serves as a screening device for uncovering symptoms, past or present, which were omitted in the earlier part of the interview.

ROS:
- A. **General:** Unusual weight gain or loss, fatigue, temperature sensitivity, mentality. Pattern of growth (record previous heights and weights on appropriate charts). Time and pattern of puberty (use Tanner Staging when appropriate).
- B. **Eyes:** Have the child's eyes ever been crossed? Any foreign body or infection, glasses for any reason. Any problems with their vision, any eye pain?
- C. **Ears, Nose, and Throat:** Frequent colds, sore throat, sneezing, stuffy nose, discharge, postnasal drip, mouth breathing, snoring, otitis, hearing, adenitis.
- D. **Teeth:** Age of eruption of deciduous and permanent; number at 1 year; comparison with siblings.
- E. **Cardiorespiratory:** Frequency and nature of disturbances. Dyspnea, chest pain, cough, sputum, wheeze, expectoration, cyanosis, edema, syncope, tachycardia.
- F. **Gastrointestinal:** Vomiting, diarrhea, constipation, type of stools, abdominal pain or discomfort, jaundice.

(continued)

BOX 1.1   OUTLINE FOR PEDIATRIC HISTORY AND REVIEW OF SYSTEMS (*continued*)

G. **Genitourinary:** Enuresis, dysuria, frequency, polyuria, pyuria, hematuria, character of stream, vaginal discharge, menstrual history, bladder control, abnormalities of penis or testes. Details of menarche and menstruation for adolescent females.

H. **Neuromuscular:** Headache, nervousness, dizziness, tingling, convulsions, habit spasms, ataxia, muscle or joint pains, postural deformities, exercise tolerance, gait.

I. **Endocrine:** Disturbances of growth, excessive fluid intake, polyphagia, goiter, thyroid disease.

J. **Hematologic:** Bruise easily, difficulty stopping bleeds, lumps under arms, neck; fevers, shakes, shivers.

K. **Rheumatologic:** Joints: pain, stiffness, swollen, variation in joint pain during day, fingers painful/blue in cold, dry mouth, red eyes, back, neck pain.

L. **Skin:** Ask about rashes, hives, problems with hair, skin texture or color, and the like.

There are differences in performing a pediatric physical examination compared with that of an adult, and it is important to gather as much data as possible. There is an agreed-upon approach to evaluation of a child. The following three recommendations will aid in the evaluation of the child. First, stay at the child's level while observing them; second, get as much history from them as possible; and third, do the exam from least distressing to most distressing.

BOX 1.2   AGE-SPECIFIC APPROACH TO THE PHYSICAL EXAM

Infant: Lying in parent/caregiver's arms, leave eyes, ears, mouth to end (least to most invasive approach), do heart/lungs when infant is quiet or sleeping, try distraction techniques with older infants.

Toddler: Minimal contact, allow to inspect equipment (i.e., stethoscope), assess heart/lungs and then head-to-toe approach.

Preschooler: Similar to the toddler, especially allow the preschooler to handle the equipment.

School Age: Respect privacy, explain steps/approach to PE beforehand.

Adolescent: Explain findings; same as school-age child, respect privacy; ask parents to leave room during part of the exam.

References

Feigelman, S. (2018). Developmental and behavioral theories. In *Nelson's textbook of pediatrics* (21st ed., pp. 117–123). Philadelphia, PA: Elsevier.

Hagan, J., Shaw, J., & Duncan, P. (2020). *Bright futures: Guidelines for health supervision of infants, children and adolescents* (4th ed.). [ebook]. https://doi.org/aappublications.org/bright-futures-guidelines

2

Pediatric Growth and Development

Kristine M. Ruggiero

INTRODUCTION

While each child grows and gains skills at their own pace, children, overall, move through milestones in a predictable manner. These concepts of growth and development happen in an expected and sequential pattern (as shown in Table 2.1). The role of the pediatric advanced practicing clinician (APC) is to monitor the major growth and developmental milestones in the areas of physical growth, cognitive development, emotional development, social development, and motor development. If a child is missing milestones, or has regressed or lost milestones, these are red flags for further evaluation and possible referral to a specialist.

OBJECTIVES

1. Identify normal patterns of physical growth and development.
2. Identify deviations from normal patterns of growth and development and recognize the importance of developmental surveillance and screening in the pediatric patient.
3. Be familiar with screening and other resources available for children with developmental delays/disabilities.

Key Points

- Any regression at any age of development or any loss of any milestone is a red flag for further developmental assessment.
- Although there are variations in patterns of growth and development, development happens in a sequential pattern (cephalocaudal development and proximodistal development; Figure 2.1).
- It is important to always follow up on any parental concerns regarding delays in growth and development in the pediatric patient.

Table 2.1

Common Developmental Milestones (Age Approximate)

Age	Physical	Gross Motor	Fine Motor	Social	Language
0–6 months	Height increases 1 in./month; Weight increases 1½ lb/month; Weight doubles in 6 months; HC increases 0.5 in./month	Rolls back to side: 3 months; Holds head erect: 4 months; Rolls front to back: 5–6 months	Voluntary grasp: 5 months	Regards a person's face: 1 month; Displays social smile and follows objects 180 degrees: 2 months; Recognizes faces: 3 months; Stranger anxiety: 6 months	Coos: 1–2 months; Laughs: 2–4 months; Makes sounds: 3–4 months; Imitates sounds: 6 months
1–3 years	Posterior fontanel closes: 2–3 months; Anterior fontanel closes: 12–18 months; Central incisors erupt: 5–7 months; Height increases 50% of birth height: 1 year; Birth weight triples: 1 year; Weight increases: 1 lb/month; HC increases by 33%	Walks without help: 15 months; Walks up and down steps placing both feet on each step: 24 months	Scribbles spontaneously: 15 months; Builds three-to four-block towers: 18 months; Jumps with both feet: 30 months	Separation anxiety peaks (peaks at 7–8 months, then again at 12–18 months; this developmental milestone occurs when they gain sense of object permanence. Resolves by age 3), ritualism, negativism, independence	States first and last name: 2½ years; Understands speech: 2 years; Speaks two- to three-word phrases and uses pronouns, 300 words: 2 years
3–6 years	Height increases 2.5 in./year; Weight increases 4-6 lbs/year; HC increases 0.5 in./year; Vision 20/20 with color vision intact around 5–6 years of age	Rides tricycle, climbs stairs alternating feet: 3 years; Skips and catches a ball: 4 years	Builds nine–ten block towers: 3 years; Laces shoes, copies a square: 4 years; Ties shoes and uses scissors well: 5 years; Prints letters, numbers, and name: 5 years	Shares toys with others, imitates caregivers	900 words: 3 years; Speaks three-to four-word sentences: 3 years; 1,500 words: 4 years; Tells stories, sings songs: 4 years; Says more than 2,000 words: 5 years; Names colors: 5 years
6–12 years	Height increases 2–3 in./year; Weight increases 4.5–6.5 lbs/year; Secondary teeth erupt; Tanner state II may begin	Rides bicycle, runs, jumps, swims	Cursive by 8 years	Develops ability to read at grade level	School relationships become important; Becomes independent from family

(continued)

Table 2.1

Common Developmental Milestones (Age Approximate) *(continued)*

Age	Physical	Gross Motor	Fine Motor	Social	Language
Adolescence	Most females have completed physical changes related to puberty by age 15, whereas most males are still gaining muscle mass and height, and sexual maturation is continuing until about 17–18 years of age			Friends become more important; More aware of social behaviors and friendships; May be influenced by peers to try risky behaviors	Cognitively has a better understanding of complex problems; Starts to develop moral ideals and to identify role models

HC, head circumference.

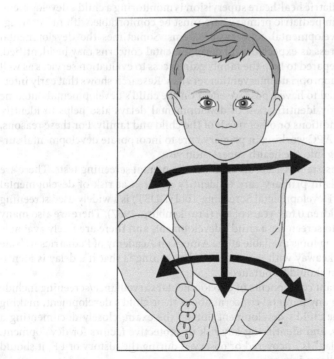

Figure 2.1 Sequence of Growth and Development. Cephalocaudal development: A progressive development of skills and abilities, which begins at the head and ends at the feet; it progresses in a vertical direction. Proximodistal development: A progressive development of skills and abilities, which proceeds from the center of the body to the periphery; it progresses in a bilateral and symmetric fashion.

CONCEPTS OF GROWTH AND DEVELOPMENT

There are three major principles of growth and development: the cephalocaudal principle, the proximodistal principle, and the orthogenetic principle. These predictable patterns of growth and development allow us to predict how and when most children will develop certain characteristics. Cephalocaudal development occurs in infancy and through early childhood and follows a head-to-toe progression. The proximodistal principle refers to development that progresses from the center of the body outward, and the orthogenetic principle states that development proceeds from the simple to more complex tasks (i.e., from a raking grasp to a refined pincer grasp).

From birth to 1 year of age, motor development and growth is quicker than any other time in a child's life. During this time, growth happens in a predictable pattern. For motor development to occur, the primitive reflexes leave, and the emergence of purposeful reactions occurs. Table 2.1 reviews some of the common developmental milestones in early childhood. Deviations in development at this early age tend to present as motor milestone delays and may signify neuromuscular, genetic, metabolic, infectious, or other abnormalities. Therefore, a careful history and physical exam (PE) is essential to try to determine the cause of the delay.

DEVELOPMENTAL SURVEILLANCE AND SCREENING

A critical aspect of pediatric healthcare supervision is monitoring a child's development. The APC who works in pediatric primary care must be comfortable with monitoring/screening for any developmental concerns/problems. Sometimes the developmental process does not progress as expected, and developmental concerns may be identified. The APC should be prepared to help the family gain access to evaluation services as well as connect them with appropriate intervention services. Research shows that early intervention has the potential to have a positive effect on the child's developmental outcome (Feigelman, 2018). Early identification of developmental delays also helps to identify associated medical conditions or other needs of the child and family. For these reasons, it is important for the APC working in primary care to incorporate developmental surveillance and screening into the health supervision visit.

Clinical impressions are less accurate than developmental screening tests. There are various screening tools in primary care to identify children at risk of developmental delays, but the Denver Developmental Screening Tool (DDST) is a widely used screening tool for examining children 0 to 6 years of age (Frankenburg, 1967). There are also many other screening tools to screen for a child's development, and there are freely available developmental screening tools available at the American Academy of Pediatrics website (AAP.org). The key takeaway with developmental screening is that if a delay is identified, further evaluation should be pursued.

In addition, important components of developmental surveillance/screening include asking and addressing any parental concerns about their child's development, making observations about the child's development during the exam, closely documenting a developmental history, and identifying any risk or protective factors for development. In addition, if a "red flag" is uncovered or observed during the history or PE, it should be documented and followed up on.

An estimate of developmental risk should be assessed early on in a child's development, and a child at risk for developmental delays should be referred for evaluation to early intervention (0–3 years of age). For children over 3 years of age, an evaluation can be completed by their local public school system.

MONITORING A CHILD'S DEVELOPMENT

Developmental Disabilities

Autism Spectrum Disorders

The APC must be proficient in identifying major developmental milestones and be able to recognize signs that signify a developmental concern or delay and in identifying when to perform further developmental testing. This chapter covers a general overview of these major concepts of growth and development, developmental surveillance at the health supervision visit, and the general approach to care of developmental disabilities, specifically autistic spectrum disorders (ASDs).

Sometimes the developmental process does not progress as expected, and developmental disabilities may be suspected. ASD is a developmental disability that can cause significant social, communication, and behavioral challenges. A diagnosis of ASD now includes several conditions that used to be diagnosed separately: autistic disorder, pervasive developmental disorder not otherwise specified (PDD-NOS), and Asperger syndrome (Centers for Disease Control and Prevention [CDC], 2019). These conditions are now all called ASDs.

An ASD is a chronic nonprogressive developmental disability involving impairments in social interaction, communication, and behavior. The CDC estimates that 1 in 68 children in the United States have autism, with the prevalence being 1 in 42 for boys and 1 in 189 for girls. These rates yield a gender ratio of about five boys for every girl (CDC, 2019). While most children present or are diagnosed with ASD around preschool or early school age, research has shown that symptoms of autism are present in infancy. Therefore, the American Academy of Pediatrics (AAP) recommends that in addition to routine developmental screening (at 9-month, 18-month, and 24- or 30-month visits), all children be screened for ASDs at their 18- and 24-month well-child checkups.

SEXUAL DEVELOPMENT

Sexual development occurs during puberty, also happens in a predictable pattern, and is defined as biologic changes that lead to reproductive ability. These changes transpire in a predictable pattern; however, the timing at which they happen varies. In males, the first sign of puberty is enlargement of the testicles, followed by penile enlargement, a height growth spurt, and pubic hair. In females, the order of pubertal events in sexual development is thelarche (breast buds), followed by a height growth spurt, pubic hair, and menarche. The Tanner staging system is used to determine where a child is in the pubertal process. Tanner stages for the male genitalia, female breasts, and male and female pubic hair are shown in Figure 2.2. Pubertal abnormalities are addressed in Chapter 13, Endocrine Abnormalities Commonly Seen in Pediatric Primary Care.

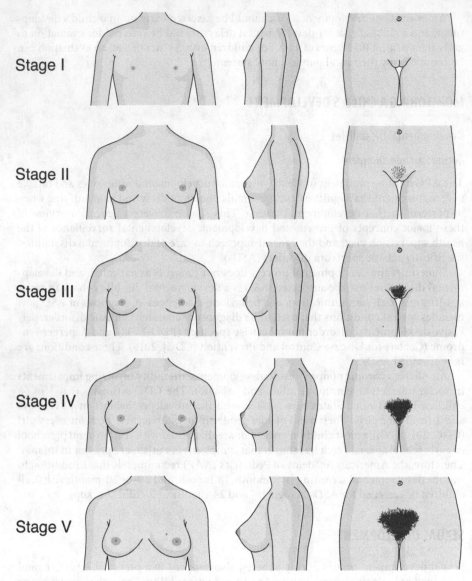

Stage I

Stage II

Stage III

Stage IV

Stage V

Figure 2.2A Tanner staging of adolescent females.

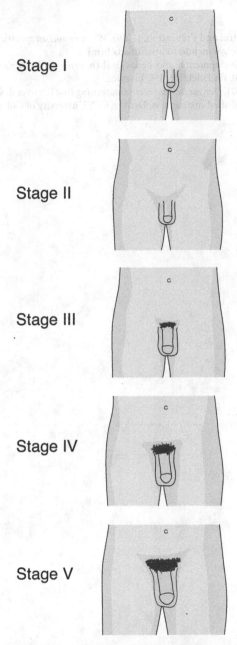

Stage I

Stage II

Stage III

Stage IV

Stage V

Figure 2.2B Tanner staging of adolescent males. In part B, testicular volume and testicular size in the longest dimension at each stage are stage I: volume 3 cc, size <2.5 cm; stage II: volume 4 cc, size 2.5–3.2 cm; stage III: volume 10 cc, size 3.6 cm; stage IV: volume 16 cc, size 4.1–4.5 cm; and stage V: volume 25 cc, size >4.5 cm.
Source: Adapted from Wikimedia Commons.

References

Centers for Disease Control and Prevention. (2019). *What is autism spectrum disorder?* Retrieved from https://www.cdc.gov/ncbddd/autism/facts.html

Feigelman, S. (2018). Developmental and behavioral theories. In *Nelson's textbook of pediatrics* (21st ed., pp. 117–123). Philadelphia, PA: Elsevier.

Frankenburg, W. K. (1967). *Denver developmental screening tool* [Denver developmental screening test: manual]. Unpublished instrument. Denver, CO: University of Colorado Medical Center.

II

Common Clinical Problems

Abnormalities of the Ears, Eyes, Nose, and Throat (EENT) Commonly Seen in Pediatric Primary Care

Michael S. Ruggiero

INTRODUCTION

Pediatric ears, eyes, nose, and throat (EENT) complaints are the most common reason for urgent care, emergency department, and primary care sick visit encounters. Millions of encounters a year are dependent on pediatric providers having a good working knowledge of these complaints. In this chapter, some of these most common complaints are discussed. Ambulatory medicine practices across the country are dependent on providers' quick and efficient recognition, workup, and treatment of these disorders. In this chapter, we will explore the most common complaints regarding the EENT. The primary focus will be on symptoms most commonly encountered in each of these systems. We will explore ear pain, nasal congestion, sinus pain, sore throat, oral ulcers/lesions, eye pain, red eye, and eye swelling.

OBJECTIVES

1. Explain the epidemiology and etiology of acute and emergent diseases of the EENT.
2. Describe the signs and symptoms of common conditions of the EENT
3. Formulate a differential diagnosis of common EENT complaints.
4. Identify patients presenting with emergent EENT disorders that require referral and/or hospital admission.
5. Explain the appropriate treatment for patients with acute ocular EENT conditions.

EAR PAIN (OTALGIA)

Ear complaints are common in children. The most notable complaint is ear pain or otalgia. Children will manifest symptoms of ear pain differently based on their age:

■ Infants may present as fussy or with inconsolable crying and swatting at ears.

- Toddlers will be more vocal and able to tell you that they have ear pain; younger ones will tend to pull at their ear.
- Preschool-age children will tend to have the vocabulary to tell you that their ear hurts. There are several causes of ear pain. In this chapter, we will focus on the most common causes.

A review of the ear's major components can help providers in the description of and in determining the cause of ear pain in children. See Figures 3.1 and 3.2 demonstrating the internal and external anatomy of the ear.

The ear is separated into three different segments: the inner, middle, and outer ear. The chief complaint of ear pain is, in general, related to the outer and middle segments.

- Since symptoms of inner ear pathology tend to be related to hearing loss and dizziness, the inner ear will be covered in Chapter 7, Common Neurologic Complaints Seen in Pediatric Primary Care.
- The middle ear comprises the tympanic membrane (TM) including the auditory ossicles (incus, malleus, and stapes) and the eustachian tube (ET).
- The outer ear comprises the pinna, which is the external auricle, and is composed of different components such as the tragus, the helix, and the fossa triangularis. The auditory canal starts at the opening of the ear and ends at the TM.

ACUTE OTITIS EXTERNA

Commonly referred to as swimmer's ear and synonymous with otitis externa (OE), acute otitis externa (AOE) is inflammation to the external auditory canal. This condition is common in children and is most prominent during the summer months.

Etiology

There are several possible causes for AOE: infectious (bacterial or fungal), dermatologic (eczematous), or even allergic. However, infectious is the most common cause in children and will be the focus of this chapter. The most common pathogenic organisms

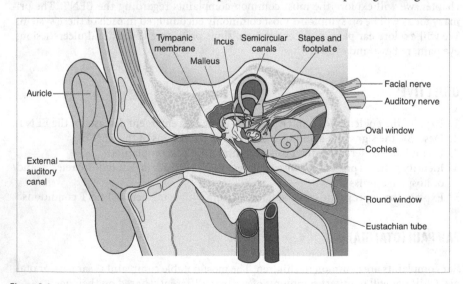

Figure 3.1 Internal anatomy of the ear.
Source: Reproduced from Myrick, K. M., & Karosas, L. M. (Eds.). (2021). *Advanced health assessment and differential diagnosis: Essentials for clinical practice.* New York, NY: Springer Publishing Company, p. 92.

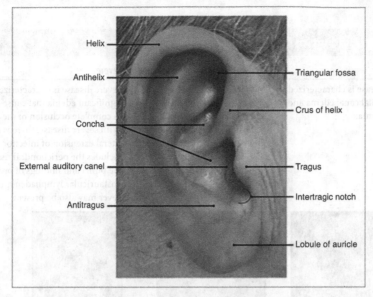

Figure 3.2 External anatomy of the ear.
Source: Reproduced from Gawlik, K. S., Melnyk, B. M., & Teall, A. M. (Eds.). (2021). *Evidence-based physical examination: Best practices for health and well-being assessment.* New York, NY: Springer Publishing Company, p. 338.

responsible for external otitis are *Pseudomonas aeruginosa* (38%), *Staphylococcus epidermidis* (9%), and *Staphylococcus aureus* (8%).

Epidemiology/Risk Factors

Risk factors that can cause trauma or infection in the ear canal include moisture in the ear from swimming or bathing, various traumas including cotton tip applicators and other objects used to clean and scratch the canal, and foreign body (FB) devices such as earphones/buds/pods and hearing aids that can scratch the ear canal and increase moisture buildup.

Focused Physical Exam Signs/Findings

Symptoms range from ear discomfort, pruritus, otorrhea, and muffled hearing to severe pain and systemic effects such as fever.

Patients will often present with a history of an itchy ear that progresses to pain with or without discharge. Pain may also be noted to radiate to the jaw on the ipsilateral side.

Classic signs of OE are swelling and erythema to the external canal, and in severe cases, this extends to the perichondral tissue of the pinna.

On exam, patients tend to have pain with insertion of the otoscopic speculum into the ear canal and can have pain with pinna pulling and tragus tugging. Classifying disease to allow for appropriate management can be accomplished with a simplified mild, moderate, and severe classification system such as the Brighton grading scheme, which grades 1–4 (Lesperance & Flynt, 2015). See Table 3.1 for severity grading for OE.

Follow-Up

1. Follow-up is not necessary in mild cases or in uncomplicated moderate cases.
2. If a wick is placed, follow up for reevaluation to see if new wick placement is necessary. Wicks should be removed or replaced within 24 to 48 hours after initial placement.
3. Anytime there is treatment failure or a referral was made.

Table 3.1

Severity Grading for Otitis Externa

Mild	Moderate	Severe
Mild disease is characterized by minimal canal edema and/or erythema.	Moderate disease is characterized by moderate edema that causes partial occlusion of the canal; however, the TM is still visible.	Severe disease is characterized by significant edema that causes near to complete occlusion of the canal. With severe disease, there is often lateral extension of infection that includes the perichondral tissue of the pinna and findings of pre- and postauricular lymphadenopathy. Fever may also be present.
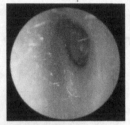	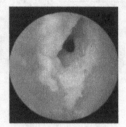	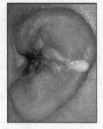
Topical acetic acid–hydrocortisone solution. Apply three to four drops to the affected ear every 4–6 hours for 7 days.	Debridement followed by ciprofloxacin 0.3% and dexamethasone 0.1% otic suspension or ciprofloxacin 0.2% and hydrocortisone 1% otic suspension.	Debridement followed by wick placement and topical + PO medications. Ciprofloxacin 0.2% and hydrocortisone 1% otic suspension + PO ciprofloxacin 10 mg/kg/dose twice daily (maximum 500 mg/dose) for 7–10 days.

Refer to otolaryngologist if:
- TM is perforated
- There are tympanostomy tubes
- Severe disease
- Immunocompromised
- Recalcitrant case

PO, by mouth; TM, tympanic membrane.

Special Considerations/Complications

Malignant (Necrotizing) Otitis Externa

While OE is generally easily treated with no significant sequelae, missing a case of malignant (necrotizing) otitis externa (MOE) is a severe and potentially fatal complication. A complication of acute bacterial OE, MOE occurs when the infection spreads from the superficial structures of the ear canal and auricle to the deeper soft tissue and bone of the jaw and temporal bone (osteomyelitis). This complication is most commonly seen in diabetics, the elderly, and the immunocompromised. There should be a high index of suspicion in those patients presenting with ear pain who are diabetic.

Symptoms

Symptoms include severe otalgia, otorrhea, and referred pain to the temporal and tempomandibular bones.

Signs

Physical examination (PE) will show granulation tissue in the external auditory canal, and there is commonly discharge as well. Fever is uncommon.

Treatment

Antibiotics should be started immediately

Don't Miss

Patients with malignant external otitis should be promptly started on antipseudo-monal antibiotics, such as ciprofloxacin 20 mg/kg/dose twice daily (not to exceed 750 mg/dose), and referred urgently to an otolaryngologist. If the otolaryngologist is unavailable for urgent consultation, then admitting a child would be appropriate.

ACUTE OTITIS MEDIA

Acute otitis media (AOM) is an acute infection of the middle ear space associated with inflammation and effusion that translates to ear pain. It is worth noting that if the pressure from the effusion is evacuated via perforation or tympanostomy tube, a child may present with no pain and only ear drainage.

Epidemiology/Risk Factors

AOM is the most common bacterial infection in children, with 75% of cases being diagnosed before the age of 5 years (Liese et al., 2014). Risk factors for increasing incidence of AOMs include smoking or exposure to secondhand smoke, bottle-feeding, pacifier use, day care attendance, and younger children (≤ 3 years old).

Etiology

AOM etiology is largely bacterial in nature, and almost all bacterial isolates are one of the following: *Streptococcus pneumonia* (the most common, comprising approximately 40% of AOM infections despite the pneumococcal vaccine), *Haemophilus influenza* (30%), *Moraxella catarrhalis* (up to 25%), and *Streptococcus pyogenese*.

Symptoms

Children will present with ear pain and sometimes a "muffled" or blocked ear. Characteristically, symptoms of upper respiratory infections or allergic rhinitis will precede the infection and the complaint of ear pain. Inflammation of the nasal mucosa and ETs leads to an accumulation of fluid in the middle ear and creates an environment conducive to bacterial growth. Parental suspicion of AOM has been shown to be one of the most sensitive and specific historical cues in diagnosing a child with AOM.

Focused Physical Exam Signs/Findings

Children presenting with isolated AOM typically present well and do not appear ill or toxic. Fever, although possibly present, has not been shown to be a predominant symptom and has a relatively low sensitivity and specificity for AOM.
Otoscopic examination is required to make the diagnosis of AOM. This includes a clear visualization of the TM in question.

Cerumen impaction and obstruction if present need to be cleared. Inspection and identification of certain TM characteristics are what confirms the diagnosis of AOM. Erythematous TM, bulging TM, cloudy or opaque TM, and middle ear effusion

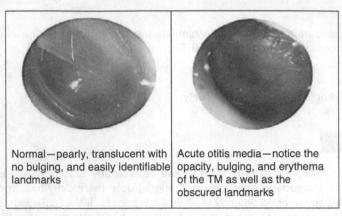

Normal—pearly, translucent with no bulging, and easily identifiable landmarks	Acute otitis media—notice the opacity, bulging, and erythema of the TM as well as the obscured landmarks

Figure 3.3 Comparison of normal TM versus AOM.

confirmed by impaired mobility of TM are all characteristics of an AOM (as shown in Figure 3.3). TM perforation may also be seen. TM perforation typically heals quickly without intervention.

Treatment

Management of pain can be accomplished with over-the-counter (OTC) analgesics. This is recommended for all children with otalgia.

- **Ibuprofen:** 10 mg/kg orally every 6 to 8 hours as needed (maximum single dose 600 mg; maximum daily dose up to 2.4 g/day)
- **Tylenol:** 10 to 15 mg/kg orally every 4 to 6 hours as needed (up to five doses not to exceed 4 g/day)

Antibiotic Treatment

Practice varies around management with antibiotic therapy or not. Table 3.2 compares immediate treatment with antibiotics versus observation with reevaluation and antibiotic therapy if the symptoms and signs worsen or fail to improve after 48 hours.

Table 3.2

How to Approach Care of a Child With AOM: Immediate Treatment With Antibiotics Versus Watch-and-Wait Approach

Immediate treatment with antibiotics:
0–24 months with AOM or children ≥2 years who
-appear toxic,
-have persistent otalgia for more than 48 hours,
-have temperature ≥102.1°F,
-have bilateral AOM or otorrhea, or
-do not have access to immediate follow-up

Observation for 48 hours is acceptable in the following:
In children ≥2 years who
-are immunocompetent with mild signs and no otorrhea
Initial observation is appropriate for 48 hours.

AOM, acute otitis media.

Table 3.3

Approach to Antibiotic Treatment of AOM		
First Line	**Second Line**	**Special Circumstances**
Amoxicillin **Age:** <3 months: 30 mg/kg/day divided into two doses per day ≥3 months: 80–90 mg/kg/day divided into two doses per day Duration: 7–10 days If less than 2 years of age or severe symptoms present, treat for 10 days	Mild allergy (delayed reaction) to penicillin/amoxicillin Second- or third-generation cephalosporin **Cefdinir** (≥6 months of age) 14 mg/kg/day divided into two doses a day **Cefpodoxime** (≥2 months of age) 5 mg/kg orally every 12 hours for 5 days; do not exceed 200 mg/dose **Cefuroxime** (≥3 months of age) 30 mg/kg per day in a divided dose every 12 hours for 10 days **Ceftriaxone** (newborns less than 2 months) 50 mg/kg IM in a single dose for 1–3 days	On antibiotics in the past 30 days Or conjunctivitis-otitis syndrome: purulent conjunctivitis with AOM that has a high risk of beta-lactamase-producing *Haemophilus influenzae* Or treatment failure-continued or worsening symptoms despite 48–72 hours of treatment
	Anaphylaxis or life-threatening reaction to penicillin or amoxicillin Azithromycin 10 mg/kg on day 1 as a single dose and then 5 mg/kg per day for days 2–5	**Augmentin** 90 mg/kg per day of amoxicillin and 6.4 mg/kg per day of clavulanate divided into two doses **IV/IM ceftriaxone** 50 mg/kg maximum 1 g/day for 3 days *If severe penicillin allergy and failed on azithromycin, refer to an otolaryngologist

IM, intramuscularly; IV, intravenous.

Follow-Up

Follow-up is typically not necessary unless there is treatment failure.

Referral

AOE tends to respond well to treatment (see Table 3.3); however, referral to an otolaryngologist (ENT) for further evaluation would be warranted if a patient fails to clear an infection despite two rounds of appropriate antibiotics or if there is recurrent infection that amounts to more than four in a 12-month span.

Special Considerations/Complications

Mastoiditis

Acute mastoiditis (AM) is an extension of AOM that can have long-term sequelae and possible mortality if missed. AM is caused when an infection of the middle ear extends and spreads to the mastoid cells and to the periosteal tissue of the mastoid.

The diagnosis is made by PE and confirmed by imaging studies such as CT scans and magnetic resonance images. In the early stage, there are no specific signs and symptoms of mastoid infection, with later progression to erythema and tenderness over the mastoid area to edema or a subperiosteal abscess with displacement of the pinna inferiorly and anteriorly. The diagnosis is based on clinical findings, including postauricular tenderness, erythema, and swelling with protrusion of the auricle (Lesperance & Flynt, 2015).

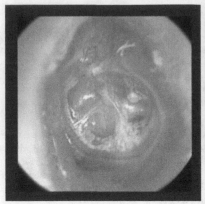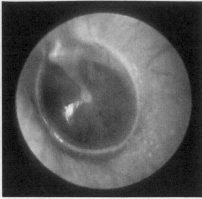

Figure 3.4 Comparison of middle ear effusion (A) versus tympanic membrane retraction (B).
Source: Wikimedia Commons. (2020, January 30). *File: Wiki TM retraction.jpg. Wikimedia Commons, the free media repository.* Retrieved from https://commons.wikimedia.org/w/index.php?title=File:Wiki_TM_retraction. jpg&oldid=391039860; Wikimedia Commons. (2020, January 30). *File: Adult Serous Otitis Media.jpg. Wikimedia Commons, the free media repository.* Retrieved from https://commons.wikimedia.org/w/index. php?title=File:Adult_Serous_Otitis_Media.jpg&oldid=391033874.

◼ EUSTACHIAN TUBE DYSFUNCTION

The ET is a narrow tube that communicates between the nasopharynx and the middle ear. The purpose of the ET is to protect the middle ear from pathogens, to ventilate the middle ear, and to help drain secretions from the middle ear cleft.

Eustachian tube dysfunction (ETD) is the inability of the ET to adequately perform these functions. This can be caused by swelling of the mucosal lining of the tube, or if the tube does not open or close properly. ETD in children is typically due to obstructive causes as a result of mucosal swelling of the nasopharynx from upper respiratory infections, allergic rhinosinusitis, or a mass effect occurring due to enlarged adenoids (Steele, Adam, & Di, 2017).

Symptoms

Symptoms include ear pain or fullness, muffled hearing, popping sounds, tinnitus, and reduced hearing; problems with balance may occur.

Focused PE Signs/Findings

Retraction of the TM or effusion without other signs of middle ear infection/AOM will be noted on PE. An effusion without evidence of infection is known as otitis media with effusion (OME).

Treatment

Treatment should be focused on the underlying etiology (see Treatment for Allergic and Viral Rhinosinusitis).

Follow-Up/Patient/Family Education

Reassurance and time are typically all that is needed for action. As obstructive causes of the viral URI resolve so will symptoms of the middle ear, and the ET function will return to normal. There are limited studies to support use of decongestants, nasal steroids, systemic steroids, and antihistamines for the treatment of ETD.

For medical management, please reference the "Nose" section of this chapter for treatment of some of the underlying contributors to ETD.

Surgical referral: If symptoms persist for greater than 90 days, then it is recommended to refer to an otolaryngologist for possible tympanostomy +/– tube placement, or tonsillectomy and adenoidectomy if chronically enlarged (Mansour, Magnan, Haeder, & Nicolas, 2014).

OTOMYCOSIS

Any recalcitrant case of bacterial otitis externa is grounds for considering otomycosis, which is a fungal infection of the external auditory canal. It is not common but should be considered if the patient is failing to improve or develops recurrent OE-type symptoms soon after resolution of previous OE treated with topical antibiotics.

Symptoms are like bacterial OE; however, on exam, there is evidence of fungal infection as shown in Figure 3.5.

Treatment

Otomycosis is treated with thorough debridement of the ear canal and then topical antifungal therapy. With young children who may not tolerate the debridement or for clinicians who are not well versed in canal debridement, a referral to an otolaryngologist is recommended. Antifungal solution is the preferred treatment. Clotrimazole 1% topical solution three to four drops into affected ear four times daily for 7 days is recommended.

TYMPANIC MEMBRANE RUPTURE

The TM separates the external canal from the middle ear. Perforation of this membrane can lead to increased risk of middle ear infection and can lead to hearing loss.

Etiology/Risk Factors

There are two main causes of a ruptured eardrum. The most common is due to inner ear infection that causes increased pressure on the inner aspect of the TM. The pressure can cause a small perforation that leads to pressure release and often pus or blood discharge from the ear.

The second is trauma due to FB, blunt trauma to the head, or barotrauma. Of the traumatic causes, the most common is due to insertion of a FB/cotton-tipped applicator to the ear canal. This type of injury is more traumatic than a perforation due to infection

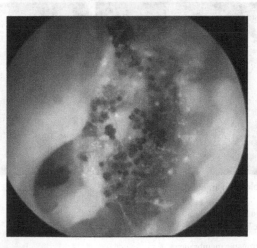

Figure 3.5 Picture of otomycosis.

and can lead to more long-term sequelae and healing issues. It is also possible to dislocate the ossicles in this type of injury that can lead to long-term hearing loss.

Symptoms

Often symptoms of a ruptured ear drum include an acute onset of ear pain (primary symptom) or a recent history of upper respiratory symptoms and/or acute otitis media. Onset of ear pain is the primary symptom. History of traumatic mechanism or, more likely, history of AOM symptoms or upper respiratory infection symptoms.

Focused PE Signs/Findings

Signs of a ruptured eardrum include discharge from the ear, either bloody if traumatic or clear or pustulant if related to serous fluid buildup due to infection. Patient may also have objective hearing loss. A visual inspection will reveal a breach in the TM. The TM may also be erythematous.

Table 3.4

Infectious Versus Traumatic Perforated Tympanic Membrane		
Type	**Infectious**	**Traumatic**
Description	Middle ear infection leads to effusion and increased pressure on the inner portion of the TM. The TM can rupture releasing pressure of the middle ear. These perforations tend to be small	Trauma is due to FB, blunt trauma to the head, or barotrauma. Of the traumatic causes, the most common is due to insertion of FB/cotton-tipped applicator to the ear canal. This type of injury is more traumatic than a perforation due to infection and can lead to more long-term sequelae and healing issues. It is also possible to dislocate the ossicles in this type of injury, which can lead to long-term hearing loss.
Treatment	Antibiotic drops safe for middle ear such as ciprofloxacin or ofloxacin until evidence of infection clears. Most TMs will repair spontaneously over 2 months.	Serial exams including audiogram.

Refer to an otolaryngologist if any of the following persists:
- Vertigo
- Incomplete healing after 2 months
- Hearing deficit once TM has healed.

FB, foreign body; TM, tympanic membrane.

Treatment

In either case, most often these can be managed with observation. In the setting of infection, antibiotic ear drops are recommended (see Table 3.4). In the case of the ruptured TM due to trauma, antibiotic medication is not recommended. Supportive care is used, and most cases will spontaneously resolve within 2 months.

EYE

The job of the pediatric advanced practicing clinician is to help maintain normal vision in their pediatric patients. Part of this is through the normal age-determined screening recommendations, but, at other times, there are acute issues that threaten a child's vision for both the short term and some indefinitely. Thus, it is the providers' responsibility to identify these issues promptly so that appropriate treatment and management can ensure the maintenance of normal healthy vision.

In this section, we will focus on some of the more common acute manifestations of ocular disorders, injuries, and diseases. Some of the most common complaints children have regarding their eyes are redness, pain, swelling, and visual changes.

A reminder to those reading this—general pediatric providers must perform a thorough eye evaluation when confronted with ocular symptoms.

Focused PE Signs/Findings

Evaluation of the eye involves thorough inspection of the eyelids and preauricular lymph nodes, visual fields, extraocular movements, and pupils including light reflex, conjunctiva, cornea, and sclera and fundoscopic examination if determined necessary. Visual acuity can be assessed using several instruments, most commonly the Snellen eye chart. If trauma is suspected, then corneal defects should be assessed using fluorescein staining and then illuminated with a Wood's lamp. This may necessitate a referral to an ophthalmologist.

Prior to reviewing common ocular symptoms encountered in the ambulatory practice, it is imperative that providers are routinely screening pediatric patients for underlying eye disease. Remember to always check for a red reflex. Screening can pick up a condition called leukocoria or a white pupillary reflex. This is an abnormal white reflection from the retina of the eye. This finding is most commonly encountered in congenital glaucoma but is also found in retinoblastoma, which is an eye cancer of the retina. A finding of leukocoria requires an urgent ophthalmology referral.

■ CONJUNCTIVITIS

Conjunctivitis is an inflammation of the conjunctiva. This is a common condition in children and can be caused by several infectious etiologies as well as irritants and allergens. Despite the cause, the condition tends to be benign.

Etiology

Conjunctivitis can be broken down into infectious causes, such as bacterial and viral, or noninfectious, such as allergic and irritative/chemical.

Viral conjunctivitis: The most common cause of conjunctivitis is viral infection. This tends to occur in tandem with other findings of viral upper respiratory infections with the most common virus being adenovirus.

Bacterial conjunctivitis: Bacterial cases tend to present with more purulent discharge and are most commonly caused by *S. pneumoniae, H. influenzae, M. catarrhalis,* and, to a lesser degree, *S. aureus. Neisseria gonorrhoeae* must be considered in diagnosis of bacterial conjunctivitis; although rare, it is sight threatening.

Allergic conjunctivitis: Allergic conjunctivitis is caused by multiple different allergens. Allergens are typically airborne and contact the eye but may be transferred from surface to eye with the hands. Allergic causes are distinguished from infectious causes in that they tend to be bilateral, affecting both eyes. Allergic conjunctivitis is more common in patients with history of seasonal or perennial allergies or atopy such as eczema.

Chemical or irritative conjunctivitis: Noninfectious or nonallergic conjunctivitis has too many possible etiologies to list in this format; however, a thorough history will typically elicit the cause of an acute exposure conjunctivitis. Chemical splash injuries, shampoos and soaps, cosmetics, hairspray, and small particles and matters cause mechanical irritation.

Toxic conjunctivitis should also be considered in which reactions usually result from chronic use of eye solutions. A careful history looking for common offending agents is important; some of these include contact solution, aminoglycoside antibiotics, antiviral agents, glaucoma medications, and topical anesthetics.

Epidemiology

Most conjunctivitis is treated by primary care providers, with 70% of all patients presenting with acute conjunctivitis initially being seen in primary care or urgent care settings. Conjunctivitis is also the most common ocular diagnosis seen in the emergency department (ED).

Prevalence of the types of conjunctivitis is seasonal. Viral conjunctivitis is most prevalent in the summer months. Bacterial conjunctivitis is most commonly diagnosed in the winter and early spring. Allergic conjunctivitis is most commonly encountered in the spring and summer months coinciding with other manifestations of seasonal allergies. The distribution of conjunctivitis diagnosed in the ED was bimodal, with the highest rates being in children younger than 7 years. Approximately 1 out of every 100 visits in primary care settings is for conjunctivitis (Ramirez, Porco, Thomas, & Keenan, 2017).

Patient and Family Education

Viral and bacterial conjunctivitis are extremely contagious, so good hand hygiene is strongly reinforced (see Table 3.5). If the patient is a contact lens wearer, contacts are not to be worn until the condition has cleared completely, and lenses worn just prior to or during the infection should be disposed of. Allergic conjunctivitis is not contagious; however, it is still recommended that contact lenses are not worn until the signs and symptoms resolve.

Additional Considerations

Neonatal conjunctivitis is an acquired condition of neonates that manifests in the first month of life. This is an infectious conjunctivitis that is commonly caused by sight-threatening pathogens. Neonates present with purulent discharge and conjunctival injection. Common pathogens are *Chlamydia trachomatis, N. gonorrhoeae,* herpes simplex, and *Escherichia coli.* Acute reaction to topical antibiotics as part of gonococcal prophylaxis should also be considered. Pediatric ophthalmologist should be consulted, so prompt treatment can ensue.

Subconjunctival hemorrhage is also a cause of a red nonpainful eye. These tend *not* to have discharge associated with them and are most commonly asymptomatic. Questioning usually elicits a history of increased venous pressure that is seen in coughing, vomiting, or Valsalva maneuver/straining. Minor trauma such as itching or rubbing

Table 3.5

Differentiating Between Viral, Bacterial, and Allergic Conjunctivitis and Treatment Considerations

	Viral	Bacterial	Allergic
Symptoms	Painless/clear discharge; gritty sensation or foreign body sensation Typically, unilateral at presentation	Painless/thick purulent discharge Typically, unilateral at presentation	Painless/clear thin discharge/itching History of allergies
Signs	Injection May have other viral symptoms such as pharyngitis, rhinitis, and fever Clear thin discharge/ excessive lacrimation Vision and visual fields preserved Follicular appearance to tarsal conjunctiva preauricular lymphadenopathy	Injection Mucopurulent unilateral or bilateral discharge, normal vision Vision and visual fields preserved	Injection Clear watery discharge Follicular appearance to tarsal conjunctiva Bullous chemosis Vision and visual fields preserved
Treatment	Self-limited Removal of CL until condition clears Dispose of CL that were worn during the condition or just prior to symptoms Can last up to 2 weeks	Removal of CL until condition clears Dispose of CL that were worn during the condition or just prior to symptoms Erythromycin ophthalmic ointment 5 mg/g 1 cm ribbon of ointment to the lower inner lid 4 times daily for 7 days. --------------- If CL wearer, ofloxacin ophthalmic solution 0.3% Days 1 and 2: Instill one drop every 4 hours in the affected eye(s) Days 3–9: Instill one drop every 6 hours in the affected eye(s)	Refrigerated artificial tears Avoidance of allergens ------------------ Antihistamines with mast cell stabilizer >2 years old Olopatadine 0.1% 1 drop per eye 2 times daily or ------------------ Vasoconstrictor with antihistamine >6 years old Naphazoline 0.25% and pheniramine 0.3% 1 drop per eye every 6 hours
Considerations	Patients with symptoms of viral conjunctivitis but who have a severe foreign body sensation and deficit in the visual acuity should be	If there is a failure to improve, the patient should be referred to an ophthalmologist	Topical allergy drops should not be used for more than 2 weeks

(*continued*)

Table 3.5

Differentiating Between Viral, Bacterial, and Allergic Conjunctivitis and Treatment Considerations (*continued*)

	Viral	Bacterial	Allergic
	suspected of having viral keratoconjunctivitis and be referred to an ophthalmologist	*Neisseria gonorrhoeae* copious purulent discharge with concurrent urethritis/cervicitis This is sight-threatening infection management **in patients with topical and systemic antibiotics**	

CL, contact lens.

Data from Abelson, M. B., Allansmith, M. R., & Friedlaender, M. H. (1980). Effects of topically applied ocular decongestant and antihistamine. *American Journal of Ophthalmology, 90*(2), 254–257. doi:10.1016/s0002-9394(14)74864-0

the eye may also be elicited in the history. Symptoms such as pain, discharge, and visual changes should cause reconsideration of diagnosis. Subconjunctival hemorrhage is a self-limited condition, and no specific treatment is necessary.

■ RED EYE

The red eye can be very dramatic; however, the condition is usually benign. Eye redness is a sign of ocular inflammation. The pediatric provider's responsibility is to identify benign versus serious causes of eye redness and manage accordingly. Some of the most common causes of red eye are conjunctivitis, iritis, scleritis, and subconjunctival hemorrhage.

■ OCULAR FINDINGS IN CHILDREN OF ABUSE

Ocular injury and findings are common manifestations of child abuse. The ophthalmologic examination is essential when evaluating young children whose injuries are suspicious of child abuse. Ocular exam findings that may suggest abuse are poorly reactive pupils, periorbital ecchymoses, subconjunctival hemorrhage hyphemia, orbital fractures, ecchymosis or laceration of the lids, hemorrhage in or about the eye, cataract or dislocated lens, and retinal detachment. Shaken baby syndrome is the deliberate, repetitive, unrestrained acceleration–deceleration of the head and neck, and a funduscopic exam may show retinal hemorrhages or retinal detachment. Trauma-related eye injuries should be evaluated by an ophthalmologist, and child protective services should be contacted. Admitting the child may be necessary for injuries.

EYELID DISORDERS

Swelling from lid abnormalities is a common occurrence in children. Seldom a medical urgency, these tend to be easily identified and treated in the ambulatory clinic setting. In this section, we will discuss a few of the most common acquired lid abnormalities, such as blepharitis, hordeolum, and chalazia.

◼ BLEPHARITIS

Blepharitis is an inflammation of the eyelid. There are two forms of blepharitis: posterior and anterior. Posterior is more common. The distinction is the location of the inflammation and structures involved. Posterior blepharitis is inflammation of the inner portion of the eyelid overlying the meibomian gland. Anterior blepharitis is inflammation at the base of the eyelashes.

Etiology

Blepharitis has several causes. The most common causes are seborrheic dermatitis, bacterial infection with *Staphylococcus*, *Corynebacterium*, or *Cutibacterium*, and irritation or allergy often due to cosmetics and contact lenses.

Symptoms

Patients tend to present after noticing that their eyelid is swollen, and they may have slight discomfort described as a foreign body sensation. This condition tends not to cause pain. Eyes may also be described as watering.

Signs

Inspection of the eye reveals erythema and swelling to the portion of the lid involved and commonly scaling or crusting.

Diagnostics

This is a clinical diagnosis, and additional testing tends to be unnecessary. Culturing eye discharge and crusting is appropriate for recalcitrant cases to investigate bacterial causes.

Treatment

Treatment begins with warm compresses and good eye hygiene. Warm moist compresses should be used two times a day for 10 to 15 minutes, and the eyelid and lashes should be cleansed following compresses with warm water and baby shampoo. The goal of the cleansing is to remove the scale and crusting and to help restore normal function of the meibomian glands. Artificial tears may also be beneficial as the film can be affected in blepharitis. For those with more bothersome symptoms or for patients who do not respond to the initial treatment outlined earlier, topical antibiotics should be added in addition to continuation of the aforementioned treatment. Erythromycin ophthalmic ointment should be used.

- ◼ **Erythromycin ophthalmic ointment** 5 mg/g
  - ◼ 1 cm ribbon of ointment to the lower inner lid four times daily for 7 days.

Follow-Up

Any case that is recalcitrant or worsening requires follow-up and referral. Even though the condition tends to be benign, it can lead to sight-altering complications due to corneal changes and damage.

Education

Often blepharitis can be a chronic condition, and good lid and lash hygiene should be practiced indefinitely to prevent future exacerbation and complications. Contact lenses should be removed until condition subsides. Chronic or recurrent cases managed by ophthalmology should consider discontinuing contact lenses.

■ **CHALAZIA**

A chalazion is a benign swelling of the eyelid. It is a result of gland blockage at the lid; the Zeis and meibomian glands are the involved glands. The glands secrete an oil substance that helps prevent tears from evaporating and aids in the tears' ability to bathe the eye.

Etiology

Chalazia can form from blockage of oil-secreting glands in the lids. This obstruction is typically caused by decreased flow due to the thickness of the oil itself or inflammation of the surrounding tissue due to infection, or it is also commonly associated with blepharitis (see earlier) where the lid inflammation impairs the oil flow. As the oil backs up in the gland, it is released into surrounding tissue causing an inflammatory response.

Symptoms

It is often asymptomatic; however, if the lesion is big enough, it can cause a foreign body sensation.

Signs

There is localized swelling in the form of a subcutaneous nodule in the lid, typically nontender or erythematous. The remainder of the eye is not involved; however, it is a sign that blepharitis may be present during the lid exam as the two conditions are often found together.

Diagnostics

Diagnostics are not necessary for diagnosis. This is a clinical diagnosis.

Treatment

Warm compresses several times a day are usually enough to clear the blockage.

Follow-Up/Referral

Uncomplicated cases do not typically require follow-up. For chalazia that do not respond to warm compresses, referral to an ophthalmologist is warranted for possible incision and drainage or glucocorticoid steroid injection.

Special Considerations

For recurrent or recalcitrant cases, one must consider a more concerning diagnosis such as basal cell carcinoma or sebaceous carcinoma. These are not common in children; however, these recurrent or prolonged cases should be referred to an ophthalmologist for further evaluation.

■ **HORDEOLUM**

A hordeolum is an acute infection of the meibomian gland. Also known as a stye, these infections cause localized swelling and erythema to the lid. There are two types of hordeola: internal that involves infection of the meibomian gland and external that is due to infection of the Zeis gland along the lash line.

Etiology

A hordeolum is an infection of either the meibomian or Zeis gland and is most commonly caused by the *Staphylococcus* species. This is a common infection. Internal hordeolum may cause a more general lid swelling as opposed to the external hordeolum that is more localized and forms a single pustule.

Treatment

Hordeolum tends to follow a benign course. Treatment consists of warm compresses two to four times daily and topical antibiotics.

- **Erythromycin ophthalmic ointment** 5 mg/g
  - 1 cm ribbon of ointment to the lower inner lid four times daily for 7 days.

Follow-Up/Referral

Most cases do not require follow-up. Patients with recalcitrant hordeolum should be referred to an ophthalmologist for incision and drainage.

Complications

Hordeolum infrequently can lead to periorbital and orbital cellulitis (see the "Orbital Cellulitis and Periorbital Cellulitis" section); these are emergencies and need to be managed promptly and aggressively.

■ LACRIMAL SYSTEM INFLAMMATION

Dacryocystitis and dacryoadenitis are two conditions that affect children and involve the lacrimal system of the eye (see Table 3.6). These conditions are less common than the aforementioned topics; however, it is common enough that providers should keep it in the differential for a swollen eye.

Dacryocystitis is inflammation of the lacrimal sac due to nasolacrimal duct obstruction. The obstruction causes swelling to the medial aspect of the eye. The obstruction is commonly caused by a congenital dacryocystocele; however, it is the subsequent infection that causes the urgent need for treatment. Patients present with localized pain redness and swelling over the lacrimal sac in the medial portion of the eye.

Dacryoadenitis is an inflammation of the lacrimal gland. The gland is in the upper lateral portion of the eye, along the brow. Inflammation of this gland tends to occur due to viral infection, such as mononucleosis, influenzas, or mumps. Bacterial causes are most commonly staph and strep. Recurrent cases should raise suspicion for underlying systemic illness such as sarcoid, lupus, and Sjogren's syndrome.

Additional Considerations

If a child presents with periorbital swelling with no signs of infection such as redness and pain, the provider should consider nephrotic syndrome that generally first presents with painless bilateral periorbital edema (see Chapter 10, Common Pediatric Renal/Urologic Disorders Seen in Pediatric Primary Care).

Any child that presents with acute vision loss or amaurosis should be emergently referred to an ophthalmologist and possibly admitted for further evaluation. The cause can be from an ocular disease such as cataract, chorioretinitis, retinoblastoma, or retinitis pigmentosa. Neurologic and systemic disorders that can affect vision are encephalopathy, vasculitis, migraine, leukemia, increased intracranial pressure, rapidly progressive hydrocephalus, or dysfunction of a ventricular shunt, drugs or toxins, or trauma. It may be caused by acute demyelinating disease affecting the optic nerves. Mass effect from gliomas of the optic nerve and chiasm are also considered (Latif et al., 2018).

Table 3.6

Signs, Symptoms, and Treatment Approach to Dacryocystitis and Dacryoadenitis

	Dacryocystitis	Dacryoadenitis
Symptoms	Pain	Pain
Signs	Tenderness, swelling, redness over the lacrimal sac located at the inferomedial aspect of the orbit	Tenderness, redness, swelling of the lacrimal gland located at the lateral one-third of the upper eyelid
Treatment	Warm compresses/massage **Amoxicillin–clavulanate** 20–40 mg/kg/day PO in three divided doses for 10 days	Warm compresses Treat underlying condition If suppurative, then antibiotics are warranted **Cephalexin** 100 mg/kg/day, divided into doses every 6 hours until signs/symptoms resolve
Referral	All patients need to see an **ophthalmologist** for management including possible nasal lacrimal duct dilation Admit patient if any signs of facial cellulitis, periorbital cellulitis, or orbital cellulitis and if fever or evidence of SIRS	All patients need to see an ophthalmologist for management including workup to diagnose possible underlying systemic disease Admit patient if any signs of facial cellulitis, periorbital cellulitis, or orbital cellulitis and if fever or evidence of SIRS

SIRS, systemic inflammatory response syndrome.

EYE PAIN

Eye pain is a red flag for an ocular and systemic condition. It is often accompanied by the red eye but can present in the setting of white sclera as well. The symptom of eye pain should be taken seriously in children and not passed off as functional eye pain or eye strain until a thorough history and eye exam has been performed. Eye pain is often the presenting symptom in vision-threatening conditions. Eye pain can be from a localized eye disorder, an ocular manifestation of an underlying systemic illness, or the result of trauma.

■ OCULAR HERPES SIMPLEX/HERPES KERATITIS

Keratitis is a common term used to infer inflammation of the cornea. Herpes simplex virus (HSV) is a common infectious cause of keratitis. This is a sight-threatening condition and needs to be treated promptly to preserve vision. Patients often present with ocular pain and visual complaints.

Etiology

Ocular manifestations of HSV infections are less likely primary manifestations of disease and more commonly represent a recurrent HSV disease, in which the virus has remained latent.

Most ocular disease is thought to represent recurrent HSV disease following the establishment of viral latency in the host rather than a primary ocular infection. Latency develops after the virus enters sensory neurons and travels to sensory ganglia, and the virus remains in ganglia for the lifetime of the host.

Epidemiology/Risk Factors

Most cases are due to latent HSV infection typically dormant in the trigeminal nerve. HSV is spread by direct contact with mucous membranes. Ocular involvement occurs in less than 5% of primary infections. For acute primary infections, the incubation from time of exposure to presentation is usually within 1 week.

Symptoms

The following are the symptoms of ocular herpes simplex/herpes keratitis: acute onset of unilateral ocular pain, visual disturbance, and thin clear discharge.

PE Signs/Key Findings

Conjunctival and corneal injection with ciliary flushing, photophobia, clear discharge, and **dendritic lesion(s)** are best seen with fluorescein staining. There may also be a cloudy cornea noted. Surrounding vesicular lesions, such as on the forehead, lid, and nose, may be noted as well.

Treatment

Due to the complexity in deciphering whether the acute presentation is epithelial disease, stromal keratitis, or endothelial, ophthalmology referral is necessary. It is important to decipher as treatment with topical glucocorticoids during active epithelial disease has been shown to worsen lesions. Topical or oral or IV antiviral mediation is a cornerstone of all HSV keratitis types. The addition of glucocorticoids is typically used in stromal and endothelial types.

- **Acyclovir ophthalmic ointment 3%:**
  - **Children ≥2 years and adolescents:**
    - Apply a 1-cm ribbon in the lower eyelid of affected eye(s) five times a day (~every 3 hours while awake) until corneal ulcer heals, and then apply a 1-cm ribbon three times daily for 7 more days.
  - **Neonates:**
    - <35 weeks' postconceptional age: acyclovir 40 mg/kg per day IV divided every 12 hours.
    - ≥35 weeks' postconceptional age: acyclovir 60 mg/kg per day IV divided every 8 hours 21 days.
  - **Infants, children, and adolescents:**
    - Oral: acyclovir 80 mg/kg/24 hr divided every 6 hours.
    - Maximum pediatric dose: 1000 mg/24 hours for 7 days (Bradley, Nelson, & Kimberlin, 2015).

Other Considerations

The exam is extremely important in the patient presenting with eye pain. Pay close attention to the eyelids and lashes. Eye pain may be the result of chronic lash irritation due to inversion of the lid margin such as in entropion or due to a roll of skin beneath the lower lashes that causes the lashes to push against the cornea epiblepharon. The term for lashes that are directed toward the cornea is trichiasis. These are serious issues as chronic irritation can cause permanent corneal scarring and visual impairment. A referral to an ophthalmologist is necessary for surgical correction.

■ UVEITIS

Uveitis is the inflammation of the uveal tract. The uveal tissue can be divided into anterior and posterior. The anterior tissues are the pigmented portion of the eye, specifically the iris and the cilia body. The posterior segment is also called the choroid, and inflammation of this region tends not to cause acute eye pain. Anterior uveitis and iritis are often interchanged terminology. This is the most common type of uveitis.

Etiology

Anterior uveitis can be idiopathic and occur due to blunt trauma or iatrogenic and caused by certain infections or underlying rheumatologic or systemic conditions. Underlying systemic conditions should be suspected in recurrent cases of uveitis. Examples of such conditions are juvenile idiopathic arthritis, ankylosing spondylitis, lupus, Crohn's/UC disease, reactive arthritis, Behcet's disease, Kawasaki disease, lupus, and granulomatosis. Infections such as toxoplasmosis, cat scratch disease, and herpes virus have been shown to cause iritis.

Epidemiology/Risk Factors

There is limited epidemiology research on uveitis in children. There are a few large multicenter studies that looked at the demographics, uveitis disease characteristics, complications, treatments, and visual outcomes in pediatric uveitis patients.

Median age at diagnosis ranged between 7 and 10 years old. The leading diagnoses were idiopathic uveitis, juvenile idiopathic arthritis–associated uveitis, toxoplasmosis, and pars planitis. Anterior uveitis was predominant. The prevalence of legal blindness as sequela was between 5% and 7% (Ramirez et al., 2017).

Focused PE Findings/Symptoms

Children with uveitis typically complain of deep ocular/eye pain, excessive tearing, and occasionally photophobia.

Signs

Conjunctival injection, particularly of the area surrounding the limbus (ciliary injection/flushing), photophobia, sluggish, or irregularly shaped pupil, can also be seen. Tender with palpation to the globe. Slit lamp findings include anterior chamber inflammatory cells and flare and occasionally keratic precipitants.

Treatment

All cases of painful eye(s) in children should be referred urgently to ophthalmology, as these can be sight-threatening conditions, and a thorough ocular evaluation that requires a slit lamp examination and dilated funduscopic exam is typically needed to rule out such conditions. The first episode of uveitis is typically treated with topical or systemic anti-inflammatory medications and cycloplegic agents. Recurrent uveitis is often associated with underlying systemic illness and requires a referral to an ophthalmologist for management of the acute ocular condition and a pediatric rheumatologist for workup of an autoimmune disorder.

EYE SWELLING

Eye swelling can take on multiple forms and be the result of several processes. The history and exam are important as the causes range from benign conditions to vision-threatening and even life-threatening conditions. In this section, we will focus on orbital and periorbital infections, eyelid swelling, and lacrimal complex pathology.

ORBITAL CELLULITIS AND PERIORBITAL CELLULITIS

Although the two conditions sound similar in name and even present in a similar fashion, orbital cellulitis is a life- and sight-threatening condition that needs to be managed aggressively, whereas periorbital cellulitis, despite needing treatment, tends to have a much more benign course without the significant sequalae of orbital cellulitis. Orbital cellulitis is an infection of the orbit or the structures behind the orbital septum. The orbital fat and muscles are the soft tissue most commonly involved. Table 3.7 describes the differences between orbital cellulitis and periorbital cellulitis, as well as treatments for both.

Etiology

Periorbital (preseptal) cellulitis is a type of facial cellulitis and is common in children. Infection typically occurs due to insect bites, trauma, or extension from other local infection such as a hordeolum or impetigo. The most common pathogens of periorbital cellulitis are *Streptococcus* and *Staphylococcus aureus*. Herpes simplex has also been implicated in periorbital cellulitis, and children will present with accompanying vesicles around the eye, forehead, nose, or eyelid.

Orbital cellulitis is a deep space infection that occurs classically from the extravasation of a bacterial sinus infection. This extension typically occurs from the ethmoid sinus. The most common pathogens are those typical of bacterial sinus infections such as *Streptococcus*, *M. catarrhalis*, *H. influenzae*, *S. aureus*, and beta-hemolytic *Streptococcus*.

Epidemiology

More common in young children (younger than 8) than in older children or adults. More common in winter months when upper respiratory infections are more prevalent. There are approximately 2,000 pediatric admissions per year for orbital/periorbital infections. Rhinosinusitis is the source of most cases of orbital cellulitis and is present in greater than 80% of cases (Latif, Mahomood, & Shah, 2018).

Follow-Up

Regarding periorbital cellulitis, in any case that is treated, the outpatient needs to have follow-up in 24 hours. Any case that is worsening or fails to respond to treatment in that 24-hour window should be admitted for inpatient management. Patients with orbital cellulitis will likely remain inpatient for a minimum of 3 days and may require repeat imaging to rule out intracranial extension. Once patients are discharged, they will require close follow-up in the ambulatory setting by either ophthalmology or primary care until symptoms resolve.

EYE TRAUMA

Eye trauma is a common injury in children and adolescents. Most trauma is minor, and the injuries are self-limited; however, approximately 30% of all blindness in children results from trauma. Boys have a higher incidence than girls, and injuries peak during adolescents. Common injuries are corneal abrasions, hyphemas, and contusions. More cornering and less common are globe rupture and orbital fractures.

Table 3.7

Differences Between and Approach to Care of Periorbital Cellulitis and Orbital Cellulitis

	Periorbital Cellulitis	Orbital Cellulitis
Symptoms	Superficial pain, difficulty seeing due to lid swelling	Deep eye pain, visual disturbance, malaise, sinusitis symptoms
Signs	Unilateral Eyelid and soft tissue swelling Erythema **Normal ocular movement** **Pain**	Unilateral Eyelid and soft tissue swelling Erythema **Proptosis** **Limitation of eye movement** febrile Ill appearing **Chemosis** Diplopia **Painful eye movement**
Diagnostics	Clinical diagnosis	**CT scan**
Treatment	Outpatient management if mild–moderate **Amoxicillin–clavulanate** (Augmentin) 45 mg/kg PO per day in divided doses every 12 hours **Plus** **Trimethoprim-sulfamethoxazole** 8-12 mg/kg PO per day in divided doses every 12 hours **Severe or with signs of SIRS*: the patient should be admitted with parenteral treatment and ophthalmology consult** Treatment for 7 days or longer if signs of cellulitis are still present	**Needs to be admitted with ophthalmology consultation** **Vancomycin** 40–60 mg/kg IV per day in three or four divided doses, maximum daily dose 4 g **Plus** **Ceftriaxone** 50mg/kg IV per dose twice a day with a maximum of 4 g/day **Plus/minus (yes if intracranial extension or chronic sinusitis or oral source of infection)** **Metronidazole** 30 mg/kg IV per day in divided doses every 8 hours Switch to PO medications once symptoms start to resolve, usually within 5 days Treatment on PO medications varies but is usually 2–4 weeks depending on severity
Complications	**Necrotizing fasciitis** Caused by beta-hemolytic *Streptococcus* Cellulitis with excessive edema and can be violaceous, +/− bullous formation. Necrosis develops, and toxic shock syndrome is common **Admit to hospital with ophthalmology consult**	**Cavernous sinus thrombosis** is a blood clot in the cavernous sinus causing **ocular pain** and swelling along with **headache** and fever Retinal venous dilatation and swelling, typically bilateral Hyperalgesia in the distribution of the fifth cranial nerve is common If orbital or subperiosteal abscess forms, these may require surgical drainage **Admit to hospital with ophthalmology consult**

*SIRS, systemic inflammatory response syndrome. Fever greater than 100.4°F (or less than 96.8°F) taken orally or rectally, tachycardic, tachypneic, elevated white blood cell (WBC) count or greater than 10% bands or depressed WBC count. IV, intravenous.

■ CORNEAL ABRASIONS

Etiology

Corneal abrasions are caused by direct trauma from either an object or finger and cause a scratch or an abrasion to the cornea. Corneal abrasion may also be caused by a foreign body on the inner surface of the lid that scratches the cornea upon each blink. These abrasions are in a linear and vertical distribution.

Symptoms

Corneal abrasions are very painful and typically cause excessive tearing and photophobia.

PE Signs/Findings

Tearing and injected sclera are common. The exam consists of instilling opthcaine to facilitate the exam and control pain. Fluorescein stain is then instilled into the eye using a Wood's lamp to highlight the fluorescein-stained abrasion (see Figure 3.6). The abrasion appears as a yellow to orange illuminated area.

Treatment

Corneal abrasion over the iris or pupil needs close follow-up and ophthalmology follow-up. Otherwise, these can be managed with topical antibiotics, and symptoms tend to improve dramatically over 24 hours. Patching is not indicated and has shown to cause more problems than benefit.

- **Erythromycin ophthalmic ointment** 5 mg/g
  - 1 cm ribbon of ointment to the lower inner lid four times daily for 7 days.

Referral

Ophthalmology referral is indicated for any metal foreign body, retained or embedded foreign body, central abrasion over the pupil, or if symptoms do not significantly improve in 24 hours or if symptoms worsen.

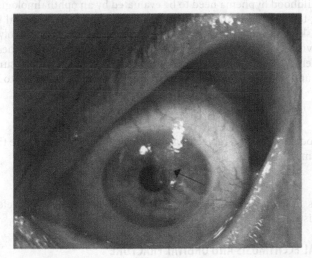

Figure 3.6 Large central corneal abrasion using a Wood's lamp to highlight the fluorescein-stained abrasion.

Source: Wikimedia Commons. (2014, December 24). *File: Human cornea with abrasion highlighted by fluorescein staining.jpg. Wikimedia Commons, the free media repository.* Retrieved from https://commons.wikimedia.org/w/index.php?title=File:Human_cornea_with_abrasion_highlighted_by_fluorescein_staining.jpg&oldid=143989910.

Complications

Any corneal abrasion that increases in pain and symptoms should be suspected of a retained foreign body or subsequent bacterial ulcer. These need to be referred to ophthalmology evaluation and treatment.

Don't Miss

During your examination for the eye, the lids need to be everted to check for a foreign body.

■ HYPHEMA

Hyphema is bleeding into the anterior chamber of the eye, the region between the iris and the cornea. Dramatic in appearance, most of these injuries are self-limiting.

Etiology

It is most commonly caused by trauma to the eye and history of a ball hitting the child in the eye. Risk factors are concomitant diagnoses of diabetes and coagulopathies, such as hemophilia.

Symptoms

Eye pain and visual impairment range from vision loss to blurry vision.

Signs

A hyphema appears as a layering of red blood cells, red fluid level, in the anterior chamber and possible anisocoria.

Treatment

All cases of childhood hyphema need to be evaluated by an ophthalmologist. Hyphema can have long-term sequelae including permanent vision loss. The goal of treatment is to reduce risk of such complications. Treatment of the hyphema involves efforts to minimize the vision-threatening sequelae, bed rest with elevation of the head of the bed to approximately 30 degrees, and an eye shield that does not place pressure on the eye itself. Aspirin and nonsteroidal anti-inflammatories should be avoided to help prevent rebleeding.

Complications

Elevated intraocular pressure, rebleeding, and corneal blood staining are the complications of hyphema.

Referral

All hyphemas (as shown in Figure 3.7) should be emergently referred to an ophthalmologist.

■ PERIORBITAL ECCHYMOSIS AND ORBITAL FRACTURE

A black eye is a common injury in children. A full eye exam is necessary to ensure that there is no globe injury. Isolated black eyes are self-limited. Treatment centers around controlling swelling and pain.

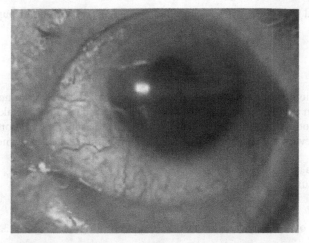

Figure 3.7 Picture of hyphema.
Source: Wikimedia Commons. (2019, August 3). *File: Hyphema - occupying half of anterior chamber of eye.jpg. Wikimedia Commons, the free media repository.* Retrieved from https://commons.wikimedia.org/w/index. php?title=File:Hyphema_-_occupying_half_of_anterior_chamber_of_eye.jpg&oldid=360451219.

Orbital Fracture

The orbit is the bony structure surrounding the eye. The most common site of fracture from blunt trauma is the orbital floor termed a blowout fracture. Orbital fractures present with pain, enophthalmos, diplopia, strabismus, and swelling and palpation tenderness. The fracture sign may entrap orbital structures, which can cause ocular motility dysfunction. Orbital fracture requires an urgent ophthalmology referral. The diagnosis is confirmed by orbital CT scan.

Treatment is typically medical and supportive such as iced compresses to the orbit and elevation of the head of the bed for the first 24 to 48 hours. Prophylactic use of broad-spectrum antibiotics is also commonly used to prevent orbital and intracranial infection. Surgery may also be indicated, further promoting the need for prompt ophthalmology evaluation.

Do not miss a penetrating or perforating globe injury. This is an emergency. Repair needs to be immediate. A penetrating or perforating corneal wound will often present

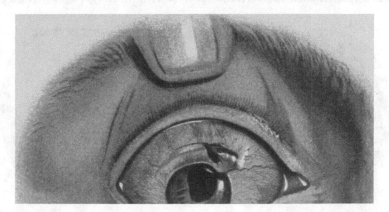

Figure 3.8 Picture of a perforating globe injury.
Source: Reproduced from Ramsay, A. M. (1907). *Eye injuries and their treatment.* Glasgow, UK: J. Maclehose; New York, NY: Macmillan.

with prolapsed iris tissue through the wound or a peaked or irregular pupil (as shown in Figure 3.8).

NOSE

Nasal congestion, rhinorrhea, and sneezing are some of the most common symptoms encountered in a pediatric setting, and nothing brings a parent or caretaker more concern than a bloody nose that seems to want to persist despite intervention. In this section, we will review some of the most common complaints related to the nose:

a. Rhinorrhea and congestion
b. Sinus pressure and pain
c. Epistaxis

A brief review of anatomy can aid in describing PE findings (see Figures 3.9 and 3.10).

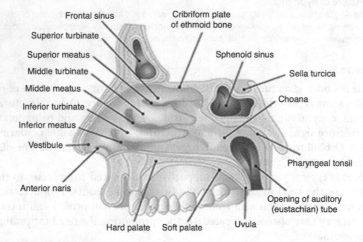

Figure 3.9 Anatomy of the internal nasal cavity.
Source: Reproduced from Gawlik, K. S., Melnyk, B. M., & Teall, A. M. (Eds.). (2021). *Evidence-based physical examination: Best practices for health and well-being assessment.* New York, NY: Springer Publishing Company, p. 342.

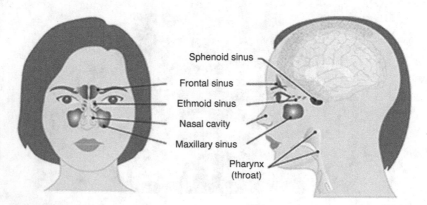

Figure 3.10 Paranasal sinuses.
Source: Reproduced from Gawlik, K. S., Melnyk, B. M., & Teall, A. M. (Eds.). (2021). *Evidence-based physical examination: Best practices for health and well-being assessment.* New York, NY: Springer Publishing Company, p. 342.

■ ACUTE BACTERIAL SINUSITIS

Sinusitis is inflammation of the tissue lining of the sinuses. Inflammation is most commonly caused by viral infections or allergens (see Rhinitis section). Inflammation of the sinuses and surrounding tissues results in impaired clearance of mucous and fluid from the sinuses, which increases the likelihood of a secondary bacterial infection, due to bacterial overgrowth. This results in signs and symptoms of acute bacterial sinusitis. In children, the maxillary and ethmoidal sinuses are the most commonly involved. While frontal sinusitis is common in adulthood, it is rare in children younger than 10 years old, as these sinuses do not pneumatize until around 8 years old.

Etiology

Bacterial sinusitis is most commonly caused by *S. pneumonia*, *H. influenzae*, and *M. catarrhalis*.

Symptoms

Symptoms include nasal congestion, cough, facial pressure, pain, malaise, fatigue and headache, purulent nasal discharge, facial pain, and/or sinus pressure.

PE Signs/Findings

Purulent nasal discharge and fever are common PE findings. Tenderness to palpation and transillumination of sinuses is of limited value in the diagnosis.

Diagnosis

Any child with purulent nasal discharge and fever should be suspected of acute bacterial sinusitis. Acute bacterial sinusitis should also be considered in children who present with 10 days of upper respiratory symptoms including rhinitis for more than 10 days and if symptoms fail to improve or continue to worsen.

Imaging is not necessary in uncomplicated, nonrecurrent, nonchronic cases of acute bacterial sinusitis. Culturing of the paranasal cavity is also not recommended for uncomplicated cases of acute bacterial sinusitis (Hawk, 2015).

Complications

Spread of infection from the sinuses to the surrounding bone and soft tissue of the orbit is the most common complication of acute bacterial sinusitis in children. These can have significant implications. These need to be recognized early and worked up and treated aggressively. These complications are most common in children younger than 5 years old.

PE Signs and Symptoms

Sign and symptoms that should raise suspicion are proptosis, ptosis, lid edema, chemosis, decreased visual acuity, periorbital swelling, and limited extraocular motion. Intracranial complications such as intracranial empyema, venous thrombosis, brain abscess, and meningitis are not as common but have a higher mortality rate and need to be treated emergently. These complications should be suspected in a child with a severe headache, photophobia, seizures, or other focal neurologic findings.

Treatment

Treatment of acute bacterial sinusitis is outlined in Table 3.8.

Table 3.8

Treating Acute Bacterial Sinusitis		
Treatment for ABS		
Uncomplicated	Immunocompromised Younger than 2 years old or recent antibiotic use (<3 months prior)	Penicillin allergy
Amoxicillin–clavulanate 45 mg/kg per day of the <u>amoxicillin</u> component orally in two divided doses (maximum daily dose 1.75 g) for 10 days	**Amoxicillin–clavulanate** 90 mg/kg per day of the amoxicillin component orally in two divided doses (maximum daily dose 4 g) for 10 days	**Mild delayed penicillin allergy** **Cefpodoxime** 10 mg/kg per day orally divided every 12 hours (maximum daily dose 400 mg) **Severe penicillin reaction** **Levofloxacin** 10–20 mg/kg/day PO every 12–24 h

ABS, acute bacterial sinusitis.

Note: Any case of nasal discharge should be evaluated for retained foreign body. Foreign bodies are often lodged in the nose in young children of toddler age. These children present with nasal pain, foul-smelling discharge, possible fever, and facial pain. Simple visualization with either an otoscope and otoscope speculum or a nasal speculum is enough.

■ NASAL CONGESTION AND RHINORRHEA (RHINITIS)

Rhinitis is an extremely common symptom throughout childhood and adolescents. Nasal congestion and rhinorrhea are caused by inflamed mucous membranes in the nose, which is termed rhinitis.

Common causes of rhinitis are of infectious and allergic etiologies.

Acute Viral Rhinitis

Often referred to as the common cold, this is the most common infection in children of all ages but especially less than 5 years of age. Some estimates have infection rates as high as 6 to 12 times per year.

Etiology

The following are the common etiologies of rhinitis: rhinovirus, influenza, coronavirus, and enterovirus.

Symptoms

Symptoms can last 10 days. Sudden onset of clear mucous production is the common symptom, which is often accompanied by other upper respiratory symptoms such as sneezing, sore throat, cough, and fever.

PE Signs/Findings

Clear rhinorrhea, inflamed nasal mucosa, cobblestoning of oropharynx, periorbital swelling, conjunctiva injection, and excessive lacrimation are the common PE findings. OME may be present as well.

Treatment

Symptoms can last for 5 to 10 days. Educating parents and children on the course and length of the symptoms reminds them that this is a self-limited course and this education is beneficial in preventing return visits for unchanged symptoms. Treatment is supportive. Antibiotics are not warranted.

Common approaches to supportive care are nasal suction; saline nasal drops, spray, or irrigation; adequate hydration; and cool mist.

For patients who do not respond and still are complaining of bothersome symptoms, the following have shown some promise:

- For children 6 years old, ipratropium nasal spray 0.06% (Atrovent) is recommended; two sprays per nostril two to three times daily.
- For children ≥12 years, ipratropium 0.06% nasal spray is recommended; two sprays in each nostril three to four times per day for 4 days
- For children ≥12 years with bothersome nasal symptoms that do not respond to supportive interventions, OTC decongestants (oral or topical) are appropriate to try.

Follow-Up

Typically not necessary.

Allergic Rhinitis

Etiology

Allergic rhinitis may be seasonal and caused by grasses and pollens, or perennial, meaning recurring, and caused by animal dander, dust, or mold. Patients with a history of atopy such as eczema and asthma are most commonly affected.

Table 3.9

Differentiating Viral Versus Allergic Rhinitis		
Rhinitis	**Viral**	**Allergic**
History	Acute <10 days	Symptoms tend to last longer and should be suspected if symptoms last greater than 2 weeks or are recurrent
History and symptoms	Acute onset, runny nose, congestion, sneezing, sore throat, ear fullness	History of asthma or eczema, seasonal recurrence, subacute or chronic symptoms, runny nose, congestion, sneezing, ear fullness, malaise, fatigue, headache
Signs	Clear rhinitis, +/−fever, +/−cervical and tonsillar lymphadenopathy	Clear rhinitis, conjunctivitis, allergic shiners
Treatment	First line: supportive, saline nasal spray/drops Second line: for <6-year-olds, ipratropium is recommended Third line: for >6-year-olds, decongestants topical or oral are recommended	First line: for >6-month-olds, nonsedating antihistamines are recommended Second line: for >2-year-olds, intranasal corticosteroids are recommended Third line: combination For <5-year-olds, intranasal steroid and PO antihistamine are recommended For >5-year-olds, intranasal steroid and antihistamine are recommended
Referral	Typically not necessary	Allergist

PE Symptoms

PE findings are very similar to those of the common cold. Chronic or recurring symptoms should prompt the provider to suspect an allergic cause of rhinitis.

In general, more systemic symptoms such as fatigue, headache malaise, conjunctivitis, and periorbital venous congestion allergic shiners suggest an allergic rhinitis.

Signs

Allergic shiners (i.e., dark areas under the eyes) suggest allergic rhinitis.

Treatment

As shown in Table 3.9, treatment varies depending on the diagnosis of viral versus allergic rhinitis. Intranasal corticosteroids are the most effective treatment and should be the first-line therapy for persistent symptoms affecting quality of life. More severe disease that does not respond to intranasal corticosteroids should be treated with second-line therapies, including oral antihistamines, decongestants, cromolyn, eukotrienes receptor antagonists, and nonpharmacologic therapies such as nasal irrigation.

MOUTH

Acute soft tissue lesions of the oral cavity are common encounters for the pediatric primary care provider. Seldom a medical emergency, these tend to elicit high anxiety and concern in patients and parents. The next paragraphs aim to help pediatric primary care providers approach these in an efficient and logical manner. The most commonly encountered lesions are thrush, herpangina, aphthous ulcers, HSV (see Chapter 9, Dermatologic Abnormalities Commonly Seen in Pediatric Primary Care), and erythema multiforme (see Chapter 9, Dermatologic Abnormalities Commonly Seen in Pediatric Primary Care).

■ APHTHOUS ULCERATIONS

Otherwise known as canker sores, aphthous ulcers are shallow ulcerations of the buccal mucosa, tongue, and gingiva.

Etiology

The exact cause of these ulcers is unknown but likely to be multifactorial. Trauma, genetic factors, nutritional deficiencies, viral and bacterial infections, medications, food hypersensitivities, hormonal or endocrine changes, and tobacco use have been thought to be causative factors associated with aphthous ulcers. However, there have been no strong correlations made. What is known is that aphthous ulcers are normally recurrent in a condition known as recurrent aphthous stomatitis, or RAS, where the patient experiences two or more outbreaks of these ulcerations per year

Epidemiology/Risk Factors

Most aphthous ulcers occur during adolescents, and recurrences resolve by early adulthood. Some studies suggest a prevalence of 20% of children will experience an occurrence. Acute outbreaks typically resolve in 1 to 2 weeks.

Symptoms

There are painful ulcers in the mouth. Pain can be exacerbated by acidic food and drink, cold or hot food and liquids, or friction from dental appliances. These tend not to have associated systemic symptoms.

Signs

Shallow round oral ulcers with erythematous border.

Diagnostics

None required. This is a clinical diagnosis.

Treatment

- Treatment centers around symptom relief, specifically pain management, until the ulcers resolve.
- Topical anesthetics are effective at relieving pain from the ulcers.
  - 2% viscous lidocaine swish and spit or combination analgesic mouthwashes such as magic mouthwash.
    - It is a combination of 2% viscous lidocaine, liquid diphenhydramine, and magnesium hydroxide used in a swish-and-spit application.
- Using ibuprofen and acetaminophen is appropriate for all ages.
  - **Ibuprofen**
  - 10 mg/kg orally every 6 hours as needed (maximum single dose 600 mg; maximum daily dose up to 2.4 g/day).
  - **Acetaminophen**
  - 10 to 15 mg/kg orally every 4 to 6 hours as needed up to five doses not to exceed 4 g/day.
- To aide in resolution of ulcers:
  - Dexamethasone elixir 0.5 mg/5 cc: 5 mL swish and spit up to four times daily.

Patient Education

Educating patients/parents to avoid hot, spicy, or acidic foods is generally an accepted first-line recommendation for preventing exacerbation of pain. A soft toothbrush and mild toothpaste are recommended.

Special Considerations

Behcet syndrome is an autoimmune vasculitis that typically presents with recurrent aphthous ulcers. Oral ulcers are often accompanied by genital ulcerations. Patients will often have multisystem symptoms such as uveitis, vasculitis, arthritis, abdominal pain, diarrhea, and constitutional symptoms such as fever and malaise. Multisystem symptoms and aphthous ulcers or three or more occurrences of aphthous ulcer outbreaks should raise suspicion for Behcet syndrome. Patients should be referred to rheumatology for confirmation and treatment.

Periodic fever with aphthous stomatitis, pharyngitis, and adenitis (PFAPA syndrome) is a benign syndrome with cyclical fever and aphthous ulcers that are accompanied by cervical adenitis and pharyngitis. This is a clinical diagnosis. Fever is cyclical and remitting. Referral to a rheumatologist is recommended despite its benign course to rule out other periodic fever syndromes.

■ HERPANGINA

Herpangina is a viral illness that presents with oral lesions and a constellation of viral illness symptoms such as high fever, headache, myalgia, and malaise. The oral lesions of herpangina are vesicular ulcerative and present on the anterior tonsillar pillars, soft palate, uvula, tonsils, or posterior pharyngeal wall.

Etiology

Herpangina is a viral illness that is caused by enteroviruses, most commonly coxsackie A virus, which is also the main cause of hand foot and mouth disease (see Chapter 9, Dermatologic Abnormalities Commonly Seen in Pediatric Primary Care).

Epidemiology

A common childhood illness, herpangina most frequently affects children younger than 10 years. Outbreaks tend to be higher in summer and early fall months.

Symptoms

Oral and pharyngeal pain, headache, and malaise are common. Typically, prior to the manifestation of oral lesions, there is a prodrome of fever and malaise.

Signs

Oropharyngeal vesicles that ulcerate within 24 hours leaving a shallow ulcer with erythematous border. Lesions are most commonly found on the pillars, soft palate, pharynx, and tonsils. Herpangina fever is generally high, sometimes as high as 104–105°F, and has been associated with febrile seizures. There are typically no other dermatologic manifestations of herpangina.

Treatment

- Herpangina is a self-limiting viral illness that is usually resolved within 2 to 5 days.
- Treatment is supportive, focusing on adequate hydration, fever management, and pain management.
- Recommendations are for use of antipyretics and analgesics such as ibuprofen and acetaminophen.
  - **Ibuprofen**
    10 mg/kg orally every 6 hours as needed (maximum single dose 600 mg; maximum daily dose up to 2.4 g/day).
  - **Acetaminophen**
    10 to 15 mg/kg orally every 4 to 6 hours as needed up to five doses, not to exceed 4 g/day.

Complications

Herpangina compilations are rare. Dehydration is the most common complication due to high fevers in combination with decreased oral intake of fluids. There have been cases of neurologic and cardiac complications associated with herpangina, such as meningitis, flaccid paralysis, and myocarditis (Messacar, Abzug, & Nelson, 2020).

Referral

Referral is seldom necessary; however, patients who are not able to maintain adequate hydration should be hospitalized. Coxsackie A virus can have multiple manifestations; albeit uncommon, providers should actively question and examine for any expression of meningitis, flaccid paralysis, or myocarditis; if these are detected, the patient should be admitted for observation and treatment.

■ OROPHARYNGEAL CANDIDIASIS

More commonly referred to as thrush, it is a common oral condition in children and typically manifests as white plaques on the oral mucosa and tongue.

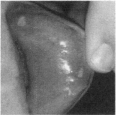
Aphthous ulcers

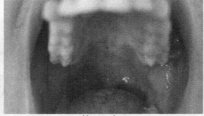
Herpangina

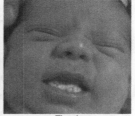
Thrush

Figure 3.11 Examples of thrush, aphthous ulcers, and herpangina.
Source: Wikimedia Commons. (2017, January 6). *File: Aphthous stomatitis.jpg. Wikimedia Commons, the free media repository.* Retrieved from https://commons.wikimedia.org/w/index.php?title=File:Aphthous_stomatitis. jpg&oldid=228811465; Wikimedia Commons. (2016, November 29). *File: Herpangina 2.JPG. Wikimedia Commons, the free media repository.* Retrieved from https://commons.wikimedia.org/w/index.php?title=File:Herpangina_2. JPG&oldid=223793992; Wikimedia Commons. (2018, April 29). *File: Thrush2010.JPG. Wikimedia Commons, the free media repository.* Retrieved from https://commons.wikimedia.org/w/index.php?title=File:Thrush2010. JPG&oldid=298940324.

Etiology

Thrush is caused by *Candida albicans. Candida* species are considered part of the normal oral flora. *Candida* overgrowth in the oropharynx can lead to thrush (as shown in Figure 3.11).

Epidemiology

Thrush is a common pediatric condition, with some studies citing up to 37% of healthy newborns being diagnosed. Risk factors include diabetes, hypothyroidism, steroid inhalers, chemotherapy, and antibiotic use.

Symptoms

Many patients with thrush are asymptomatic; others may have pain with chewing and swallowing.

Signs

White plaques appear on the oral mucosa and tongue. Scraping of the white plaques will leave an erythematous base that sometimes will bleed.

Diagnosis

This is generally a clinical diagnosis; however, in cases that are less clear or in recurrent cases, scrapings can be cultured or a KOH preparation can be performed in office.

Treatment

- In bottle-fed infants, it is assumed that the bottles, nipples, and pacifiers are contaminated. New items or sterilization of existing items need to be performed.
- For infants who are breastfeeding, treatment of mother's nipple/breast should be considered. The recommendation is topical clotrimazole or miconazole, applied between feedings and wiped away prior to feeding.

Complications

While most cases of thrush are benign and managed quite easily, cases that are recalcitrant to treatment or children who present with multiple recurrent cases should be tested for immunodeficiency.

Table 3.10

Nystatin Treatment and Dosing in Newborns, Infants, Toddlers, and Older Children	
Newborns and Infants (0–12 months)	**Toddler and Older (1+ years old)**
Nystatin solution 100,000 units using dropper to each inner cheek every 6 hours; treat for 2–3 days past resolution of lesions	**Nystatin solution 200,000–300,000 units** using dropper to each inner cheek every 6 hours; treat for 2–3 days past resolution of lesions
Immunocompromised or if it does not resolve with nystatin **Fluconazole** 3 mg/kg, once a day for 7 days	Immunocompromised or recalcitrant to nystatin Day 1 **Fluconazole** 6 mg/kg PO once daily Days 2–7 **Fluconazole** 3 mg/kg PO

There are also rare times when oral cases of candidiasis can disseminate. Children who have cases of thrush who present with systemic symptoms of sepsis, development of other skin lesions, and fever should be evaluated for disseminated cases.

Follow-Up

Follow-up in mild cases responding to treatment is unnecessary. Follow-up in severe cases or in cases where newborn and infant feeding was interrupted due to oral lesions is necessary.

Referral

Any recalcitrant case to treatment is outlined in Table 3.10. In any recurrent cases in which immune deficiency is suspected and in the case of disseminated candidiasis, hospital admission is warranted.

THROAT (OROPHARYNX)

■ PHARYNGITIS/TONSILLITIS/PHARYNGOTONSILLITIS

Pharyngitis, or sore throat, is a common childhood illness. It is the second most common acute infection seen in the pediatrics and family medicine practice. Sore throat is a more prominent chief complaint encountered in the pediatric patient population, specifically of school-age children.

Don't Miss

It is important to note that tonsillitis and pharyngitis are used interchangeably in this chapter with the main distinction being that tonsillitis occurs when the primary area of swelling and erythema involves the actual tonsils.

Etiology

Most causes are infectious with the clear majority caused by viruses. Viruses are responsible for 70% of sore throats in children aged 5 to 16 years and closer to 95% of sore throats in children younger than 5 years old. The viruses that are responsible for pharyngitis are the same that cause most viral upper respiratory infections, such as adenoviruses, enteroviruses, rhinoviruses, coronaviruses, and parainfluenza viruses. Some

Table 3.11

Differentiating and Treating Common Causes of Acute Pharyngitis

	Viral	GABHS	Mononucleosis	Epiglottitis	Peritonsillar abscess
Symptoms	Sore throat Rhinitis Congestion Fatigue Laryngitis Cough	Sore throat Fever Headache Abdominal pain Nausea/vomiting	Sore throat Fever Fatigue	Sore throat Fever **Dysphagia** Dyspnea	Unilateral sore throat Fever Neck pain
Signs	Erythematous oropharynx/ tonsils +/– tonsillar swelling Low-grade fever Nasal discharge conjunctivitis	Erythematous oropharynx/ tonsils Tonsillar swelling Exudates Cervical adenopathy Rash (scarlatiniform)	Erythematous oropharynx Exudates **Posterior cervical lymphadenopathy** Enlarged spleen/ liver	Ill appearing Labored breathing **Drooling** Tripod position Muffled voice Stridor **Distressed**/anxious Hyperextended neck	Anxious Trismus Sniff position **Muffled voice** **Unilateral tonsillar swelling** Uvular deviation
Diagnostics	Not required	+ rapid strep test Or + throat culture *– rapid strep tests should be confirmed with throat culture	+ Monospot (heterophile antibody) **Lymphocytosis** Elevated LFTs *If negative monospot, but clinically suspicious, send for confirmation labs EBV IgM and IgG VCA	**Prompt transfer to an emergency medical center** Laryngoscope in ICU Or Lateral neck x-ray in hypertension to look for thumb sign	Imaging Intraoral US CT scan MRI Needle aspiration

(continued)

Chapter **3** Abnormalities of the Ears, Eyes, Nose, and Throat (EENT) Commonly Seen in Pediatric Primary Care

Table 3.11

Differentiating and Treating Common Causes of Acute Pharyngitis (continued)

	Viral	GABHS	Mononucleosis	Epiglottitis	Peritonsillar abscess
Treatment	Supportive and symptomatic care **Ibuprofen** 10 mg/kg orally every 6 hours as needed (maximum single dose 600 mg; maximum daily dose up to 2.4 g/day) **Acetaminophen** 10–15 mg/kg orally every 4 to 6 hours as needed up to 5 doses not to exceed 4 g/day	**Penicillin VK** Children ≤27 kg: 250 mg three times daily for 10 days Children >27 kg and adolescent 500 mg three times daily for 10 days **Penicillin allergy (mild)** **Cephalexin** 40 mg/kg/day divided every 12 hours for 10 days, maximum dose: 500 mg/dose **Penicillin allergy (severe)** **Azithromycin** 12 mg/kg/dose once daily for 5 days; maximum dose: 500 mg/day Rheumatic fever Risk significantly reduced by treating GABHS *PSGN **Risk is not influenced by antibiotic treatment of the primary infection**	Supportive care Rest Avoid contact sports until splenomegaly resolves and asymptomatic Ibuprofen for fever and sore throat Consider corticosteroids in patients who have severe throat pain or significant tonsillitis Rash may develop if given ampicillin or amoxicillin **Monitor for splenic rupture pericarditis encephalitis**	**Secure airway intubation** ICU Antibiotics **Ceftriaxone** 50–100 mg/kg per day once daily or in two divided doses Maximum daily dose 2 g **plus** **Vancomycin** 40–60 mg/kg per day in three to four divided doses Maximum daily dose 2 g **Prompt transfer from ambulatory practice to a medical center** **Keep patient calm** This is rare because of HIB vaccination	**Needle aspiration** or **I-D** Empiric IV antibiotics **Ampicillin–sublactam** 50 mg/kg q6 hr with maximum single dose of 3g **Or** **Clindamycin** 13 mg/kg per q8 hr with maximum single dose of 900 mg **Transfer to ED** **Or** **Otolaryngology** The setting for needle aspiration or I +D needs to ensure the ability to manage airway complications Ambulatory practice settings are generally not suitable

EBV, Epstein–Barr virus; GABHS, group A beta-hemolytic *Streptococcus*; US, ultrasound; VCA, viral capsid antigen.

fewer common causes of viral pharyngitis are influenza A and B and mononucleosis. High fever, fatigue, and cervical adenopathy should prompt the provider to strongly consider infectious mononucleosis as the cause of the patient's symptoms.

The most common bacterial cause of sore throat is group A beta-hemolytic *Streptococcus* (GABHS). Some less common bacterial causes are groups C and G *Streptococcus* and *N. gonorrhoeae*. Presentation is similar among all of these. Presentation is most likely to include sore throat, pharnygotonsillar exudate, and fever in the absence of cough and rhinitis. GABHS is the most common of the bacterial infections, and a rapid strep test is the first line in distinguishing these. A rapid strep test is a rapid antigen detection test (RADT). All rapid tests that are negative for GABHS should be followed by a throat culture. The throat culture is not only a confirmation test but also used to identify the other aforementioned causes of pharyngotonsillitis. Treatment should be geared toward the pathogen isolated from culture (see Table 3.11).

A common noninfectious cause of acute pharyngitis is postnasal drip from rhinitis either infectious or allergic. More chronic sore throats may be caused by gastroesophageal reflux, smoking or secondhand smoke exposure, or perennial allergic rhinitis (Miriam, Celestin, & Hussain, 2004).

Epidemiology

Pharyngitis is most commonly encountered in the winter and early spring months. Transmission of pathogens occurs because acute pharyngitis occurs mostly through contact with nasal discharge and oral secretions. Acute pharyngitis accounts for approximately 13 million ambulatory care visits, or 1% to 2% of all ambulatory care visits, in the United States annually. The incidence peaks in childhood and adolescence with approximately 50% of all cases occurring before age 18 years.

Complications

Epiglottitis and suppurative infections of the neck, such as a peritonsillar abscess, need to be considered when a child presents with acute pharyngitis. Both are life-threatening conditions and should not be managed in an ambulatory practice setting. Patients should be transferred promptly to a hospital setting preferably with access to pediatric critical care specialists.

Referral

As described earlier, any case of deep space infection such as PTA or a case of epiglottis needs to be emergently transferred to a hospital setting.

Ambulatory referral to an otolaryngologist should be considered in any child who has a recalcitrant case of pharyngotonsillitis despite appropriate intervention, recurrent infections ≥7 per year, and obstructive symptoms such as snoring, choking, or obstructive sleep apnea.

References

Abelson, M. B., Allansmith, M. R., & Friedlaender, M. H. (1980). Effects of topically applied ocular decongestant and antihistamine. *American Journal of Ophthalmology, 90*(2), 254–257. doi:10.1016/s0002-9394(14)74864-0

Bradley, J. S., Nelson, J. D., & Kimberlin, D. K. (2015). *Nelson's pocket book of pediatric antimicrobial therapy* (21st ed.). Philadelphia, PA: Lippincott Williams & Wilkins.

Hawk, L. (2015). AAP releases guideline on diagnosis and management of acute bacterial sinusitis in children one to 18 years of age. *American Family Physician, 89*(8), 676–681.

Latif, A., Mahomood, S., & Shah, A. (2018). Asad Latif and Syed Mahmood Ali Shah ophthalmology. *American Journal of Ophthalmology, 185*, 185–191.

Lesperance, M., & Flynt, P. (2015). *Pediatric otolaryngology*. Philadelphia, PA: Elsevier Saunders.

Liese, J. G., Silfverdal, S., Giaquinto, C., Carmona, A., Larcombe, J. H., Garcia-Sicilia, J., & Roselund, M. (2014). Incidence and clinical presentation of acute otitis media in children aged <6 years in European medical practices. *Epidemiology and Infection, 142*(8), 1778–1788. doi:10.1017/S0950268813002744

Mansour, S., Magnan, J., Haidar, H., & Nicolas, K. (2014). *Tympanic membrane retraction pockets*. Retrieved from https://link.springer.com/book/10.1007/978-3-319-13996-8

Messacar, K., Abzug, M. J., & Nelson, N. (2020). *Nelson textbook of pediatrics* (21st ed.). Philadelphia, PA: Elsevier.

Miriam, V., Celestin, N., & Hussain, A. (2004). *American family physician*. Brooklyn, NY: State University of New York-Downstate Medical Center.

Ramirez, D. A., Porco, T. C., Thomas, M., & Keenan, J. (2017). Epidemiology of conjunctivitis in US emergency departments. *JAMA Opthalmology, 135*(10), 1721–1729. doi:10.1001/jamaophthalmol.2017.3319

Steele, D., Adam, G. P., & Di, M. (2017). *Tympanostomy tubes in children with Otitis Media*. Rockville, MD: Agency for Healthcare Research and Quality (US). Retrieved from https://www.ncbi.nlm.nih.gov/books/NBK447521/

Abnormalities of the Respiratory System Commonly Seen in Pediatric Primary Care

Michael S. Ruggiero

INTRODUCTION

Respiratory illnesses have a number of clinical manifestations with the most common being cough and breathlessness. Respiratory disease is a major cause of mortality and morbidity worldwide, with infants and young children being the most vulnerable. The spectrum of disease ranges from acute infections to chronic noncommunicable diseases. Viral infections of the airway are a frequent cause of hospitalization in children, and pneumonia remains a major cause of childhood mortality and the leading infectious cause of death in children, responsible for over a million childhood deaths a year.

Asthma is the most common noncommunicable pulmonary disease in children. This chapter will focus on the most common causes of acute cough and acute breathlessness in children.

OBJECTIVES

1. Identify common causes of acute cough in children.
2. Recognize the child in acute respiratory distress.
3. Discern between the viral and bacterial causes of acute cough.
4. Explain the treatment and management of children diagnosed with croup, whooping cough, bronchiolitis, influenza, and the common cold.
5. Identify signs and symptoms, workup, and appropriate treatment associated with community-acquired pneumonia (CAP).
6. Describe the management of a child who presents with an acute asthma exacerbation.
7. Explain the criteria for transfer to an emergency medical center for a child presenting with an acute asthma exacerbation.

Key Points

- A proper physical examination and history are required to efficiently and effectively diagnose a child with pulmonary complaints.

(continued)

(continued)

- Clothing should be removed from the upper half of the child's body so that the thorax may be inspected; proper draping is appropriate in teens to help preserve modesty.
- Providers must observe respiratory patterns and respiratory effort in order to pick up subtleties of early respiratory distress.
- Remember to closely look for intercostal and substernal retractions and nasal flaring as these are findings consistent with increased effort of respiration and signs of underlying pulmonary illness and possible respiratory distress.
- Rate of breathing is also important as tachypnea is an important sign of respiratory distress and early sign of imminent respiratory failure.
  - Respiratory rates should be taken for a full minute via auscultation and preferably with the patient calmly at rest. See Table 4.1 for age-appropriate respiratory rates.

Table 4.1

Age-Appropriate Respiratory Rates

Age	Normal Respiratory Rate, breaths/minute
<3 months	34–57
3–6 months	33–55
6 to <9 months	31–52
9 to <12 months	30–50
12 to <18 months	28–46
18 to <24 months	25–40
2 to <3 years	22–34
3 to <4 years	21–29
4 to <6 years	20–27
6 to <8 years	18–24
8 to <12 years	16–22
12 to <15 years	15–21
15–18 years	13–19

COUGH

■ BRONCHIOLITIS

Bronchiolitis is a common and potentially serious lower respiratory tract disorder in infants and children. Bronchiolitis is an inflammation of the lower respiratory tract's bronchioles and is most commonly caused by a viral infection. It affects infants and young children most commonly, with many cases occurring within the first 2 years of life.

Etiology

Bronchiolitis is caused by viral etiologies, with RSV being the most common. Although the exact mechanism is unclear, it is likely that direct viral cytotoxic injury has a role in the pathogenesis of RSV infections. This leads to necrosis of the epithelial cells of the small airways, and the sloughed cells and mucus cause plugging of the bronchioles that leads to hyperinflation and atelectasis.

Epidemiology/Risk Factors

Bronchiolitis affects infants and young children, most commonly under 2 years of age. It is estimated that more than 57,500 hospitalizations and 2.1 million outpatient visits are associated with RSV infections each year in U.S. children younger than 5 years. Babies born prematurely (at or before 35 weeks) and who are 6 months of age or less at the beginning of RSV season are at increased risk of RSV infection.

Prevention

Synagis (palivizumab) is not a vaccine, but it is an injection containing virus-fighting antibodies to infants and children at risk for RSV infection and should be given every 28 to 30 days during the RSV season.

Consider Synagis (palivizumab) for children who have

- bronchopulmonary dysplasia (BPD);
- chronic lung disease of prematurity (CLDP);
- hemodynamically significant congenital heart disease (HS-CHD); and
- premature infants (born at or before 35 weeks; Box 4.1).

BOX 4.1 WHEN TO CONSIDER SYNAGIS INJECTIONS

First year of life during the RSV season, if:

Hemodynamically significant heart disease

Preterm with chronic lung disease of prematurity

Second year of life (younger than 24 months at time of RSV) during the RSV season, if:

Chronic lung disease requiring treatment (e.g., supplemental oxygen, steroid therapy)

Congenital heart disease

RSV, respiratory syncytial virus.

Symptoms, focused physical exam (PE) signs/findings, lab tests/diagnostics, and treatment of bronchiolitis can be found in Table 4.2.

Cough is the most common pediatric symptom managed by pediatric practitioners. Most coughs are caused by acute viral infections, with the most common diagnosis being "upper respiratory tract infection." Most coughs in children are caused by undifferentiated acute respiratory tract infections, but some common causes have a clear diagnostic syndrome, such as croup, whooping cough, pneumonia, and bronchiolitis. Asthma is another common cause of cough; however, this will be covered further along in this chapter, under Dyspnea/Shortness of Breath.

The next few sections will explore some of the most common causes of cough in children. Cough due to a viral respiratory infection is sometimes referred to as the common cold, which is typically the most common cause of acute cough; however, other forms of viral respiratory illnesses are common in children, and identifying and differentiating them is important as each has their own set of possible complications.

■ LARYNGOTRACHEOBRONCHITIS

Laryngotracheobronchitis (LTB), otherwise known as croup, is the swelling of the larynx, trachea, and bronchi, leading to inspiratory stridor and a barking cough. This is a common cause of an acute cough in children, specifically those younger than 5 years.

Etiology

Viruses are responsible for croup, with parainfluenza virus being the predominant cause isolated in 75% of patients. Less common viral etiologies include influenza A and B, adenovirus, respiratory syncytial virus (RSV), rhinovirus, and enterovirus.

Epidemiology

Most common in young children and infants, croup is a major cause of hospitalization of children in the United States (Smith, McDermott, & Sullivan, 2018). Peak occurrence is in the fall and winter and affects approximately 3% of children aged 6 months to 3 years. Each year in the United States, croup accounts for 7% of hospitalizations for fever and/or acute respiratory illness in children.

Symptoms, signs, and treatment of croup are outlined in Table 4.2.

■ PERTUSSIS

Pertussis, also known as whooping cough, is an acute bacterial respiratory tract infection that often presents with its classic paroxysmal cough. Some studies report that up to 17% of patients who develop a cough lasting longer than 2 weeks have pertussis.

Etiology

Whooping cough is a highly contagious disease caused by the bacteria *Bordetella pertussis* and rarely other *Bordetella* species. It is an infection of the trachea and the bronchi, as it affects the ciliated tissue of the airway.

Epidemiology/Risk Factors

The reported incidence of pertussis is 8.5 cases per 100,000 persons in the overall population. In infants, the incidence is considerably higher (88.7 per 100,000). Most cases of pertussis are in children under the age of 1 year. Pertussis is a relatively common cause of respiratory tract infection in infants, children, adolescents, and adults, especially in those who are under-immunized or not immunized. Therefore, prevention is key, and the recommendation is still for age-related vaccination of pertussis, which is given as the DTaP (diphtheria, tetanus, and acellular pertussis) vaccine at months 2, 4, 6, and 15 and at year 4.

Symptoms, focused PE signs/findings, lab tests/diagnostics, and treatment of pertussis can be found in Table 4.2.

■ PNEUMONIA

Pneumonia is an inflammation of the lung tissue that is typically due to infection. Pneumonia remains a common cause of cough in children.

Etiology

The presumed infectious cause(s) of pneumonia in children varies by age, as shown in Table 4.3. For instance, viruses cause a significant percentage of CAP infections, especially in children younger than 2 years; however, the prevalence of viral pneumonia decreases with age. *Streptococcus pneumonia* is the most common bacterial cause of

Table 4.2

Clinical Manifestations, Workup, and Treatment of Common (Nonpneumonia) Causes of Cough in Children

	Croup	Bronchiolitis	Whooping Cough	Viral URI (Common Cold)	Influenza
Symptoms	**Cough** Low-grade fever Coryza Cough more pronounced at night and with crying	**Cough** Low-grade fever Congestion Difficulty feeding	**Three stages:** **Catarrhal** Runny nose Sore throat Mild cough **Paroxysmal** Coughing spells Posttussive emesis **Convalescent** Intensity and frequency of coughing spells gradually diminish	**Nasal congestion** Sore throat Sneezing Fever Cough	**Fever (>100.4°F)** **Headache** **Myalgia** Cough Sore throat Rhinorrhea
Focused PE signs/ findings	**Barking cough** **Inspiratory stridor** Hoarseness Tachypnea	**Wheezing** **Inspiratory crackles** Increased respiratory effort Severe cases: **Cyanosis** **Apnea** Tachypnea	**Three stages:** **Catarrhal** Rhinitis Mild cough Fever **Paroxysmal** Coughing spells Inspiratory whoop **Convalescent** Frequency of coughing spells gradually diminishes	**Rhinitis** Pharyngeal erythema	**Fever** Rhinitis Pharyngitis
Lab tests/ diagnostics	Clinical diagnosis	PCR of nasopharyngeal secretions The chest is hyperinflated on x-ray	Pertussis cultures or PCR	Clinical diagnosis	Clinical diagnosis that can be confirmed by testing Rapid flue antigen test Or Rapid molecular assays, if available

(continued)

Chapter **4** Abnormalities of the Respiratory System Commonly Seen in Pediatric Primary Care

Table 4.2

Clinical Manifestations, Workup, and Treatment of Common (Nonpneumonia) Causes of Cough in Children (continued)

	Croup	Bronchiolitis	Whooping Cough	Viral URI (Common Cold)	Influenza
Treatment	*All cases:* Dexamethasone 0.6 mg per kg for one dose (maximum 16 mg) *Moderate/severe:* Nebulized racemic epinephrine 2.25%. Dose 0.05 mL/kg with maximum dose 0.5 mL. The medication should be diluted to 3 ml total volume with normal saline. **If repeat dose is necessary, consider transferring to inpatient/hospital setting.**	Supportive care Suctioning of secretions Maintain proper hydration Ibuprofen and Tylenol for fever **Ibuprofen** 10 mg/kg orally every 6 hours as needed (maximum single dose 600 mg; maximum dailydose up to 2.4 g/day) **Acetaminophen** 10–15 mg/kg orally every 4–6 hours as needed, up to five doses, not to exceed 4 g/day	Supportive care Maintain proper hydration *<6 months of age:* **Azithromycin** 10 mg/kg per day in a single dose for 5 days *≥6 months:* **Azithromycin** 10 mg/kg in a single dose on day 1 (maximum 500 mg); then 5 mg/kg per day (maximum: 250 mg) on days 2–5 *Postexposure prophylaxis for household/close contacts:* Azithromycin Dosage same as for treatment	Supportive care Treatment for viral rhinitis (see Chapter 3, Abnormalities of the Ears, Eyes, Nose, and Throat Commonly Seen in Pediatric Primary Care) Ibuprofen and Tylenol for fever and sore throat **Ibuprofen** 10 mg/kg orally every 6 hours, as needed (maximum single dose 600 mg; maximum daily dose 2.4 g/day) **Acetaminophen** 10–15 mg/kg orally every 4–6 hours, as needed; up to 5 doses, not to exceed 4 g/day	**Antiviral treatment is recommended for:** Children younger than 5 years Immunocompromised Sickle cell Renal and liver disease Asthma/pulmonary disease Neuromuscular disorders Severe disease **Medication dosage** *Infants ≤8 months:* **Oseltamivir** Oral: 3 mg/kg/dose twice daily for 5 days *Infants ≥9 months:* **Oseltamivir** 3.5 mg/kg/dose PO twice daily for 5 days *Children and Adolescents:* Oseltamivir

Consider	All severe cases should be hospitalized	All cases of infants younger than 6 months with pertussis should be hospitalized.	Apnea is a common complication of RSV	Antibiotics are not part of the treatment for viral URI	≤15 kg: PO: 30 mg twice daily >15–23 kg: PO: 45 mg twice daily >23–40 kg: PO: 60 mg twice daily >40 kg: PO: 75 mg twice daily for 5 days Consider hospitalizing; Any patient younger than 6 months Severe illness Progressive illness Hypotensive Lethargy Cyanosis Hypoxia Respiratory distress Dehydration
	Must distinguish croup from epiglottitis (see Chapter 3, Abnormalities of the Ears, Eyes, Nose, and Throat Commonly Seen in Pediatric Primary Care)	Do not return to school until after 5 days of antibiotics or until it has been 21 days since the onset of symptoms.			

Repeated observations are necessary to adequately assess disease severity, because examination findings may vary.

Despite the diagnosis, the children should be hospitalized and monitored if they display any of the following: toxic appearance, poor feeding, depressed level of consciousness, or dehydration.

Any of the following signs of respiratory distress: nasal flaring; intercostal, subcostal, or suprasternal retractions; tachypnea (see rates by age in Table 4.1), dyspnea; or cyanosis apnea SpO$_2$ (oxygen saturation) <95%.

Definitions:

Mild croup: occasional barky cough, no stridor at rest, mild or no retractions

Moderate croup: frequent barky cough, stridor at rest, and mild-to-moderate retractions, but no or little distress or agitation

Severe croup: frequent barky cough, stridor at rest, marked retractions, significant distress and agitation

Impending failure: depressed level of consciousness, stridor at rest, severe retractions, poor air entry, cyanosis, or pallor

PCR, polymerase chain reaction; PE, physical exam; RSV, respiratory syncytial virus; URI, upper respiratory infection.

CAP in children overall and is the prime bacterial pathogen in children aged 3 months to 5 years, but the most likely bacterial pathogens in school-aged children (older than 5 years) are *Mycoplasma pneumonia* and *Chlamydia pneumoniae* (Shah, Bachur, Simel, & Neuman, 2017). It is also worth noting that several studies have found that mixed viral and bacterial infection accounts for 30% to 50% of CAP infections in children.

For newborns, infants, and children who have a neuromuscular diagnosis that may impair swallowing, if they have been intubated or are on a ventilator, aspiration pneumonia should be considered, and they should be screened for pathogens, such as *Staphylococcus*, *Klebsiella*, *Bacteroides* spp., and anaerobic *Streptococcus* and *Pseudomonas* species.

Epidemiology/Risk Factors

Pneumonia is also a major cause of childhood mortality, and the leading infectious cause of death in children, responsible for over one million childhood deaths per year. Pneumonia can be categorized as CAP or hospital-acquired (nosocomial). In this chapter, we will focus on CAP as it is far more common, except for newborns in which nosocomial pneumonias are common.

Table 4.3

Most Common Pathogens of Pneumonia Based on Age	
Age	Pathogens
Less than 1 week	Group B *Streptococcus*, enteric gram-negative bacilli, HSV
1 week to 3 months	*Streptococcus pneumoniae*, Chlamydia trachomatis, RSV, parainfluenza, adenovirus, influenza
3 months to 5 years	*S. pneumoniae*, *Mycoplasma* and *Chlamydia pneumoniae*, RSV, parainfluenza, adenovirus
5–18 years	*C. pneumoniae*, *M. pneumoniae*, *S. pneumoniae*

HSV, herpes simplex virus; RSV, respiratory syncytial virus.

Symptoms

There are several symptoms common to pneumonia; however, none are pathognomonic or uniquely specific to pneumonia. Chief complaints typically involve any combination of cough, fever, loss of appetite/anorexia, dyspnea, and pleuritic chest pain. Less common findings are abdominal pain and headache.

In a multicenter study that included 2,358 children <18 years old, with median age of 2 years, who were hospitalized with radiographic evidence of pneumonia, 95% had cough, 90% had fever, 75% had anorexia, and 70% had dyspnea (Seema, Derek, Williams, & Arnold, 2015).

Focused PE Signs/Findings

Just like symptoms, there are many common findings in patients presenting with pneumonia; however, none are overly sensitive or specific for pneumonia. Clinical signs on examination may be any combination of the following: cough, tachypnea, fever, hypoxia, retractions, nasal flaring, decreased breath sounds, wheezing, bronchial breath sounds, bronchophony, tactile fremitus, and crackles. The World Health Organization uses the combination of fever and cough as strongly suggestive of pneumonia in the pediatrics; however, this approach has not shown to be a strong predictor of radiographically confirmed pneumonia.

Research has shown that the presence of at least two (out of three) of these signs (tachypnea, reduced oxygen saturation, and fever) is associated with a high risk of pneumonia, whereas the absence of all three make pneumonia unlikely (Ebell, 2010).

Lab Tests/Diagnostics

Mild pneumonia is a clinical diagnosis. Confirmatory testing with a **chest x-ray** is definitive. An infiltrate on chest radiograph confirms the diagnosis. All children with moderate-to-severe disease (see findings suggestive of severe pneumonia under the following heading, "Referral") should have an x-ray.

Treatment

Outpatient management of CAP is treated with empiric antibiotics based on likely pathogen and age (see Table 4.4). Any x-ray-confirmed pneumonia should be treated as there is no way to reliably distinguish between viral and bacterial causes of pneumonia in a clinic setting. All patients should be reevaluated 48 to 72 hours after the initiation of treatment to reassess the empiric treatment. For example, if a patient who is treated based on age and likely pathogen is placed on a Macrolide for coverage of an atypical pneumonia and is still symptomatic, the addition of amoxicillin to cover a typical pathogen is an acceptable next step. The same would be true for a patient initially covered for a typical bacterium (*S. pneumoniae*) who does not improve after 48 to 72 hours; a Macrolide could be added.

Table 4.4

Outpatient Management of Community-Acquired Pneumonia			
Age	First-Line Treatment	Mild PCN Allergy	Type 1/Severe PCN Reaction or Allergic Reaction to First-Line Treatment
≤6 months	Children 6 months old or younger suspected of having pneumonia should be hospitalized.		
6 months to 5 years Likely is typical bacterial pneumonia	Amoxicillin 90 mg/kg per day in two or three divided doses (maximum 4 g/day)	Cefdinir 14 mg/ kg per day in two divided doses (maximum 600 mg/ day)	Azithromycin 10 mg/ kg on day 1 followed by 5 mg/kg daily for 4 more days (maximum 500 mg on day 1 and 250 mg thereafter)
≥5 years Likely atypical	Azithromycin 10 mg/kg on day 1 followed by 5 mg/ kg daily for 4 more days (maximum 500 mg on day 1 and 250 mg thereafter)		

PCN, penicillin.

Data from Seema, J., Derek, J., Williams, S., & Arnold, S. R. (2015). Community-acquired pneumonia requiring hospitalization among U.S. children. *New England Journal of Medicine, 372*, 835–845. doi:10.1056/ NEJMoa1405870; Shah, S. N., Bachur, R. G., Simel, D. L., & Neuman, M. I. (2017). Does this child have pneumonia? The rational clinical examination systematic review. *Journal of the American Medical Association, 318*, 462–471. doi:10.1001/jama.2017.9039

Referral

Patients who present with clinical features of severe pneumonia should be admitted. Clinical findings that suggest severe pneumonia are any of the following:

- Fever greater than 101.3°F
- Respiratory distress: tachypnea, retraction, grunting, nasal flaring
- Cyanosis
- Altered mental status
- Hypoxic SpO$_2$ <94%

VIRAL UPPER RESPIRATORY INFECTION

Otherwise known as the common cold, upper respiratory infection (URI) is the most common cause of an acute cough in children. Cough is mainly due to rhinitis and post-nasal drip (see Chapter 3, Abnormalities of the Ears, Eyes, Nose, and Throat Commonly Seen in Pediatric Primary Care). Over-the-counter cough and cold medications are commonly used. Evidence of efficacy of these medications for children with URI is lacking. Because of the known risk for unintentional overdose of these medications, their use is not recommended in children under the age of 4.

Etiology

Common viral pathogens include rhinovirus, coronaviruses, influenza, enterovirus, and parainfluenza viruses.

Signs, symptoms, and treatment of viral URI can be found in Table 4.2.

DYSPNEA/SHORTNESS OF BREATH

Dyspnea is a frequently presenting complaint in the outpatient pediatric setting. One of the most common causes of shortness of breath in children is asthma. The following section will focus on the identification, workup, and treatment of the acute asthma exacerbation.

ASTHMA

Asthma is a chronic inflammatory disease of the airways, defined as airway obstruction that is reversible either spontaneously or with the use of medication. Children present with obstructive symptoms/dyspnea, episodic wheezing, and cough. Although asthma is a chronic disease, it is often the acute exacerbations that bring children into the ambulatory practice for evaluation.

Etiology

The development of asthma is thought to be multifactorial with genetic predispositions and environmental triggers being the likely contributing factors. The obstructive pathophysiology is due to bronchial hyperresponsiveness, leading to hypersecretion of mucus, smooth muscle constriction, and inflammatory cell infiltrate. It is this bronchial hyperresponsiveness that allows viral and environmental triggers to manifest as acute exacerbations.

Asthma exacerbations are an exaggerated lower airway response to an environmental exposure, most commonly viruses. Viral infections are the most common trigger of an acute asthma exacerbation, triggering up to 85% of acute asthma exacerbations. Other common causes are allergens, pollutants, or medications, such as aspirin. Sports-induced asthma exacerbations occur from repetitive rapid deep breathing.

Epidemiology/Risk Factors

It is estimated that 6 million children under 18 years of age are living with asthma in the United States. Some risk factors for the development of asthma have been identified as a positive family history and a history of allergies and/or atopy.

Symptoms

Pediatric patients often present with complaints of breathlessness, anxiety, cough, and chest pain.

PE Signs/Key Findings

The first part of the evaluation is always the assessment of the severity of the dyspnea. As stated previously in this chapter, any signs of acute respiratory distress should prompt consideration of transfer to the emergency department (Table 4.2). Patients with severe refractory moderate distress should also be transferred to an emergency medical center.

Frequent findings of an acute asthma exacerbation are tachypnea, hypoxia, wheezing, accessory muscle use, retractions, and prolonged expiratory phase. The patient tends to appear anxious and in distress. Identifying patients in severe distress is imperative to avoid respiratory arrest. Categorizing the acute exacerbation will help guide in the management of the child (Table 4.5).

Diagnostics

Asthma exacerbations are largely a clinical diagnosis supported by the following tests: SpO_2 <95% and peak expiratory flow (PEF) <80%.

Treatment for chronic and acute asthma can be found in Table 4.6.

Table 4.5

Categorizing Severity of Acute Asthma Exacerbation

Signs and Symptoms	Mild	Moderate	Severe
Breathlessness	With activity, not at rest Can speak in full sentences Can lie flat	While at rest Speaks in phrases Prefers sitting	While at rest Infant will stop Speaks in single words Sits upright
Alertness	May be anxious or agitated	Usually agitated and/or anxious	Usually agitated and/or anxious
Respiratory rate (see Table 4.1)	Tachypneic	Tachypneic	Tachypneic
Chest retractions and/or nasal flaring	No	Commonly	Usually
Wheezing	End expiratory Mild to moderate	Loud through exhalation	Loud inspiratory and expiratory
Percent predicted Peak expiratory flow (%)	≥70%	~40–69%	<40%
SpO_2 (room air at sea level)	>94%	92–94%	<92%

Table 4.6

The Outpatient Management of an Acute Asthma Exacerbation in Children

Treatment	Mild	Moderate	Severe
All patients Short-acting beta-agonist (SABA; albuterol)	Nebulized or MDI **Albuterol nebulized** 0.15 mg/kg per dose (minimum 2.5 mg, maximum 5 mg/dose) every 20–30 minutes for three doses Or **Albuterol by MDI with spacer** (90 mcg/puff) Weight-based dosage: ■ 5–10 kg: 4 puffs ■ 10–20 kg: 6 puffs ■ >20 kg: 8 puffs every 20–30 minutes for three doses Use spacer. Add mask in children younger than 4 years.	Nebulized or MDI **Albuterol nebulized** 0.15 mg/kg per dose (minimum 2.5 mg, maximum 5 mg/dose) every 20–30 minutes for three doses Or **Albuterol by MDI with spacer** (90 mcg/puff) Weight-based dosage: ■ 5–10 kg: 4 puffs ■ 10–20 kg: 6 puffs ■ >20 kg: 8 puffs Use spacer. Add mask in children younger than 4 years.	**(Call 911 for transfer to emergency medical center and begin treatment, including supplemental oxygen until EMS arrives.)** Nebulized or MDI **Albuterol nebulizer** 0.15 mg/kg per dose (minimum 2.5 mg, maximum 5 mg/dose) every 20–30 minutes for 3 doses, then 0.15–0.3 mg/kg (maximum 10 mg) every 30 minutes to 4 hours as needed Or **Albuterol by MDI with spacer** (90 mcg/puff) Weight-based dosage: ■ 5–10 kg: 4 puffs ■ 10–20 kg: 6 puffs ■ >20 kg: 8 puffs Use spacer. Add mask in children younger than 4 years. **If failed to respond to SABA, consider adding epinephrine** 1 mg/mL (also labeled 1:1000) 0.01 mg/kg IM or SC, if no evidence of anaphylaxis (maximum 0.4 mg/dose = 0.4 mL of 1 mg/mL solution). May be repeated every 10–20 minutes for three doses.

All patients if available Anticholinergic	Ipratropium bromide nebulizer solution (250 mcg/mL) <20 kg to 250 mcg/dose ≥20 kg to 500 mcg/dose Every 20 minutes for three doses, then as needed Ipratropium bromide MDI with spacer (18 mcg/puff) 4–8 puffs every 20 minutes as needed for up to 3 hours. Use spacer; add mask in children younger than 4 years.	Ipratropium bromide nebulizer solution (250 mcg/mL) <20 kg to 250 mcg/dose ≥20 kg to 500 mcg/dose Every 20 minutes for three doses, then as needed Ipratropium bromide MDI with spacer (18 mcg/puff) 4–8 puffs every 20 minutes as needed for up to 3 hours. Use spacer; add mask in children younger than 4 years.	Ipratropium bromide nebulizer solution (250 mcg/mL) <20 kg to 250 mcg/dose ≥20 kg to 500 mcg/dose Every 20 minutes for three doses, then as needed Ipratropium bromide MDI with spacer (18 mcg/puff) 4–8 puffs every 20 minutes as needed for up to 3 hours. Use spacer; add mask in children younger than 4 years.
Steroids	If no improvement after initial SABA treatment or a history of frequent exacerbations Dexamethasone 0.6 mg/kg (maximum 16 mg/day) by mouth, IM, or IV Or Prednisone 1–2 mg/kg (maximum 60 mg/day) by mouth for the first dose	Dexamethasone 0.6 mg/kg (maximum 16 mg/day) by mouth, IM, or IV Or Prednisone 1–2 mg/kg (maximum 60 mg/day) by mouth	Dexamethasone 0.6 mg/kg (maximum 16 mg/day) by mouth, IM, or IV Or Prednisone 1–2 mg/kg (maximum 60 mg/day)
Transfer to ED Or Discharge home	If good response, discharge home on SABA and +/− steroids. If failed to have adequate response after SABA and steroids, transfer to emergency medical center.	If good response after one to three doses of SABA and dose of steroid, discharge home on SABA and steroids. Prednisone 0.5–1 mg/kg twice daily for 3–10 days. If incomplete response or symptoms worsen, transfer to emergency medical center	Arrange transfer to emergency medical center immediately upon presentation. Begin treatments while waiting for EMS. This includes supplemental oxygen.

(continued)

Table 4.6

The Outpatient Management of an Acute Asthma Exacerbation in Children (continued)

Treatment	Mild	Moderate	Severe
The primary criterion for referral to the ED is any one of the following: 1. Severe presentation 2. Lack of response to inhaled albuterol and oral glucocorticoids 3. Incomplete response to inhaled albuterol and oral glucocorticoids 4. Worsening symptoms and signs			
Discharge home: after treatment, observe for 60 minutes with all of the following: SpO_2 >94% on room air, normal rate of respirations and heart rate, diminished or absent wheezing, absent retractions, and increased aeration			

EMS, emergency medical service; IM, intramuscular; IV, intravenous; MDI, metered dose inhaler; SC, subcutaneous.

FOREIGN BODY ASPIRATION

In any child presenting with acute cough, you must consider foreign body (FB) aspiration. Generally, children above the age of 4 years can alert a parent and medical provider to this; however, in youngerchildren, you must depend on the reported history of parents and caregivers, the exam, and imaging.

Unfortunately, children aged 6 months to 4 years are at highest risk of FB aspiration, so an accurate patient account is often lacking.

Complete obstructions will typically lead to on-site first aid and emergency medical service (EMS). The ambulatory practice is more likely to encounter children who are brought in due to a suspicion of FB aspiration with symptoms of partial obstruction. Cough, wheezing, and respiratory distress are common in partial obstructions.

Auscultation may result in asymmetric breath sounds or localized wheezing. Imaging can be performed as well. Typically, an inspiratory and forced expiratory x-ray is performed. Forced expiratory films in children need to be performed with a medical provider physically compressing the child's stomach as they exhale. Positive findings show mediastinal shift or hyperinflation. Also, the object may be seen on x-ray if it is radiopaque.

Positive radiographic findings or strong clinical suspicion requires the child to be admitted for hospital evaluation and treatment.

Bronchoscopy is the recommended diagnostic and therapeutic approach. Even children with minor symptoms who have aspirated an FB to the lower respiratory tract should be treated in this fashion as failure to remove the FB can lead to abscess formation or long-term inflammatory changes, such as bronchiectasis.

References

Ebell, M. H. (2010). Clinical diagnosis of pneumonia in children. *American Family Physician, 15*(82), 192–195.

Seema, J., Derek, J., Williams, S., & Arnold, S. R. (2015). Community acquired pneumonia requiring hospitalization among U.S. children. *New England Journal of Medicine, 372*, 835–845. doi:10.1056/NEJMoa1405870

Shah, S. N., Bachur, R. G., Simel, D. L., & Neuman, M. I. (2017). Does this child have pneumonia? The rational clinical examination systematic review. *Journal of the American Medical Association, 318*, 462–471. doi:10.1001/jama.2017.9039

Smith, D. K., McDermott, A. J., & Sullivan, J. F. (2018). Croup: diagnosis and management. *American Family Physician, 97*(9), 575–580.

5

Cardiac Abnormalities Commonly Seen in Pediatric Primary Care

Allea Scifo and M. T. Parsons

INTRODUCTION

Heart murmurs, palpitations, and syncope are frequently seen problems by pediatric advanced practicing clinicians (APCs) and oftentimes can be assessed and treated without a referral to a pediatric cardiologist. Additionally, as pediatric APCs, we are expected to provide anticipatory guidance and play a vital role in the prevention of cardiovascular disease, which is a leading cause of morbidity and mortality in the adult population. Identifying pediatric cardiac issues such as hypertension and dyslipidemia and their causes in the pediatric period and counseling on prevention is also a key role of the pediatric APCs in primary care.

OBJECTIVES

1. Discuss common cardiology symptoms and findings that often initially present in the pediatric primary care setting.
2. Differentiate between cardiac and noncardiac causes of chest pain in pediatric patients.
3. Recognize the various types of palpitations commonly seen in pediatric patients and the appropriate treatments.
4. Help to work up, identify, and treat hypertension and dyslipidemia in the pediatric period.
5. Understand common causes of and identify innocent/functional heart murmurs from pathologic murmurs and know when to refer to a pediatric cardiologist.
6. Understand common causes of pediatric chest pain and reasons for referral to a pediatric cardiologist.
7. Become proficient with history taking in the patient with syncope and palpitations to determine if a concerning arrhythmia is suspected.
8. Provide anticipatory guidance to the pediatric cardiac patient and family.

ABNORMAL HEART SOUNDS/HEART MURMURS

Shortly after birth, the ductus arteriosus closes and pulmonary vascular resistance begins to fall. As a result, shunting lesions such as ventricular and atrial septal defects (VSD, ASD) will not necessarily be heard for a few days following delivery as opposed to obstructive lesions such as aortic stenosis (AS) or pulmonary stenosis (PS), which are typically heard at birth. Closure of the ductus arteriosus can also be associated with coarctation of the aorta.

Etiology

Heart murmurs are a common finding when auscultating the pediatric heart. Heart murmurs are extra or abnormal sounds made by turbulent blood flowing through the heart. Murmurs are graded on a scale of one to six based on how loud they are. One means a very faint murmur. Six means a murmur that is very loud.

It is estimated that up to 72% of all children will have a heart murmur heard through-out the course of their infancy and childhood (Farr, Downing, Riehle-Colarusso, & Abarbanell, 2018). It is important to note that murmurs are turbulence of blood flow and can occur with illnesses, especially in the febrile pediatric patient; therefore, close follow-up when a child is feeling better is imperative.

Types of murmurs include the following:

- **Systolic murmur:** a heart murmur that occurs when the heart contracts
- **Diastolic murmur:** a heart murmur that occurs when the heart relaxes
- **Continuous murmur:** a heart murmur that occurs throughout the heartbeat

Epidemiology/Risk Factors

To differentiate a normal from an abnormal heart murmur, a thorough cardiovascular assessment is critical. Murmurs heard in the first few days and weeks of life are more likely to represent cardiac disease as compared with murmurs heard during childhood.

Symptoms

Heart murmurs, or abnormal heart sounds, may be common in normal, healthy children. These are called functional or innocent heart murmurs and are a normal finding that is not associated with any adverse symptoms. Causes of this type of murmur include infection, fevers, anemia, and hyperthyroidism.

Abnormal or pathologic heart murmurs are heard in infants and children with structural abnormalities. These abnormal structures cause blood to flow turbulently through the heart structures and produce a murmur. A child with congenital heart disease (CHD) may have varying symptoms depending on the problem or structural defect but indicators can range from no symptoms to symptoms of respiratory distress, sweating, poor feeding, poor growth, cyanosis, pallor, and syncope.

Focused Physical Exam Signs/Findings

A comprehensive history including gestational age, fetal exposures, feeding history, and growth patterns is essential in differentiating a normal murmur from a congenital heart defect. Physical examination (PE) includes palpation of the chest to assess for increased precordial impulse and thrills that are associated with more severe heart defects. An auscultative exam determines murmur grading (I–VI), murmur location, and at what time in the cardiac cycle the murmur is heard. Auscultative skills are known to increase in accuracy over the course of one's training and career. Becoming comfortable and proficient in differentiating normal from abnormal murmurs takes time and practice. Determining adequate perfusion and strong femoral pulses is an important piece to the cardiac exam. Absent femoral pulses can indicate coarctation of the aorta and resultant poor perfusion.

Lab Tests/Diagnostics

Electrocardiograms (EKGs) are helpful in determining cardiac rhythms, frontal plane axis, atrial enlargement, and ventricular hypertrophy, but routine screening EKGs and chest x-rays are probably not helpful (Chen, Riehle-Colarusso, Yeung, Smith, & Farr, 2018). If the decision to refer has been made, it is best to leave testing to the cardiologist. Table 5.1 shows the common types of murmurs and when referral should be made to cardiology.

Table 5.1

Common Types of Murmurs and When to Refer to Cardiology in a Pediatric Primary Care Setting			
Type of CHD:	**Functional/ Innocent Murmur**	**Shunting/ Pulmonary Over Circulation**	**Obstructive Lesions**	**Cyanotic/Complex**
Level of Care/ Referral Required?	No referral necessary	Referral required	Referral required	Urgent/emergent care should be sought
	Still's murmur Grade II and softer, musical, vibratory quality. Louder with increased cardiac output such as fever/anemia.	**PDA** Continuous murmur at the LUSB radiates to the left clavicle. Does not resolve with position changes. May be associated with bounding peripheral pulses.	**AS** Harsh grade II–IV systolic murmur at RUSB. Grating sound. May have associated systolic ejection click. Louder murmur associated with more stenosis.	**TOF** Harsh systolic murmur grade II–III heard at left sternal border with radiation to base. Cyanosis correlates with degree of pulmonary stenosis. May develop cyanotic spells necessitating emergent care.
	PPS Grade I–II soft murmur in infants at the base— radiates to axillae and infra scapular region.	**VSD** Holosystolic murmur heard at left lower sternal border. Intensity is variable based on size. Large defects— associated with poor feeding and FTT.	**PS** Harsh grade II–IV. Heard best at LUSB. Degree of stenosis may worsen over the course of few months of life.	**Epstein's anomaly of the tricuspid valve** Soft systolic murmur crested by tricuspid regurgitation. Cyanosis from right to left shunting across atria. Severe forms diagnosed in utero/ neonatal time frame.

(continued)

Table 5.1

Common Types of Murmurs and When to Refer to Cardiology in a Pediatric Primary Care Setting (*continued*)

Type of CHD:	Functional/ Innocent Murmur	Shunting/ Pulmonary Over Circulation	Obstructive Lesions	Cyanotic/Complex
	Venous hum Soft, low-frequency, continuous murmur heard best at the clavicular region in thin young children. Best heard when sitting upright. Murmur obliterates with neck reposition and jugular compression.	**ASDs** Low-frequency systolic ejection murmurs grade I–II. Second heart sound is widely or fixed split. Rarely associated with cardiac symptoms. Can be associated with frequent pneumonias.	**CoA** Murmur heard best in back. Weak or absent femoral pulses. Upper extremity BP is greater than lower extremity BP. May be associated with respiratory distress and cardiovascular shock.	**Complex CHD disease** diagnosed in utero or during the neonatal time period. *Rarely seen in ambulatory care.* **Tricuspid atresia Pulmonary atresia Transposition of the great arteries Single ventricle physiology HLHS**

AS, aortic stenosis; ASD, atrial septal defect; BP, blood pressure; CHD, congenital heart disease; CoA, coarctation of the aorta; FTT, failure to thrive; HLHS, hypoplastic left heart syndrome; LUSB, left upper sternal border; PDA, patent ductus arteriosus; PPS, peripheral pulmonary artery stenosis; PS, pulmonary stenosis; RUSB, right upper sternal border; TOF, tetralogy of Fallot; VSD, ventricular septal defect.

Don't Miss

Murmurs are common in pediatrics, and most are benign. Thorough history and PE will determine the need for referral to a cardiologist. Testing done in the community setting is often not helpful.

Murmur referral guidelines for any newborn with a murmur for assessment to a pediatric cardiologist would include (see Table 5.1) the following:

- Any holosystolic murmur
- Murmurs louder than a grade III in childhood
- Any diastolic murmur
- Any murmur with intensity at the left upper sternal boarder
- Any presence of an abnormal second heart sound; either widely split or loud
- Any early- or midsystolic click
- The presence of a murmur and diminished femoral pulses

Treatment

Treatment is variable based on the diagnosis. Innocent murmurs require no intervention. Treatment of congenital heart disease is based on the defect. Treatment may range from close monitoring without intervention to surgical repairs. The cardiology team will determine a treatment plan.

Follow-Up/Patient/Family Education

In the child diagnosed with an innocent murmur, it is important to provide reassurance that the heart is normal and encourage healthy heart lifestyles. Children diagnosed with a CHD are living longer, and while the type of defect may impose no limitations, there may be some limitations on the child (varies depending on type of CHD). Supporting the patient and family is key when caring for pediatric patients (Ruggiero, Hickey, Leger, Vessey, & Hayman, 2018).

ACUTE RHEUMATIC FEVER

Epidemiology/Risk Factors

It is the most common cause of acquired heart disease in the world and is associated with group A beta-hemolytic streptococcal (GABHS) infections. It is most often seen in underdeveloped countries and occurs in 2 to 3% of patients with untreated GABHS pharyngitis; it is not generally seen in children under age 5 and mostly affects school-age children/adolescents. There is thought to be a genetic predisposition that makes a person more susceptible when exposed to GABHS infections.

Symptoms/Clinical Manifestations

- It generally presents within weeks of a group A streptococcal (GAS) tonsillopharyngitis.
- Cardiac: tachycardia, new murmur, pericardial friction rub, gallop, tachypnea, irregular pulse, chest pain, pulmonary edema.
  - Most often involves the endocardium and especially affects the mitral and aortic valves.
- Joints: migratory arthritis of large joints, that is, ankle, knees, wrists, elbow—pain occurs at rest and worsens with movement; painful to touch; and may be red/swollen.
- Neurological: chorea (involuntary writhing/purposeless movements that cease when asleep), personality changes.
- Skin: erythema marginatum (pink/faint red, nonpruritic rash involving the trunk and sometimes limbs; face is spared).
- Subcutaneous nodules (rare finding): small nodules most often on elbows, knees, wrists, occipital bones, and over vertebrae.
- Low-grade fever (Gleason et al., 2012).

Diagnosis

Modified Jones Criteria is used for diagnosis; this was most recently updated in 2015. This fever may present with multiple findings several weeks after GABHS infection.

- **Five major manifestations:**
  1. Carditis and valvulitis (can be subclinical)
  2. Arthritis (typically migratory and involves the large joints)
  3. CNS involvement (chorea)
  4. Subcutaneous nodules (less common)
  5. Erythema marginatum

- **Four minor manifestations:**
  1. Arthralgia
  2. Fever

3. Elevated acute phase reactants (ESR/CRP)
4. Prolonged PR interval (abnormal atrioventricular conduction is common—first-degree block is most common with ARF)

- Diagnosis requires two major manifestations or one major plus two minor in a patient with recent history of known GAS infection

Differentials

KD, myocarditis, congenital heart disease, endocarditis, JRA

Labs/Tests

- Throat culture should be sent for patients with fever, sore throat, malaise to rule out GAS
- CBC to evaluate anemia and elevated white count, ESR/CRP for inflammation, antistreptolysin O titer
- EKG and echocardiogram (cardiology consult would obtain)
- CXR

Don't Miss

- Diagnosis is made clinically; prompt diagnosis and treatment are important.
- Ensure importance of follow-up and education.

Treatment

- Primary prevention by recognizing and treating upper respiratory GAS infections
- IM benzathine penicillin G and oral penicillin V or amoxicillin are drugs of choice; use cephalosporin (clindamycin) for penicillin allergy
- Refer to cardiology; all patients should have cardiac evaluation even in the absence of cardiac symptoms
- **Secondary prevention:** long-term antibiotics

CARDIOMYOPATHIES

■ DILATED CARDIOMYOPATHY

DCM is characterized by left ventricular dilation and dysfunction resulting in decreased cardiac output and CHF.

Etiology/Epidemiology

Annual incidence of DCM is 0.57 per 100,000 children. DCM is idiopathic in more than 60% of cases. Other causes may be primarily due to familial gene mutations or myocarditis. Secondary causes of DCM include neuromuscular, metabolic, or mitochondrial disorders or chemotherapy exposure to anthracycline.

Symptoms

May have insidious onset in cases of familial DCM and neuromuscular disorders (Duchenne and Becker muscular dystrophy).

Infants: fatigues easily during feeds, irritability, tachypnea, diaphoresis, poor weight gain, failure to thrive

Young children: abdominal pain, nausea, vomiting, poor appetite, fatigues easily, chronic cough, wheeze (symptoms may be mistaken for gastroenteritis or asthma)
Older children: exercise intolerance, dyspnea on exertion, abdominal pain from hepatomegaly and low cardiac output, wheezing, chest pain, palpitations, syncope

Focused PE

About 75% to 80% of children present with signs and symptoms of HF such as tachycardia, syncope, pulmonary crackles, weak peripheral pulses, and hepatomegaly. They may have a gallop rhythm or soft systolic murmur from mitral or tricuspid regurgitation.

Differential Diagnosis

In new cases of DCM, other causes that are potentially correctable should be ruled out prior to making a diagnosis of primary dilated cardiomyopathy.

- Considerations such as anomalous origin of a coronary artery or early-onset atherosclerotic disease (although very rare) should be excluded.
- Consider recent viral illness and likelihood of an acute inflammatory process (myocarditis).
- Consider and exclude any systemic disorders that DCM can be secondary from neuromuscular, metabolic, and mitochondrial disorders or postchemotherapy exposure.

Don't Miss

Findings that should raise suspicion of HF include a gallop rhythm, tachycardia out of proportion to other symptoms, abdominal pain complaints in the setting of hepatomegaly, altered systemic perfusion, and EKG abnormalities.

CXR and laboratory tests (e.g., brain natriuretic peptide) can help differentiate HF from noncardiac conditions.

Treatment

Treatment includes referral to a specialist with a pediatric cardiac transplant program and advanced cardiac therapies. Medical therapy is initiated with the goal of improving heart function, preventing disease progression, and managing symptoms of CHF. It prevents complications such as arrhythmias, thrombosis, and end-organ damage. Diuretics, ace inhibitors, angiotensin receptor blockers, aldosterone antagonists, beta-blockers, and antiplatelet agents are the preferred drugs. Cardiac transplantation/mechanical support acts as a bridge to transplant.

Family Education

Refer to genetic counseling. In familial dilated cardiomyopathy, genetic testing should start with the index case. If a known gene mutation responsible for DCM is identified in the index case, then all first-degree relatives may be tested to identify asymptomatic or undetected disease.

■ HYPERTROPHIC CARDIOMYOPATHY

HCM is defined as the presence of a hypertrophied, nondilated ventricle in the absence of another disease that creates a hemodynamic disturbance that can produce the same magnitude of wall thickening (i.e., hypertension, aortic valve stenosis, catecholamine secreting tumors, hyperthyroidism [Colan, 2019]).

Etiology

HCM is the second most common cardiomyopathy, occurring at a rate of 0.47 cases per 100,000 children. It is most often diagnosed during infancy and adolescence (commonly with pubertal growth spurt). Cardiac sarcomere gene mutations occur in 40% to 60% of cases, which are inherited in an autosomal dominant fashion.

Many children who are diagnosed with HCM are leading normal healthy lives. The most feared complication is the risk of sudden cardiac death due to ventricular arrhythmias; this risk is ~1% per year.

(Colan et al., 2007)

Symptoms

It is often nonspecific; unless there is a known family history, HCM is unlikely to be the initial consideration:

- May be asymptomatic until a murmur is heard at a well-child visit
- Chest pain
- Dyspnea on exertion
- Fatigue
- Presyncope/syncope (often during or immediately following physical activity/exertion)
- Palpitations
- CHF

Focused PE/Findings

Murmur

- Due to left ventricular outflow tract obstruction (develops due to positioning of the septal hypertrophy that obstructs blood flow exiting the left ventricle)
- May be due to mitral regurgitation (systolic anterior motion of the mitral valve)

In addition to a positive family history of sudden death or HCM, other findings on PE may include dysmorphic features (which may suggest underlying syndrome [HCM seen in Noonan's, Friedrich ataxia, Pompe disease]) and ventricular arrhythmias.

Lab Tests/Diagnostics

Refer to a cardiovascular geneticist; genetic testing can be arranged for first-degree relatives of the index case (if they are known to have a positive familial mutation).

EKG: Potential EKG findings include left axis deviation, deep Q waves in the inferior and lateral leads, left atrial or biatrial enlargement, and/or deeply inverted T-waves in the midprecordial leads.

- A small number of patients with HCM may even have a normal EKG (therefore, EKG alone cannot rule out HCM).
- Cardiac MRI: Used for delineating anatomy and left ventricular outflow tract obstruction, also for detecting presence of myocardial scarring, which may play a role in a person's risk of ventricular arrhythmias.

Diagnosis

Patients are often referred to cardiology for further evaluation due to new murmur auscultated at a well-child visit, family history screening of a first-degree relative, or an abnormal EKG and echocardiogram; +/− cardiac MRI: Hallmark finding is left ventricular (LV) wall thickening without other identifiable cause (i.e., hypertension, valve disease, or other obstruction).

Differentials

Left ventricular hypertrophy (LVH) is due to other causes such as hypertension, athletic heart syndrome, endocrine diseases (i.e., maternal gestational diabetes), valvar or aortic stenosis, rheumatic and immunological diseases, and underlying disease associated with HCM (Noonan's syndrome, Fredrich's ataxia, RASopathies).

Don't Miss

Children with syncope during exercise and chest pain on exertion require prompt referral to a cardiologist. Although patients with HCM are at risk of sudden cardiac death due to a fatal arrhythmia, the risk of this is ~1% per year. HCM may be familial; refer all first-degree relatives for a phenotype screening with a cardiologist (especially in all cases of HCM, DCM, RCM)—you cannot rule out HCM by the presence of a normal EKG.

Treatment

While there is no cure for the disease, medications are prescribed for management of symptoms (beta-blockers, calcium channel blockers) to reduce outflow tract obstruction and alleviate associated symptoms of dyspnea. Surgical myectomy may be another treatment modality.

Risk stratification for ventricular arrhythmias: The cardiologist will monitor the child and perform risk stratification testing annually to determine the risk of life-threatening arrhythmias. This is calculated through a series of Holter monitors, stress testing, cardiac MRI, echocardiograms, and prior history of sudden death in a first-degree relative with HCM. The cardiologist will then refer to an electrophysiologist for consideration of an implantable cardioverter defibrillator (ICD). ICD implantation (referral made by the cardiologist) is performed if the child is determined to be at high risk for ventricular arrhythmias.

Family Education

Genetics do play a role in HCM; however, not all cases are found to be familial. Refer to a cardiovascular genetics specialist to discuss testing and potentially identify other family members. Genetic testing may be offered if the index case is found to have a positive familial gene mutation. Lifelong follow-up with a cardiologist is required. Children are encouraged to lead as normal of a life as possible. Although recommendations against playing competitive sports are made, avoiding all physical activities entirely promotes an unhealthy sedentary lifestyle, which may lead to acquiring cardiovascular disease as an adult. Children with HCM are preload dependent; teach careful precautions to avoid dehydration.

CHEST PAIN

Fifty percent of children believe their chest pain is cardiac in nature when rarely chest pain complaints represent true cardiovascular anomalies (American Heart Association, 2019). While heart problems can cause chest pain, chest pain is more likely related to noncardiac causes in children, including pains from pulled muscles or sports-related injury, pain related to asthma or cough, and pain due to infections such as pneumonia. Usually, if the pain is caused by anything serious, there will be other signs. A careful history and PE can easily provide reassurance or confirm reasons for referral.

Etiology/Epidemiology

The pediatric APC is frequently asked to assess complaints of pain. After headache and abdominal pain, the third most common "pain" confronted in the school-aged child is pain in the chest. Over the course of the past few decades, referrals for complaints of chest pain have increased.

Symptoms

Benign chest pain in children often occurs at rest, is characterized by a sharp midsternal anterior pain, and does not radiate to the arm or neck. Musculoskeletal pain is easily reproduced with palpation and will exacerbate with deep inspiration. Other benign and common causes of chest pain in children are pulmonary, that is, reactive airway disease, pleuritic, and pneumonias. Gastrointestinal (GI) complaints are also often the cause of chest pain. GI issues can include esophagitis, gastritis, peptic ulcer, and foreign body ingestion, and are often described as a burning pain occurring at night in a recumbent position.

Cardiac manifestation of chest pain is either ischemic, inflammatory, or arrhythmogenic and are tremendously rare in children. The symptoms seen in Table 5.2 would require referral to a cardiologist.

Table 5.2

Symptoms in a Pediatric Patient Requiring a Referral to a Cardiologist		
Exertional Chest Pain/Ischemic Pain	**Chest Pain in the Setting of Fever**	**Pain Associated With Abnormal Heart Rhythm**
Heavy, pressure, and squeezing pain that only occurs with exertion and exacerbated with increased physical activity.	Myocarditis Crushing midsternal pain Tachycardia Poor perfusion Needs emergent assessment in ED	Heart rates exceeding 200 bpm can be associated with arrhythmia and cause chest discomfort.
Pain usually radiated to left arm, neck, back, and jaw.	Pericarditis Pain with recumbent position Pain refers to shoulder Pain associated with postviral illness and improves with NSAIDs	Pain associated with syncope can be associated with cardiomyopathy.
Pain is relieved by rest.		
Pain can be caused by anomalous left and right coronary arteries, pulmonary hypertension, or severe left-sided obstructive disease such as AS or hypertrophic cardiomyopathy. Additionally, complications from coronary aneurysm from previous history of Kawasaki disease. Illicit drug use, i.e., cocaine, can cause ischemia.		

AS, aortic stenosis; NSAIDs, nonsteroidal anti-inflammatory drugs.

Focused PE

Noncardiac chest pain is consistent with normal cardiac examination and, in some cases, reproducible chest pain upon palpation to the costochondral junctions. Myocarditis should be suspected in the patient with a hyperdynamic precordial impulse, fever, tachycardia, poor perfusion, and possibly a gallop rhythm. This patient needs ED assessment. A friction rub can be heard in the patient with pericarditis. An irregular heart rhythm may be auscultated in the patient with an arrhythmia.

Lab Tests/Diagnostics

A screening EKG is helpful in ruling out rhythm disorders and ventricular hypertrophy seen in hypertrophic cardiomyopathy (HCM). A chest x-ray is helpful if a pulmonary process is suspected.

Troponins are recommended if chest pain is associated with a fever and tachycardia and are usually obtained in the ED setting. If a strong suspicion of cardiac etiology is present, then a referral should be made with testing ordered by the pediatric cardiologist.

Differentials

See Table 5.3.

Table 5.3

Common Causes of Pediatric Chest Pain	
Noncardiac Chest Pain/Occurs at Rest	Cardiac Chest Pain
Musculoskeletal	Occurs with exercise/possible coronary abnormality
Gastroesophageal reflux	Occurs with fever, tachycardia, and altered perfusion/myocarditis
Pneumonia/asthma	Arrhythmia

Don't Miss

- Any child with chest pain, fever, and tachycardia should be considered to have myocarditis and referred to ED or a pediatric cardiologist for urgent assessment.
- Exertional chest pain can indicate an anomalous coronary artery. A referral to a pediatric cardiologist should be made. An echocardiogram should be obtained by a cardiologist to examine cardiac anatomy, coronary artery origins, and ventricular function.

Treatment

Treatment of chest pain depends on its cause. Pediatric patients with obvious etiology of their noncardiac chest pain should be treated accordingly. Musculoskeletal chest pain should be treated with reassurance, rest, and nonsteroidal anti-inflammatory drugs (NSAIDs).

Cardiac causes of chest pain, including myocarditis, requires inpatient hospitalization. Some cases respond to intravenous immunoglobulin (IVIG). Ventricular dysfunction is treated with inotropic support and, in some cases, extracorporeal membrane oxygenation (ECMO). Patients can suffer long-term ventricular dysfunction following an episode of myocarditis. Some children are left without any long-term sequela. Exercise is restricted for 6 months following an episode of myocarditis.

Surgical intervention for anomalous coronary arteries is recommended in some cases. This depends on the coronary artery course and is determined after more thorough testing such as cMRI or cCT scanning.

CHILDHOOD OBESITY

Obesity is defined as body mass index (BMI) greater than or equal to the 95th percentile, and overweight is a BMI in the 85th to 94th percentile for age and sex. The risk of CVD mortality increases two- to threefold higher if BMI is in the overweight or obese category during adolescence compared with youth with a normal weight. One-third of children and adolescents in the United States are either overweight or obese. Once identified, children should be followed and screened for associated cardiovascular risk factors.

Don't Miss

Insulin resistance, dyslipidemia, and hypertension can be seen in polycystic ovary syndrome (PCOS), considered in females with irregular menses.

Treatment

- Multiple methods and graduated approach are generally required.
- Education on improvements in dietary quality, reduction in caloric intake, promoting physical activities that the child or family enjoys, pharmacotherapy, and bariatric surgery for severe cases is required.
- Refer to counseling and nutrition; consider participation in a local weight reduction program that combines nutrition, behavioral changes, and physical activity.
- Consider associated contributing factors such as underlying endocrine cause (i.e., hypothyroidism, Cushing's syndrome) and associated syndromes (Prader–Willi and Beckwith–Wiedemann).

Family Education/Patient Resources

Refer to the Obesity Society Patient pages (https://www.obesity.org/information-for -patients/); start with small changes, positive reinforcement, and encourage activities. Refer patient to a nutritionist or other health coach/counselor for better eating habits.

DYSLIPIDEMIA

Prior research has suggested that elevated cholesterol can occur at a very young age, and children with dyslipidemia may have evidence of arterial fatty streaks, which may later progress to atherosclerosis.

Screening

Early identification and control of dyslipidemia will reduce overall risk and severity of cardiovascular disease in adulthood.

Etiology

Dyslipidemia often begins during childhood and follows children into adulthood, and may contribute to the development of early atherosclerosis and premature cardiovascular disease (CVD). Identifying patients with dyslipidemia during childhood and adolescence, early education, and improvements in lipid profile may reduce the risk of developing these complications.

Dyslipidemia occurs with altered lipoprotein metabolism, which can result in high total cholesterol, high low-density lipoprotein cholesterol (LDL-C), high non–high-density lipoprotein cholesterol, high triglycerides, and low high-density lipoprotein cholesterol.

Epidemiology/Risk Factors

High-risk factors for developing atherosclerosis and early CVD during childhood include dyslipidemia, obesity, diabetes, hypertension, and family history of premature CVD.

Other conditions with increased CVD risk include the following: familial hypercholesterolemia, chronic kidney disease, KD, childhood cancer, certain types of CHD (i.e., coarctation, aortic stenosis, transposition of the great arteries, and congenital anomalies of the coronary arteries), cardiomyopathy, chronic inflammatory disorders (systemic lupus erythematosus [SLE], juvenile idiopathic arthritis [JIA]), HIV infection, and some psychiatric disorders.

If a patient has one or more of these risk factors, begin screening when first identified.

- Children without any known risk factors should have an initial lipid screening once during the ages of 9 to 11 and 17 to 21 years.
- Lipid screening is not recommended from the ages of 12 to 16 years as pubertal changes can affect sensitivity and specificity.
- Fasting or nonfasting lipid profiles can be obtained for screening (confirm findings with a fasting lipid profile if abnormalities are present).
- Screening should not be limited to only those with risk factors (you end up missing children with real disease, increasing chances that diagnosis will not be picked up until later and missing early opportunities for treatment and education).

Diagnosis

Requires confirmation testing with fasting lipid profiles obtained on two separate occasions 2 weeks to 3 months apart.

Don't Miss

Consider patients at risk for CVD on an annual basis.

Treatment

- Dietary and lifestyle modifications should begin at the first abnormal result (not after being diagnosed).

- Consider secondary causes for patients with borderline or abnormal screening: diabetes, nephrotic syndrome, hypothyroidism, pregnancy, liver disease, medications (glucocorticoids, isotretinoin, antiretrovirals).
- Very high cholesterol (LDL-C of 250 or higher)—refer to a pediatric lipid specialist as they may have severe primary hyperlipidemia (e.g., familial hypercholesterolemia).
- Treatment with statins is reserved for high-risk patients and those who do not respond to lifestyle changes.
- Refer to the AHA Scientific Statement (2019) for specific treatments and algorithms on treatment.

DYSPNEA

Noncardiac causes of dyspnea such as a pulmonary or psychiatric origin should be ruled out. Dyspnea of cardiac origin is most commonly due to heart failure (HF).

■ HEART FAILURE

Diagnosis of HF in children can be difficult as presenting symptoms (such as respiratory distress, abdominal pain, nausea, vomiting, poor appetite, and failure to thrive) are often nonspecific and most often have noncardiac causes (Uri et al., 2019).

Etiology/Epidemiology

Pediatric causes of HF fall into physiologic categories.

Symptoms

Infants: fatigues easily during feeds, irritability, tachypnea, diaphoresis, poor weight gain, failure to thrive
Young children: abdominal pain, nausea, vomiting, poor appetite, fatigues easily, chronic cough, wheeze (symptoms may be mistaken for gastroenteritis or asthma)
Older children: exercise intolerance, dyspnea on exertion, abdominal pain from hepatomegaly and low cardiac output, wheezing, chest pain, palpitations, syncope

Focused PE

- **Tachycardia** from physiologic response due to decreased cardiac output
- **Poor perfusion:** cool/mottled extremities, decreased capillary refill, hypotension
- **Pulmonary congestion:** tachypnea and retractions, wheezing, and rales (in older children)
- **Systemic congestion:** the most common finding of systemic venous congestion is hepatomegaly

Diagnostics

Chest Radiography

- It looks for pulmonary vascular congestion (pulmonary edema and pleural effusion common).
- Cardiomegaly on chest x-ray (CXR) may be identified due to the following causes:
  - Large left to right shunts with volume overload
  - Left ventricular dilation in dilated cardiomyopathy (DCM)
  - Biatrial enlargement with restrictive cardiomyopathy
  - Ventricular dilation in myocarditis
  - Pericardial effusion

ECG

- ST segment and T wave abnormalities with cardiomyopathies and myocarditis
- Increased QRS voltages meeting criteria for ventricular hypertrophy (can be seen in HCM/DCM)
- Biatrial enlargement with restrictive cardiomyopathy
- Deep Q wave in inferior and lateral leads (I, aVL, and V5–V6) with ST segment and T wave changes (suggestive of a myocardial infarct, consider anomalous left coronary arising from the pulmonary artery [ALCAPA] and HCM).
- Atrial, junctional, or ventricular tachycardia or frequent atrial or ventricular ectopy is suggestive of arrhythmia as an underlying cause of ventricular dysfunction or may represent a complication up to date.

Echocardiography

- Primary modality to assess ventricular size and function; will delineate anatomy to determine if the child has a structurally normal heart or underlying congenital heart disease

Laboratory Tests

Brain natriuretic peptide: It is useful for assessing the severity of HF and response to therapy by tracking trends over time, and it "can help discriminate between cardiac disease and noncardiac causes of HF symptoms (e.g., pulmonary disease)" (Koulouri, Acherman, Wong, Chan, & Lewis, 2004).

Troponin: "Cardiac troponin I and troponin T are sensitive biomarkers for myocyte injury. Troponin levels are elevated in myocarditis and myocardial ischemia. Among children presenting with left ventricular dysfunction, an elevated troponin level may suggest acute myocarditis rather than dilated cardiomyopathy" (Koulouri et al., 2004, p. 121).

Serum chemistries (electrolytes, blood urea nitrogen, creatinine, and liver function tests)

- Hyponatremia may be seen in children with severe HF.
- Renal impairment may be a contributing factor for HF or exacerbate preexisting failure.
- Baseline electrolytes prior to initiating diuretic therapy and angiotensin-converting enzyme (ACE) inhibitors avoid potential side effects of these drugs.
- Liver function tests may be elevated due to hepatic congestion.

Differentials

Edema: May have other etiologies such as a renal failure and lymphatic system dysfunction.

Don't Miss

One of the first complaints/signs of HF in adolescents with dilated cardiomyopathy are abdominal complaints.

Treatment

HF treatment is managed by a cardiac team. The long-term treatment of CHF in children includes digoxin, diuretics, and afterload reduction with ACE inhibitors. Palliative surgical treatments have shown some benefit. Heart transplant can also be an option for HF but carries its own risks.

HYPERTENSION

Hypertension in childhood and adolescence contributes to premature atherosclerosis and the early development of cardiovascular disease; therefore, early identification and treatment are necessary. The initial important component in managing this disease process is distinguishing between primary and secondary hypertension and aggressively treating the underlying cause in secondary hypertension. In 2017, the American Academy of Pediatrics published revised guidelines for screening and managing high blood pressure for children and adolescents. Definitions according to this most recent publication are summarized in Table 5.4 (Flynn et al., 2017).

Table 5.4

Pediatric Hypertension Guidelines		
Definitions	**Children Aged 1–13 Years**	**Children Aged 13 and Over**
Normal BP	SBP and DBP are both less than the 90th percentile	Less than 120/80
Elevated BP	Elevated blood pressure: SBP and/or DBP are greater than or equal to the 90th percentile but lower than the 95th percentile *or* 120/80 mmHg to less than the 95th percentile, whichever is lower	Elevated BP: SBP 120–129 mmHg with a DBP less than 80 mmHg
Stage 1 hypertension	SBP and/or DBP greater than or equal to the 95th percentile +12 mmHg, or 130/80 to 139/89 mmHg, whichever is lower	BP between 130/80 and 139/89 mmHg
Stage 2 hypertension	SBP and/or DBP is greater than or equal to 95th percentile +12 mmHg, or greater than or equal to 140/90 mmHg, whichever is lower	BP greater than or equal to 140/90 mmHg

BP, blood pressure; DBP, diastolic blood pressure; SBP, systolic blood pressure.

Source: Data from Flynn, J. T., Kaelbe, D., Baker-Smith, C. M., Blowey, D., Carroll, A., Daniels, S. R., . . . Urbina, E. M. (2017). Clinical practice guideline for screening and management of high blood pressure in children and adolescents. *Pediatrics, 140*(3). doi:10.1542/peds.2017-1904

Etiology/Incidence

Evaluation begins with determining between primary and secondary causes of hypertension, identifying comorbid risk factors, and referring for appropriate treatment and to specialists due to the identified secondary cause.

- Primary hypertension (no identified cause) is most often asymptomatic and occurs with associated comorbidities such as obesity, insulin resistance, hyperlipidemia, or obstructive sleep apnea. Patients may also have strong family history.
- Secondary hypertension (underlying cause can be identified) most often presents with symptoms of an underlying disease.
  - Renal and renovascular disease is the most common secondary cause; have a high suspicion for this in hypertensive children less than 6 years of age (Flynn et al., 2017).
  - Cardiac and neurological symptoms of hypertension include headache, stroke, seizure, visual disturbances, chest pain, syncope, and shortness of breath

(note these are not specific to any one cause—but these patients have a higher likelihood having secondary cause [Gleason, Shaddy, & Rychik, 2012]).

- Screen for signs/symptoms of conditions requiring emergent treatment: elevated intracranial pressure (ICP), coarctation of the aorta (CoA), and acute renal failure.

History/PE

- Retinal exam: vascular lesions due to chronic hypertension; papilledema in increased ICP.
- Weight loss, anorexia, irritability, epistaxis, neonatal history of umbilical lines, and strong family history of hypertension often correlate.

Diagnostics

- Diagnosis of hypertension is made when repeat blood pressure values are greater than or equal to 95th percentile on three separate visits; it is important to analyze BP data from multiple visits over time prior to making a diagnosis.
- Measurements should be taken in the right arm to verify that cuff size is appropriate.
  - Bladder length should be 80% to 100% of the arm circumference, and width should be at least 40% (Weaver, 2019).
- Ambulatory blood pressure readings may be helpful in providing better accuracy of blood pressure trends throughout day and night.
- Evaluations for end-organ damage that may be ordered by specialists:
  - Echocardiogram to assess left ventricular hypertrophy in response to chronic hypertension (assesses LV mass, geometry, and function)
  - EKG is not recommended as it is not sensitive enough to reliably identify LVH
  - Retinal exam
  - Renovascular imaging
- Labs: serum electrolytes, blood urea nitrogen and creatinine, complete blood count (CBC), urinalysis, renal ultrasound (<6 years of age with abnormal urinalysis or renal function).
- Other tests: A1c and aspartate transaminase and alanine transaminase, lipid panel, glucose (in obese patients); may also consider TSH, drug screening (if concern is present), or sleep study (AAP, 2017).

Differential Diagnosis Due to Underlying Secondary Causes

- **Cardiac:** Coarctation, anemia, patent ductus arteriosus (PDA), arteriovenous fistula, Turner's syndrome, Williams syndrome.
  - **CoA:** A discrete narrowing in the lumen of the aorta causing obstruction to blood flow and increasing afterload in the left ventricle. As a result, there is higher blood pressure proximal to the obstruction and lower blood pressure distally.
    - **Etiology:** 4% to 6% of CHD occurs in 4 per 10,000 births and is more common in males; 5% to 15% of girls with CoA have Turner's syndrome (Flynn et al., 2017).
    - **Symptoms:** Hypertension, murmur, decreased lower extremity pulses, diminished or delayed femoral pulses (brachial–femoral delay), can present at any age (more severe forms occurring during newborn period and milder forms occurring throughout childhood).
    - **Newborns:** Symptoms may be masked until after PDA closure and then present with CHF and shock if severe.

- ▫ **Children/adolescents:** Asymptomatic, upper extremity hypertension, +/− murmur.
- ▫ **Murmur:** Heard best over at left upper sternal border and between scapulae on back; may also be heard continuous murmur due to collateral blood flow.
- ▫ **Treatment:** Refer to cardiology, surgical, or transcatheter repair.
- **Renal:** Renal parenchymal disease, renal artery stenosis or thrombosis, reflux nephropathy, obstructive uropathy.
- **Endocrine/metabolic:** Cushing syndrome, hyperthyroidism, hyperaldosteronism, insulin resistance.
- **Others:** Drug-induced pain, elevated ICP, neurofibromatosis, collagen vascular disease, pheochromocytoma, Wilms' tumor, neuroblastoma, lupus (Gleason et al., 2012).

Don't Miss

- Patients with a repaired coarctation are at risk for hypertension throughout life.
  - Hypertension can be a manifestation of recoarctation even after successful repair; evaluation should be assessed by using four extremity BP measurements for these patients in addition to echocardiography (AAP, 2017).
  - Keep in mind that normally BP is 10 to 20 mmHg higher in the lower extremities than in the upper; therefore, if a leg BP is lower than the arm BP or if femoral pulses are weak/absent, coarctation should be strongly considered.
- BP should be checked in all children and adolescents ≥3 years of age at every healthcare encounter if they have obesity, are taking medications known to increase BP, have renal disease, or have history of repaired coarctation or arch obstruction or diabetes.

Treatment

The goal is to reduce long term morbidities and mortalities from prolonged hypertension.

- Reduce blood pressure to below the 90th to 95th percentile and reduce LVH.
- Lifestyle changes should be attempted first before starting pharmacotherapy depending on severity:
  - Refer to nutrition.
  - Increase physical activity; suggest activities for whole family to enjoy.
- Medications: Reserved for patients with secondary hypertension, symptomatic hypertension, and evidence of end-organ damage or diabetes, or who fail lifestyle modifications.
  - ACE inhibitor, calcium channel blocker, diuretics—start lowest possible dose and slowly titrate.
- Aggressively treat reversible secondary hypertension.

KAWASAKI DISEASE

Etiology

Kawasaki disease (KD) is characterized by an acute vasculitis in early childhood and predominantly affects children <5 years of age. If untreated, complications of coronary artery aneurysms may occur in 20% to 25% of cases. It has been reported as the leading cause of acquired heart disease in children in developed countries.

Epidemiology/Risk Factors

Estimated incidence in North American is 25 cases per 100,000 children younger than 5 years of age, with the highest risk in Asian children. Coronary artery aneurysms account for 5% of acute coronary syndromes in adults less than 40 years of age.

Classic KD is diagnosed based on the presence of fever for at least 5 days, together with at least four out of five clinical features:

1. Red, cracked lips, strawberry tongue, and/or erythema or oropharynx
2. Bilateral bulbar conjunctivitis without exudate
3. Diffuse maculopapular rash, especially in diaper area
4. Erythema and edema of hands and feet during acute phase (desquamation of fingers/ toes occurs late phase)
5. Cervical lymphadenopathy (greater than or equal to 1.5 cm diameter) and usually unilateral

Diagnosis of incomplete (or atypical KD) should be considered in any child with a prolonged and unexplained fever with fewer than four out of the five principal findings.

Labs

KD is nonspecific, and while there are no specific diagnostic labs to confirm a diagnosis of KD, a CBC with diff, erythrocyte sedimentation rate (ESR), and C-reactive protein (CRP) should be drawn.

- Leukocytosis is typical during acute phase, anemia (normochromic and normocytic), ESR, and CRP will be elevated and take about 8 weeks to return to normal.

Differentials

Infections—strep/staph, Steven Johnson's syndrome, drug reactions, toxic shock syndrome, viral exanthems, juvenile rheumatoid arthritis (JRA), rheumatic fever, measles.

Don't Miss

- Treatment should begin as early as possible to avoid long-term damage and prevent coronary aneurysm complications.

Treatment

The goal is to reduce inflammation and arterial damage during the acute phase and prevent thrombosis if coronaries are involved.

- Refer to cardiology and serial echocardiograms for evaluation of coronary artery aneurysm.
- High-dose IVIG with aspirin as early as possible and ideally within the first 10 days of onset of fever.
- IVIG administration during acute phase has been shown to reduce the prevalence of coronary artery abnormalities.

Follow-Up/Family Education

- Education surrounding the serious nature of the disease and the necessity of a follow-up with a pediatric cardiologist should be provided. ASA may be continued indefinitely for those with coronary artery aneurysms.
- Complications: Coronary artery aneurysms and therefore increased risk of thrombosis, stenosis, and resultant myocardial infarction can develop valvular heart

disease, pericarditis, myocarditis, pericardial effusion, CHF, liver dysfunction, and the development of other vascular aneurysms (not isolated to the heart).

■ With long-term aspirin use, recommend the flu shot, given the association of Reye's syndrome between flu-like viral illnesses and aspirin.

■ Ibuprofen may interfere with antiplatelet effects of aspirin and therefore should be avoided.

Don't Miss

■ Any child with chest pain, fever, and tachycardia should be considered to have myocarditis and referred to ED or a pediatric cardiologist for urgent assessment.

■ Exertional chest pain can indicate an anomalous coronary artery. A referral to a pediatric cardiologist should be made. An echocardiogram should be obtained by a cardiologist to examine cardiac anatomy, coronary artery origins, and ventricular function.

Treatment

Treatment of chest pain depends on its cause. Pediatric patients with obvious etiology of their noncardiac chest pain should be treated accordingly. Musculoskeletal chest pain should be treated with reassurance, rest, and nonsteroidal anti-inflammatory drugs (NSAIDs).

Cardiac causes of chest pain, including myocarditis, requires inpatient hospitalization. Some cases respond to intravenous immunoglobulin (IVIG). Ventricular dysfunction is treated with inotropic support and, in some cases, extracorporeal membrane oxygenation (ECMO). Patients can suffer long-term ventricular dysfunction following an episode of myocarditis. Some children are left without any long-term sequela. Exercise is restricted for 6 months following an episode of myocarditis.

Surgical intervention for anomalous coronary arteries is recommended in some cases. This depends on the coronary artery course and is determined after more thorough testing such as cMRI or cCT scanning.

PALPITATIONS

Etiology/Epidemiology

Most complaints of palpitations are benign in children and adolescents. Palpitations can be described as a forceful, rapid, or irregular heartbeat perceptible to the child/adolescent. The most common pediatric cardiac rhythm finding presenting to EDs is sinus tachycardia (seen in about 50% of children who complain of an arrhythmia; Jain & Sami Chaouki, 2018).

Sinus tachycardia has many causes and is regarded as a symptom of another problem. Some of the many causes of sinus tachycardia include the following:

■ Fever
■ Anemia
■ Hyperthyroidism
■ Pain

- Dehydration
- Anxiety

Supraventricular tachycardia (SVT) is a common arrhythmia seen in all ages; babies through adolescents. It is rarely an ominous arrhythmia and oftentimes is associated with discomfort but rarely requires emergent care. The diagnosis is made by EKG findings, so it is important to refer any baby, child, or adolescent with heart rates in the 200 bpm range to the ED for diagnosis and treatment.

Symptoms

Children with palpitations complain of a forceful and rapid heart rate. Palpitations and tachycardia that has a sudden onset and abrupt cessation with associated shortness of breath and possible dizziness may represent an arrhythmia, specifically SVT. Palpitations associated with chest pain and syncope require emergent care.

Dizziness, fatigue, and syncope may be a result of bradycardia. If this is the case, consider Lyme disease, and obtain an EKG to determine if heart block is present.

Focused PE/Findings

The PE in the child complaining of palpitations begins with a detailed history determining the onset of complaints, duration, and intensity of palpitations. It is important to ascertain if the symptoms occur at rest and if any triggers exist. It is important to determine if dizziness and syncope occur. Family history for inherited arrhythmia such as long QT syndrome, Brugada syndrome, and cardiomyopathy is essential to determine.

When assessing infants, it is important to ascertain whether there have been feeding difficulties or hyperirritability, which suggests a rhythm abnormality.

The PE includes accurate vital signs and a thorough cardiac examination. An irregular rhythm may represent premature atrial or ventricular beats. Occurring in isolation, these beats are generally benign.

Diagnostic Testing

An EKG can determine the cardiac rhythm and assess for any ectopic or abnormal beats. The presence of a shortened PR interval and a delta wave is consistent with Wolff–Parkinson–White syndrome (WPW), which predisposes one to have SVT.

A complete blood count and thyroid function testing should be obtained in the child with persistent tachycardia.

Differentials

- Sinus tachycardia is consistent with rates under 160 bpm, with gradual onset and gradual cessation. Consider the source of tachycardia.
- SVT is consistent with rates exceeding 160 bpm. An abrupt onset with abrupt cessation of tachycardia is a hallmark of SVT. It is sometimes associated with shortness of breath and dizziness and rarely associated with syncope.
- Premature atrial or ventricular contractions; Isolated early beats that feel more forceful and sometimes bothersome to patients.
- More ominous rhythm disturbances usually result in syncope. Family history of long QT syndrome or Brugada syndrome is also considered.

- Consider common conditions predisposing one to sinus tachycardia such as fever, anemia, dehydration, hyperthyroidism, anxiety.
- Obtain screening EKGs when tachycardia abruptly starts and stops.
- Consider obtaining EKG when heart rates are slow to determine if heart block is present. If so, consider Lyme testing and referral to cardiology.
- Preexcitation and delta wave on EKG are consistent with WPW. Referral to cardiology is necessary.
- Atrial and ventricular premature beats, in isolation, are not worrisome. EKG testing is diagnostic of ectopy. If frequent, then referral to cardiology is suggested.

Treatment

SVT is always more symptomatic than sinus tachycardia (see Table 5.5). With sinus tachycardia, the P waves and T waves are separate. With SVT, they are together. Vagal maneuvers can typically break SVT (see Figure 5.1).

Table 5.5

Distinguishing Sinus Tachycardia and Supraventricular Tachycardia		
Heart Rate (bpm)	**Sinus Tachycardia**	**Supraventricular Tachycardia**
Infant	<220	>220
Child	<180	>160 (at rest)
Onset	Gradual	Abrupt
Physical exam	Signs of underlying cause (e.g., fever, hypovolemia)	Infants may have signs of CHF (e.g., edema, rales, hepatomegaly)
EKG	Presence of p waves in I/aVF	P waves absent/abnormal, inverted p waves in II/III/aVF
Cardiac monitoring	Variability in rate with changes in stimulation or treatment (IVF)	Minimal variability with changes in stimulation
CXR	Small heart and clear lungs, unless underlying cause related to pulmonary infection	Signs of pulmonary edema may be present (usually seen in infants, not older children)
Treatment	In patients who are hemodynamically stable, in older children, vagal maneuvers include bearing down (Valsalva maneuver), blowing into an occluded straw, or assuming a head-down position for 15–20 seconds Carotid massage and orbital pressure should **not** be performed in children Vagal maneuvers are successful in 60%–90% of cases First-line pharmacologic therapy is adenosine in children	In patients who are hemodynamically stable, attempt vagal maneuvers (shown in Figure 5.1) to terminate the tachyarrhythmia **Vagal maneuvers:** These maneuvers should be performed while the EKG is continuously monitored If no improvement, adenosine is given

CHF, congestive heart failure; CXR, chest x-ray; EKG, electrocardiogram; IVF, in vitro fertilization.

Source: Data from Manole, M. D., & Saladino, R. A. (2007). Emergency department management of the pediatric patient with supraventricular tachycardia. *Pediatric Emergency Care, 23*(3), 176–185. doi:10.1097/PEC.0b013e318032904c, p. 183.

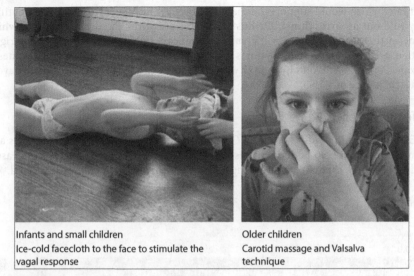

Infants and small children	Older children
Ice-cold facecloth to the face to stimulate the vagal response	Carotid massage and Valsalva technique

Figure 5.1 Treatment of SVT in pediatric patients.

SYNCOPE

Etiology

Syncope is a symptom presenting with an abrupt, transient, complete loss of consciousness (LOC) with a rapid and spontaneous recovery caused by cerebra hypoperfusion (Shen et al., 2017).

Symptoms

Syncope that occurs during restful times with a prodrome consistent with dizziness, pallor, visual alteration, diaphoresis, nausea, and brief LOC is typically consistent with vasovagal syncope (VVS; see Table 5.6). Usually, a trigger occurs that stimulated the vagus nerve, which causes peripheral vasodilation, bradycardia, and resultant syncope. Common triggers are pain, dehydration, standing for a prolonged period, anxiety, fear, and hair grooming; VVS is common in adolescents and more common in girls and frequently seen when a parent has had a history of similar events.

Syncope associated with exertion or following palpitations should be considered dangerous. Inherited cardiomyopathies and certain rhythm abnormalities such as catecholaminergic polymorphic ventricular tachycardia can occur with exertion. Other dangerous arrhythmias can cause syncope as well as ventricular tachycardia, atrial fibrillation, and Torsade's de pointes (seen in patients with long QT syndrome). Syncope that has no prodrome, occurs with exercise, or follows palpitations should be referred urgently to a cardiologist for a thorough assessment and workup.

Syncope associated with tonic–clonic movements and associated with postictal behavior should be considered seizure activity.

Focused PE Signs/Finding

Examination of the heart is typically normal in patients with syncope, be it vasovagal or caused by rhythm disorders. There may be an orthostatic change in blood pressure or heart rate, which would support the diagnosis of VVS, although this would not defini- tively rule out an arrhythmia. Orthostatic blood pressures should be obtained while supine, sitting, or standing. An increase in the heart rate upon assuming an upright position, greater than 30 bpm, supports orthostatic intolerance and vasovagal dizziness/ syncope. Patients with joint hyperlaxity seen in some connective tissue disorders have a greater incidence of VVS.

Lab Tests/Diagnostics

An EKG is helpful in ruling out long QT syndrome and WPW. Oftentimes, EKGs are normal and do not help with diagnosis. Some children with anemia have an increased incidence of VVS; therefore, a screening CBC may be helpful if anemia is suspected.

Differentials

Table 5.6

Common Causes of Syncopal Episodes in the Pediatric Patient		
Vasovagal Syncope	**Arrhythmia**	**Seizure**
Occurs at rest with trigger.	Can occur during exertion or increased emotional state.	Aura can occur prior to LOC.
Prodrome is consistent with dizziness, pallor, diaphoresis, visual and auditory disturbance, and nausea.	Typically, no prodrome or complaints of abrupt onset of tachycardia.	Syncope is associated with tonic–clonic movements and "stiffening" of body.
Generally, brief LOC with syncope occurs in swooning manner. No seizure activity, no postictal behaviors.	Syncope is abrupt and can be associated with injury.	Hypersomnolence or postictal behavior following LOC.
	Family history is important to obtain.	

LOC, loss of consciousness.

Don't Miss

- Syncope with exertion requires an urgent/emergent referral.
- Syncope that occurs at rest, with prodrome, following typical triggers is usually vasovagal and can be improved with increasing one's fluid and salt intake, exercis- ing routinely and decreasing one's anxiety.
- Syncope with seizure activity needs a neurologist referral.

Treatment

Treatment depends on identifying the cause of the syncope. Patients should follow up based on outlined points in Don't Miss.

Follow-Up/Patient Education

Education is key in preventing injury and subsequent events.

References

American Academy of Pediatrics. (2017). *New pediatric blood pressure guidelines identify more kids at higher risk of premature heart disease.* https://newsroom.heart.org/news/new-pediatric-blood-pressure-guidelines-identify-more-kids-at-higher-risk-of-premature-heart-disease?preview=95c375a65d6dfcae5eb60d3b1222cbeb

American Heart Association. (2019). *Commonly asked questions about children and heart disease.* Retrieved from https://www.heart.org/en/health-topics/congenital-heart-defects/congenital-heart-defects-tools-and-resources/commonly-asked-questions-about-children-and-heart-disease

Chen, M., Riehle-Colarusso, T., Yeung, L. F., Smith, C., & Farr, S. L. (2018). Children with heart conditions and their special health care needs—United States. *MMWR Morbidity and Mortality Weekly Report, 67*(38), 1045–1049.

Colan, S. (2019). Hypertrophic cardiomyopathy in childhood. *Heart Failure Clinics, 6*(4), 433–444. doi:10.1016/j.hfc.2010.05.004

Colan, S. D., Lipshultz, S. E., Lowe, A. M., Sleeper, L. A., Messere, J., Cox, G. F., . . . Towbin, J. A. (2007). Epidemiology and cause-specific outcome of hypertrophic cardiomyopathy in children: Findings from the Pediatric Cardiomyopathy Registry. *Circulation, 115*(6), 773–781. doi:10.1161/CIRCULATIONAHA.106.621185

Farr, S. L., Downing, K. F., Riehle-Colarusso, T., & Abarbanell, G. (2018). Functional limitations and educational needs among children and adolescents with heart disease. *Congenital Heart Disease, 13*(4), 633–639. doi:10.1111/chd.12621

Flynn, J. T., Kaelbe, D., Baker-Smith, C. M., Blowey, D., Carroll, A., Daniels, S. R., . . . Urbina, E. M. (2017). Clinical practice guideline for screening and management of high blood pressure in children and adolescents. *Pediatrics, 140*(3). doi:10.1542/peds.2017-1904

Gleason, M., Shaddy, R., & Rychik, J. (2012). *Pediatric practice cardiology.* New York, NY: McGraw Hill.

Jain, P. G., & Sami Chaouki, A. (2018). The use of electrocardiography in the emergency department. *Clinical Pediatric Emergency Medicine, 19*(4), 317–322. doi:10.1016/j.cpem.2018.12.001

Koulouri, S., Acherman, R. J., Wong, P. C., Chan, L. S., & Lewis, A. B. (2004). Utility of B-type natriuretic peptide in differentiating congestive heart failure from lung disease in pediatric patients with respiratory distress. *Pediatric cardiology, 25*, 341–346. doi:10.1007/s00246-003-0578-0

Manole, M. D., & Saladino, R. A. (2007). Emergency department management of the pediatric patient with supraventricular tachycardia. *Pediatric Emergency Care, 23*(3), 176–185. doi:10.1097/PEC.0b013e318032904c

Ruggiero, K. M., Hickey, P. A., Leger, R. R., Vessey, J. A., & Hayman, L. L. (2018). Parental perceptions of disease-severity and health-related quality of life in school-age children with congenital heart disease. *Journal for Specialists in Pediatric Nursing, 23*(1), 1–10. doi:10.1111/jspn.12204

Shen, W. K., Sheldon, R. S., Benditt, D. G., Cohen, M. I., Forman, D. E., Goldberger, Z. D., . . . Yancy, C. W. (2017). 2017 ACC/AHA/HRS guideline for the evaluation and management of patients with syncope: A report of the American College of Cardiology/American Heart Association Task Force on Clinical Practice Guidelines and the Heart Rhythm Society. *Journal of the American College of Cardiology, 70*(5), e39–e110. doi:10.1016/j.jacc.2017.03.003

Uri, K. A., Singh, H., Denifield, S. W., Cabrera, A. G., Dreyer, W. J., Tunuguntla, H. P., & Price, J. F. (2019). Use missed diagnosis of new-onset systolic heart failure at first presentation in children with no known heart disease. *Pediatrics, 208*, 258–264.e3. doi:10.1016/j.jpeds.2018.12.029

Weaver, D. J. (2019). Pediatric hypertension: Review of updated guidelines. *Pediatrics in Review, 40*, 354–358. doi:10.1542/pir.2018-0014

Common Gastroenterologic Conditions Seen in Pediatric Primary Care

Kristine M. Ruggiero

INTRODUCTION

Gastrointestinal (GI) complaints are commonly seen in pediatrics, and abdominal pain is one of the most common symptoms seen by the pediatric advanced practicing clinicians (APCs). Abdominal pain may be acute or chronic (at least three episodes within 3 months) and are often due to gastroenteritis, constipation, or a viral illness. The GI system plays an essential role in the child's growth and development, and because the GI system is so complex, the challenge is to recognize those children who require immediate evaluation for potentially life-threatening condition. This chapter provides a review of developmental aspects of the GI system in common pediatric GI disorders.

OBJECTIVES

1. Examine how to evaluate abdominal pain in a pediatric patient.
2. Examine common conditions of the GI system in the pediatric patient.
3. Identify and choose appropriate common diagnostic and laboratory testing for abdominal disorders and appropriate clinical workup for common conditions of the GI system.
4. Differentiate between acute and chronic abdominal pain, and those disorders requiring immediate attention, and develop a differential diagnosis based on age and symptoms.
5. Formulate a plan for evaluation and management of the pediatric patient with abdominal pain.
6. Understand the causes and frequency of acute and chronic abdominal pain in childhood.

ABDOMINAL PAIN

Determine whether the pain is acute or chronic and whether a medical, surgical, or non-organic disorder is most likely. If the patient is an adolescent female, you must consider genitourinary pathology and a pelvic exam should also be performed.

The age of the child can help focus the differential diagnosis. In infants and toddlers, clinicians should consider congenital anomalies and other causes, including malrotation, hernias, Meckel's diverticulum, or intussusception. In school-age children, appendicitis, constipation, functional abdominal pain, and infectious causes of pain such as gastroenteritis and colitis should be considered. In female adolescents, clinicians should consider pelvic inflammatory disease, pregnancy, ruptured ovarian cysts, or ovarian torsion. Please see Chapter 10, Common Pediatric Renal/Urologic Disorders Seen in Pediatric Primary Care, for more information on those conditions.

Physical assessment for acute abdominal pain should be comprehensive and include a patient's vital signs (which may be unstable in a patient with acute abdominal pain), a detailed abdominal examination (including noting appearance), and overall hydration status of a patient as well as presence or absence of a fever (suggests infection, urinary tract infection [UTI], pneumonia, gastroenteritis). Features that should be noted on abdominal exam include abdominal distention, which may be the result of an obstruction, and presence or absence of bowel sounds and intensity (i.e., increased bowel sounds present in bowel obstruction of gastroenteritis and decreased bowel sounds noted in appendicitis). A focused extra-abdominal examination (such as flank pain seen in pyelonephritis, erythematous pharynx seen in pharyngitis, or jaundice seen in hepatitis) should also be performed, noting any additional clinical findings.

■ ABDOMINAL MASSES

Focused PE Signs/Key Findings

A complete PE should be performed in children with abdominal masses, noting the quadrant of the abdomen affected, what organ is most likely affected, and the characteristics of the abdominal mass, including the following:

1. Is it hard or soft?
2. Is it mobile or nonmobile?
3. Does it cross the midline?
4. Is it tender with palpation or not?
5. Pay attention to the general condition of the child, including signs of metastatic disease such as weight loss and enlarged lymph nodes.
6. In addition, on PE, auscultate the heart and lungs, examine extremities for any swelling, and perform a full neuro exam to rule out any nervous system involvement. The patient's blood pressure should be obtained and may be elevated in certain abdominal masses, specifically in Wilms tumor or neuroblastoma.

Lab Tests/Diagnostics

An US should be obtained, which will show the location of the mass and whether it is solid or cystic.

Depending on these results, further lab studies include a CBC, urinalysis, and tumor markers.

Imaging studies such as plain radiography of chest and abdomen, contrast radiography of the GI tract, CT, MRI, angiography, and scintigraphy are recommended.

Differentials

See Table 6.1 for etiology by age of malignant abdominal masses.

Table 6.1

Age-Related Etiology of Malignant Abdominal Masses	
Age	**Malignant Cause of Mass**
Neonate (0–1 month)	Neuroblastoma
Infant (0–12 months)	Neuroblastoma
	Hepatoblastoma
	Teratoma
Child (1–12 months)	Neuroblastoma
	Wilm's tumor
	Leukemia
	Lymphoma
	Hepatoblastoma
Adolescent (13–18 months)	Ovarian neoplasm
	Neuroblastoma
	Lymph
	Hepatocellular carcinoma

Don't Miss

The following mnemonic was developed by the American Cancer Society to help clinicians remember the early warning signs of childhood cancer (Pollock, Krischer, & Vietti, 1991):

- **C**ontinued, unexplained weight loss
- **H**eadaches without vomiting in the morning
- **I**ncreased swelling or persistent pain in bones or joints, sometimes accompanied by limping
- **L**ump or mass in abdomen, neck, or elsewhere
- **D**evelopment of a whitish appearance in the pupil of the eye or sudden changes in vision
- **R**ecurrent fevers not caused by infections
- **E**xcessive bruising or bleeding (often sudden)
- **N**oticeable paleness or prolonged tiredness

Treatment

If the abdominal mass is suspected to be malignant (based on the history, PE findings, and lab and imaging studies), then the pediatric APC should immediately refer the patient to a pediatric oncologist for further evaluation and initiation of treatment.

Follow-Up/Patient/Family Education

Not all abdominal masses are cancerous, but optimal treatment of childhood cancer requires a high level of suspicion by the primary care pediatric APC. If any of these findings are worrisome to the APC, further evaluation and early referral to the pediatric oncologist should occur immediately.

■ APPENDICITIS

Etiology/Epidemiology

This is the most common indication for abdominal surgery in childhood. Appendicitis results from bacterial invasion of the appendix. Appendicitis occurs most frequently in children between the ages of 10 and 15 years. Less than 10% of patients are younger than 5 years of age. The incidence of perforation and diffuse peritonitis is higher in children younger than 2 years of age. Research shows appendicitis is more common in the United States due to a low-fiber diet.

Symptoms

Associated symptoms include loss of appetite, nausea, vomiting fever, diarrhea, and diffuse periumbilical pain. Pain located in right lower quadrant (RLQ) is a hallmark sign, and pain generally moves from the periumbilical area to RLQ as the parietal peritoneum becomes inflamed.

Focused Physical Exam Signs/Findings

Physical exam (PE) findings include the following:

- **Blumberg sign:** This is rebound tenderness at McBurney's point. Guarding, rebound tenderness, and obturator and psoas signs are commonly found.
- **Psoas/obturator sign**: The increased abdominal pain while raising the patient's right leg with the knee flexed and rotating the leg internally at the hip indicates a positive obturator sign.
- **Rovsing's sign:** Pressure over the descending colon causes pain in the RLQ. On rectal exam, tenderness suggests inflamed posterior appendix.

Lab Tests/Diagnostics

A moderately elevated white blood cell count (absolute neutrophilic leukocytosis) with a left shift is often seen.

- Also obtain complete blood count (CBC) and urinalysis if appendicitis is suspected.
- Always perform pregnancy test in females.
- Perform abdominal ultrasound (US) first in pediatric and pregnant patients.
- Perform abdominal CT scan in adults or pediatric patients without a diagnostic US.

Differentials

See Table 6.2.

Don't Miss

- While the most common cause of acute abdominal pain is viral gastroenteritis, it is important for the APC to work through the differential carefully as not to miss appendicitis.
- Appendicitis is the most common indication for abdominal surgery in childhood.
- The appendix tends to perforate 36 hours after pain begins.

Treatment

The following are the treatment recommended for appendicitis: emergent surgical consult, laparoscopic appendectomy, or CT-guided drainage of abscess.

Table 6.2

Causes/Differentials of Acute and Chronic Abdominal Pain			
Acute: **Most Common**	**Acute:** **Less Common**	**Chronic:** **Most Common**	**Chronic:** **Less Common**
Appendicitis	Incarcerated hernia	Functional abdominal pain (IBD, abdominal migraine)	Mittelschmerz
Diet	Gallbladder disease	Constipation	Parasitic infection
Food poisoning	Hepatitis	Lactose intolerance	Endometriosis
Gastroenteritis	Intussusception		IBD
Mesenteric lymphadenitis	Pelvic inflammatory disease		UTI
Pharyngitis	Renal stones		Sickle cell disease
UTI			

IBD, inflammatory bowel disease; UTI, urinary tract infection.

Follow-Up/Patient/Family Education

It is important to educate the family and patient about perioperative care, the need for pain medication, and maintaining nothing by mouth (NPO) status. Postoperative care includes early ambulation, advancement of diet, wound care, and monitoring for infection.

■ INTUSSUSCEPTION

Intussusception is the most common abdominal emergency affecting children under 2 years old (Lloyd & Kenny, 2004). It is usually the result of a viral illness that causes intestinal swelling and causes one portion of the intestine to slide up into the next like a telescope, causing a mechanical bowel obstruction by blocking the flow of fluids and food through that area. Other less common causes of intussusception include a polyp or tumor.

Symptoms

Symptoms of intussusception include paroxysmal abdominal pain demonstrated by sudden, loud crying that comes and goes every 15 to 20 minutes, vomiting, and stool mixed with blood and mucus, which gives the characteristic "currant jelly" stool appearance.

Focused PE Signs/Key Findings

- Focal tenderness, especially in the right or mid-upper abdomen
- Lethargy
- Palpable "sausage-shaped" mass, vertically oriented in the right mid- or upper quadrant
- Dance's sign—scaphoid RLQ

Lab Tests/Diagnostics

US will identify the intussusception. Nonoperative reduction under US or fluoroscopic guidance is diagnostic but will also reduce the intussusception. A small percentage of people may have spontaneous resolution of the intussusception.

Differentials

See Table 6.2. Rectal bleeding and vomiting should include Meckel's diverticulum, bacterial colitis, and malrotation and/or volvulus.

> **Don't Miss**
>
> Have a high index of suspicion in children 3 months to 5 years.

Treatment

Approach to treatment depends on the severity of symptoms:

- In patients who have no evidence of bowel perforation and normal vital signs, nonoperative reduction under ultrasonographic or fluoroscopic guidance using hydrostatic or pneumatic pressure by enema is the treatment of choice for an infant or child with ileocolic intussusception who is clinically stable.
- In acutely ill patients or patients with signs or symptoms of perforation, surgical intervention is recommended.

Follow-Up/Patient/Family Education

Education should be provided to patients and families regarding the risk that intussusception can recur. Evidence shows that approximately 10% of children will have recurrence of intussusception after successful nonoperative reduction. Approximately half of the recurrences are within the first 72 hours after nonoperative reduction. Many institutions admit the child for a 12- to 24-hour observation period due to the risk for recurrence, but literature is mixed as admitting the patient for observation does not prevent a further recurrence (Kwon et al., 2019).

CONSTIPATION

Etiology/Epidemiology

Constipation affects up to 30% of children and accounts for an estimated 3 to 5% of all visits to the pediatricians (Robin et al., 2018). The peak prevalence is in the preschool age child with up to 95% of constipation cases being due to functional constipation in otherwise healthy children. Functional constipation is often the result of a painful or unpleasant experience with defecation that the child wants to avoid repeating. This may prompt the child to avoid doing it again, leading to stool-withholding behaviors that promotes constipation.

Symptoms

Functional constipation describes persistently difficult, infrequent, or incomplete defecation without evidence of an anatomic cause and is frequently defined by the "Rome IV" diagnostic criteria, which requires the presence of at least two of six criteria describing stool frequency, hardness, and size; fecal incontinence; or stool retention. Symptoms should be present for 1 month in infants and toddlers and for 2 months in older children (Benninga et al., 2016; Up to Date, 2019).

Focused PE Signs/Key Findings

Abdominal distention and fullness.

Lab Tests/Diagnostics

None.

Differentials

Organic causes of constipation such as HD and celiac disease, which only account for about 5% of the total constipation, should be ruled out. In addition, the large protein in cow's milk can sometimes cause constipation in infants and young children, and if suspected, it should be ruled out by an elimination diet.

Don't Miss

Functional constipation accounts for most cases of constipation after the neonatal period.

Treatment

Begin a bowel clean-out and then a bowel maintenance program. For children with mild chronic constipation, dietary changes alone may benefit.

For children with fecal impaction, first action should always be treating the disimpaction with oral and/or rectal medication. Stool softeners such as docusate salts reduce surface tension enhancing the incorporation of water into the stools, softening them. Stimulants, such as senna, have direct effects on GI smooth muscle stimulating intestinal motility. Prolonged use can lead to dependence. Enemas and suppositories cause direct bowel distension and produce an evacuation reflex in most people.

Follow-Up/Patient/Family Education

Treatment around constipation should always combine family education and behavioral modification (routine, scheduled toileting) to improve treatment outcomes.

■ HIRSCHSPRUNG'S DISEASE

Also known as aganglionic megacolon, it is the lack of nerve innervation along a segment of the wall of the colon. There can be varying degrees of severity depending on the location in the colon and the amount of the colon affected. HD is one of the most common causes of constipation in the newborn period.

Symptoms

- Onset of symptoms in the first week of life
- Delayed passage of meconium (first meconium passed after 48 hours of life)
- Constipation (especially in the first 6 months of life)
- Vomiting (especially bilious vomiting)

Focused PE Signs/Key Findings

- Abdominal pain/distension
- No stool present in the rectal vault on digital rectal exam, or an explosion of gas and liquid stool may occur following the digital rectal exam

Lab Tests/Diagnostics

A plain abdominal x-ray will be the first step and will show if there is any stool in the rectum as well as an airless rectum, and for patients presenting with an acute abdomen, it will show an obstruction.

Differentials

Toxic megacolon, constipation, failure to thrive, and disorders of the ileus in the new-born period.

Don't Miss

Can be associated with other anomalies, such as Down syndrome.
    HD is being diagnosed in the first few months of life, and fewer and fewer children are presenting to primary care with HD.

Treatment

Barium enema can give the diagnosis and reduce the intussusception. Rarely, surgery is needed if patients present with signs and symptoms of an acute abdomen at presentation or in cases in which a barium enema cannot reduce the intussusception.

Follow-Up/Patient/Family Education

If a child requires surgery for HD, postsurgical care should be paid to the perineum area, as many children will have loose stool output after surgery.

■ MALROTATION AND VOLVULUS

Malrotation is an anomaly of intestinal fixation and rotation and is not a problem in itself. It is estimated that nearly 1 in 100 people have some form of improper rotation or fixation. Intestinal volvulus is a twisting of the intestine around the mesentery and can result in obstruction of the proximal bowel. Because the mesentery is involved, possible complications include vascular compromise and bowel necrosis.

Symptoms

- **Infants:** Intestinal malrotation should be suspected in an infant who presents with bilious emesis, abdominal tenderness associated with hemodynamic deterioration (Shalaby, Kuti, & Walker, 2013).
- **School-age and adolescent children:** Abdominal pain is the most common presenting symptom, which may present as abrupt or as chronic intermittent pain over weeks or months. In addition, it may be associated with intermittent vomiting, chronic diarrhea, malabsorption, and failure to thrive.
- Any vomiting in patients with known anomalies associated with intestinal malrotation should raise concern for malrotation.

Focused PE Signs/Key Findings

See the "Abdominal Pain" section.

Lab Tests/Diagnostics

Plain radiograph is the initial assessment. Upper GI series is the gold standard for making the diagnosis of malrotation. Barium enema was historically the procedure of choice but it has several limitations, including missing the diagnosis depending on the location. US can help determine the diagnosis of malrotation as it can determine the orientation of the mesenteric vessels, but should not be considered the definitive imaging choice.

Don't Miss

Recurrent volvulus is relatively infrequent (less than 10%) but must always be considered.

Up to 62% of children with an intestinal malrotation have another associated anomaly such as follows (Up to Date, 2019):

- Congenital diaphragmatic hernia
- Major congenital cardiac anomalies
- Abdominal wall defects
- VACTERL: Vertebral, anal, cardiac, tracheoesophageal, renal, and limb

Treatment

An acutely ill child with the presumed diagnosis of volvulus, when time is critical, requires urgent operative intervention even at the expense of full resuscitation.

In patients with malrotation without volvulus or obstruction, urgency is somewhat less.

Laparoscopic procedure is effective for nonurgent malrotation patients.

Follow-Up/Patient/Family Education

Once a patient has malrotation, they have abnormal intestinal rotation for the rest of their lives. It is a chronic condition, and families must be educated to that point.

■ MECKEL'S DIVERTICULUM

Meckel's diverticulum is a small pouch of the wall of the small intestine. Most people who have Meckel's are asymptomatic, with a prevalence of about 3% in the general population.

Half of all patients who do have symptoms from Meckel's diverticulum are children under the age of 10 years, and the majority are under the age of 2 years (Up to Date, 2019).

Symptoms

- Intestinal bowel obstruction leading to acute abdominal pain
- GI bleeding/presence of blood in stool (black or red)
- Constipation (due to blockage in the intestine)
- Not passing gas

Focused PE Signs/Key Findings

See the "Abdominal Pain" section.

Lab Tests/Diagnostics

"Meckel scan"—a small amount of radioactive material is passed through a peripheral IV prior to the scan.

US or CT scan can also show Meckel's diverticulum.

Don't Miss

The Rule of Twos is the classic description of the essential features of Meckel's diverticulum. It states Meckel's occurs in approximately 2% of the population with a male-to-female ratio of 2:1 and is located within 2 feet from the ileocecal valve and can be 2 inches in length.

Treatment

If a patient is symptomatic, surgery to remove the diverticulum is the treatment.

Follow-Up/Patient/Family Education

The patient and family are reassured that after recovery, resection of Meckel's diverticulum generally has no effect on GI functioning or nutrition.

DIARRHEA

■ GASTROENTERITIS

Most cases of gastroenteritis are self-limiting and do not require hospitalization; however, many parents of pediatric patients (especially younger infants and children) will seek medical treatment in an ambulatory or urgent care setting.

Etiology

Acute viral gastroenteritis is the most common cause of gastroenteritis. The diagnosis is made by the characteristic history of diarrhea that does not contain gross blood or mucus with or without vomiting, fever, or abdominal pain and with the presence or absence of findings more characteristic of acute abdomen or other conditions associated with diarrhea (Up to Date, 2019).

Epidemiology/Risk Factors

Viral gastroenteritis occurs throughout the year, with fall and winter being the most common times of year. It is often transmitted by the fecal–oral route. Illness usually begins 12 hours to 5 days after exposure and generally lasts for 3 to 7 days.

Symptoms

Acute gastroenteritis is a clinical syndrome often defined by increased stool frequency (e.g., greater than or equal to three loose or watery stools in 24 hours or several loose/watery bowel movements that exceed the child's usual daily number by two or more)

Table 6.3

Important Focused Physical Exam Findings Seen in Acute Gastroenteritis

VS: In severe dehydration, VSs may show a decreased BP and/or a rapid weak pulse.

HEENT: Sunken anterior fontanels, sunken eyes (seen in moderate to severe dehydration), and dry mucous membranes (seen in dehydration).

Neck: Any nuchal rigidity or other meningeal signs (not seen in gastroenteritis) should seek further evaluation for meningitis.

Chest: Deep respirations (may indicate acidosis seen in severe dehydration).

Abdomen: Hypoactive or hyperactive bowel sounds can be seen in gastroenteritis. Any abdominal distension or other signs and symptoms of acute abdomen should be further evaluated and are not commonly seen on PE for acute gastroenteritis.

Skin: Cool, mottled, poor capillary refill, and decreased turgor are all clinical findings seen in moderate to severe dehydration.

BP, blood pressure; HEENT, head, eyes, ears, nose, and throat; PE, physical exam; VS, vital sign.

with or without vomiting, fever, or abdominal pain. Acute viral gastroenteritis is caused by viral pathogens.

Focused PE Signs/Key Findings

The history and PE should focus on determining the severity of illness, mainly dehydration, and ruling out other causes of diarrhea and/or vomiting that require definitive therapy (i.e., meningitis, acute abdomen, appendicitis). These disorders can often be confused with acute gastroenteritis in the first 24 to 48 hours of symptoms.

Body weight may indicate degree of dehydration.

Fever is often present in gastroenteritis (temperature over 100.4°F for patients less than 3 months of age or temperature over 102.2°F in patients over 3 months of age), but temperature tends to be elevated more in bacterial causes of gastroenteritis (particularly over 104°F; Table 6.3).

Lab Tests/Diagnostics

Lab tests are not usually necessary but are necessary in children who require intravenous (IV) hydration therapy for moderate to severe dehydration or, if other disorders need to be excluded based on clinical findings, then a CBC with differential and a CHEM 7 may be ordered. In patients with an abnormal CBC, this may show anemia, thrombocytopenia (in conditions like hemolytic uremic syndrome), or an elevated eosinophil count like in parasitic gastroenteritis or an elevated band count seen in bacterial gastroenteritis. An elevated C-reactive protein may indicate inflammatory bowel disease (IBD) and should be further evaluated. Stool studies, especially for *Clostridium difficile*, may be indicated especially in patients on antibiotic therapy who are having persistent diarrhea.

Differentials

The most common causes of emesis and/or diarrhea include viral gastroenteritis. Other causes of gastroenteritis include bacterial or parasitic gastroenteritis. Focused PE and clinical findings should differentiate between gastroenteritis and other potential causes of vomiting and diarrhea, which can include the following:

- Acute abdomen (e.g., appendicitis, bowel obstruction, toxic megacolon)
- UTI
- Meningitis
- Sepsis
- Diabetes ketoacidosis (DKA)
- CNS mass
- Hemolytic uremic syndrome (HUS)
- Celiac disease

Don't Miss

It is important to rule out other causes of vomiting and diarrhea, specifically causes of acute abdomen, using a good history and PE.

Partial bowel obstruction or dysmotility may present with diarrhea.

In children less than 6 months of age, especially when diarrhea presents in the first few days to weeks of life, congenital causes should be considered.

Treatment

Supportive therapy (encouraging fluids at home) and IV hydration therapy to replenish any fluid loss, if needed, is recommended. Anti-diarrheal pharmacologic therapy commonly used in pediatric primary care includes bismuth subsalicylate (Pepto-Bismol), which adsorbs extra water in large intestine, as well as toxins. Use caution in children <3 years of age.

Follow-Up/Patient/Family Education

If only supportive therapy was required, follow-up is typically not indicated. If the patient was admitted or required an escalated level of care, or the parent or family had difficulty with supportive therapy, then a follow-up phone call would be indicated.

DYSPHAGIA

■ GASTROESOPHAGEAL REFLUX VERSUS GASTROESOPHAGEAL REFLUX DISEASE

To implement best evidence-based practices, an important concept for the general pediatric APC in the management of acid reflux is distinguishing between clinical manifestations of gastroesophageal reflux (GER) and gastroesophageal reflux disease (GERD) in infants, children, and adolescents and identifying who can be managed in a primary care setting and who requires referral to a gastroenterologist.

GERD is the most common esophageal disorder in children of all ages. With GER, there is movement of gastric contents back up through the lower esophageal sphincter (LES) into the esophagus. While GER is a common physiologic occurrence in all infants, this becomes pathologic GERD when infants and children have adverse symptoms from ongoing reflux, leading to esophagitis-related symptoms or extraesophageal presentations such as respiratory problems, nutritional deficits, and/or failure to thrive.

Table 6.4

Assessment and Management of Gastroesophageal Reflux and Gastroesophageal Reflux Disease

	Infants	Toddlers	Children/Adolescents
GER symptoms	**Infant reflux** becomes evident in the first few months of life, peaks at 4 months, and resolves in up to 88% by 12 months and in nearly all by 24 months. "**Happy spitters**" are infants who have recurrent regurgitation *without* exhibiting discomfort or refusal to eat and failure to gain weight.	A toddler may sometimes spit up after meals but demonstrates no negative effects from this (no weight loss).	Children and adolescents with GER may have some regurgitation after meals, especially large meals or meals with acidic foods; however, if this is a frequent occurrence or they are having negative consequences from the reflux (i.e., heartburn, vomiting, cough), this should be looked into further.
GERD signs and Symptoms	Feeding refusal Dystonic neck posturing/arching (Sandifer syndrome) Apnea spells Apparent life-threatening events Poor weight gain/failure to thrive Typical/atypical crying and/or irritability usually after feeding Wheezing, stridor Sleep disturbance	Toddlers with reflux typically cry after meals and show sleep disturbance Recurrent pneumonia Anemia Dental erosion Chronic cough Chronic nasal congestion Sore throat/laryngitis Significant dental problems (due to erosion of teeth from acid)	Heartburn Vomiting Regurgitation Halitosis Esophagitis Esophageal stricture Barrett esophagus Laryngeal/pharyngeal inflammation Recurrent pneumonia Anemia Dental erosion Chronic cough Chronic nasal congestion Dental problems
Key findings/key points	Immaturity of the lower esophageal sphincter function is manifested by frequent transient lower esophageal relaxations, which lead to the flow of gastric contents into the esophagus.	Symptoms tend to be after meals, similar to infants but often to a lesser degree.	Symptoms tend to be chronic, waxing, and waning, but completely resolving in no more than half of all cases.

(*continued*)

Chapter **6** Common Gastroenterologic Conditions Seen in Pediatric Primary Care

Table 6.4

Assessment and Management of Gastroesophageal Reflux and Gastroesophageal Reflux Disease (continued)

	Infants	Toddlers	Children/Adolescents
Lab tests/ diagnostics	**Esophageal pH and impedance monitoring:** Esophageal reflux can be quantified by monitoring esophageal pH (pH probe) and/or impedance (MII). Ideally, they should be measured on the same device and recorded for 24 hours. **However, these studies rarely are useful in evaluating GER or establishing the diagnosis of GERD in infants.** Esophageal pH monitoring can also be used to assess the adequacy of acid suppression therapy. **Radiographic studies:** While an upper GI series is not routine in the evaluation of GERD, it can be useful to rule out other organic causes of GERD especially if infants present with bilious vomiting or poor weight gain, an upper GI series may be helpful to identify anatomic abnormalities such as malrotation. **Pyloric ultrasonography:** Not routinely done in patients suspected of GERD; however, in infants with a history of projectile vomiting for the first few months. This test should be performed to rule out pyloric stenosis. **Endoscopic studies:** Upper endoscopy may be of diagnostic benefit in infants who have not responded to empiric clinical trials and/or those children who are suspected of having dietary protein intolerance that remains problematic despite dietary elimination. When endoscopy is performed, biopsies of the esophagus, stomach, or duodenum should be taken because they can reveal clinically significant diseases even when the gross appearance of the mucosa is normal.		
Differentials (should consider all differentials listed for all ages)	• Antral web • Eosinophilic esophagitis • *Helicobacter pylori*–associated gastritis • IBD • Peptic ulcer disease • Tracheoesophageal fistula • Food allergies	• Intestinal motility disorders, including achalasia, collagen–vascular disorders (e.g., systemic sclerosis) • Acute/chronic gastritis • Food allergies • Eosinophilic esophagitis • Esophageal motility disorders	Same as toddlers, and also consider the following: • *Helicobacter pylori* infection • Hiatal hernia • Intestinal malrotation • Pediatric duodenal atresia and stenosis surgery • Peptic ulcer disease
Treatment	Nonpharmacologic: - Providing small frequent feeds, often thickened with cereal - Upright positioning after feeding - Elevating head of bed - Prone positioning (infants >6 months)	Nonpharmacologic: - Diet that avoids tomato and citrus products, fruit juices, peppermint, chocolate, and caffeine-containing products - Smaller more frequent meals - Relatively lower fat diets (lips slow gastric emptying)	Nonpharmacologic: - Similar to toddler recommendations - Focus on proper eating habits - Avoidance of foods that exacerbate reflux

Mild or intermittent symptoms of GERD that do not respond to lifestyle changes:

H2 blockers:
Cimetidine:

Children:

30–40 mg/kg per day divided into four doses
Not to exceed adult dose of 400 mg twice daily

Famotidine:

Children:

1 mg/kg per day, divided into two doses
Not to exceed adult dose of 20 mg/dose twice daily

PPI:

If symptoms are recalcitrant to H2 blockers, PPI can be considered

Omeprazole:

Children ≥1 year:

1 mg/kg daily
May increase to 1 mg/kg twice daily if needed for symptomatic improvement
Not to exceed adult dosing of 20 mg once daily

Mild or intermittent symptoms of GERD that do not respond to lifestyle changes:

H2 blockers:
Cimetidine:

Children:

30–40 mg/kg per day divided into four doses
Not to exceed adult dose of 400 mg twice daily

Famotidine:

Children:

1 mg/kg per day, divided into two doses
Not to exceed adult dose of 20 mg/dose twice daily

PPI:

If symptoms are recalcitrant to H2 blockers, PPI can be considered

Omeprazole:

1 mg/kg daily
May increase to 1 mg/kg twice daily if needed for symptomatic improvement
Not to exceed adult dosing of 20 mg once daily

Pharmacotherapy is not indicated for infants with uncomplicated reflux.

In the event that an infant has esophagitis or failure to thrive due to reflux, PPIs may be indicated but should be used with caution.

Omeprazole:

3 kg to <5 kg: 2.5 mg once daily
5 kg to <10 kg: 5 mg once daily
10 kg to <20 kg: 10 mg once daily
≥20 kg: 20 mg once daily

Patient/family education

Recommendations to parents can include the following:

- Avoid giving your child foods that make symptoms worse (e.g., chocolate, peppermint, and fatty foods).
- Raise the head of your child's bed by 6–8 inches (e.g., by putting blocks of wood or rubber under two legs of the bed or a Styrofoam wedge under the mattress). Do **not** raise the head of an infant's crib or bed.
- Help your child to lose weight, if they are overweight (ask your child's doctor or nurse for advice on how to do this).
- Keep your child away from cigarette smoke.
- Have your child avoid lying down for a few hours after a meal (**Up to Date, 2019**).

GER, gastroesophageal reflux; GERD, gastroesophageal reflux disease; IBD, inflammatory bowel disease; MII, multichannel intraluminal impedance; PPIs, proton pump inhibitors.

Source: Up to Date. (2019). *Pediatric gastroenterology.* Retrieved from https://www.uptodate.com/contents/table-of-contents/pediatrics/pediatric-gastroenterology

- Remember the distinction between "physiologic" GER and "pathologic" GERD in infancy and childhood is determined not only by the number and severity of the reflux episodes (pH monitoring), but also by the presence of reflux-related complications (see Table 6.4).
- Neurologically challenged children are one group who are recognized to be at an increased risk for GERD. A low clinical threshold is important in the early identification and prompt treatment of GERD symptoms in these individuals.
- Acid suppression therapy early in life is associated with an increased risk of fracture in childhood, according to a retrospective study; the risk appeared to increase with duration of acid suppression therapy; providers should be more judicious in prescribing acid-suppressing medication (Medscape, 2019).
- **When to refer:** GERD should not be assumed to be the primary problem in infants and children present with a history of emesis. Emesis is associated with many disorders, and these should be ruled out if emesis is accompanied by other warning signs, including bilious or forceful vomiting (as in pyloric stenosis), hematemesis, vomiting and diarrhea, abdominal tenderness and distension, onset of vomiting after 6 months, fever and lethargy associated with vomiting, hepatosplenomegaly, and seizure disorder.

Treatment

Goals of medical therapy are to decrease acid secretion and reduce gastric emptying time.

Nonpharmacologic: See Table 6.4.

Pharmacologic management: This includes first-line antacids, commonly used in the school-age child, and over-the-counter (OTC) medications. Common antacids include aluminum hydroxide and magnesium hydroxide. In addition, first-line therapy consists of histamine H2 antagonists (e.g., nizatidine, cimetidine, ranitidine, famotidine). Proton pump inhibitors (PPIs) are seen in second-line therapy and are more effective in treating symptoms of GERD and include lansoprazole, omeprazole, esomeprazole, dexlansoprazole, rabeprazole sodium, pantoprazole.

Acid-suppressing medications have a limited role in treatment and are *not* valuable in treating children less than 1 year of age with uncomplicated GER.

When treating an infant with GERD, a trial of acid-suppressing medications should be prescribed for a 2-week period, and a scheduled follow-up exam should be established. In addition, when weaning a patient from a PPI (after approximately 6 months of prescribed therapy), try to switch to an H2 agonist for approximately 2 weeks and then wean the dose to avoid reflux rebound.

Surgical intervention such as fundoplication is required in only a very small minority of patients with GERD (when rigorous medical therapy has failed or when complications of GERD pose an increased risk of mortality [i.e., history of frequent aspiration pneumonias]). In a Nissen fundoplication, a portion of the upper stomach is wrapped around the lower esophagus to "tighten" the lower esophageal junction to limit reflux of contents back up into the esophagus.

EMESIS

■ GASTROENTERITIS (SEE ALSO "GASTROENTERITIS" UNDER THE "DIARRHEA" SECTION)

When a child is vomiting with or without diarrhea, parents will often call the clinic asking if they should bring their child in to be seen by a medical provider. It is important to discern if a patient requires medical treatment in an office setting or can be managed at home. Indications for a medical visit would include (Matson & O'Ryan, 2019, p. 8) the following:

- The patient is an infant (< 6 months) or has weight <8 kg
- A temperature of ≥38°C (100.4°F) for infants or of ≥39°C (102.2°F) for children 3 months to 36 months
- Visible blood in stool (melena)
- Frequent and substantial volumes of diarrhea
- Persistent vomiting or diarrhea for greater than 7 days
- Multisystem compromise, cardiovascular instability (refer directly to ED)
- Inability of the caregiver to administer, or failure of the child to tolerate or respond to, oral rehydration therapy at home
- Underlying immunodeficiency or condition complicating the treatment or course of illness (i.e., metabolic disease, diabetes mellitus)
- Caregiver's report of moderate to severe dehydration

■ PYLORIC STENOSIS

Infantile hypertrophic pyloric stenosis (IHPS) is a disorder of young infants caused by hypertrophy of the pylorus, which can progress to near-complete obstruction of the gastric outlet, leading to forceful vomiting.

Etiology

Multifactorial but can involve genetic predisposition and environmental factors.

Epidemiology/Risk Factors

IHPS occurs in approximately 2 to 3.5 per 1,000 live births and is more common in males than females (Benninga et al., 2016). This is more common in firstborn children (30%–40%), usually presents around 3 to 5 weeks of age, and is rare after 12 weeks of age. Moreover, prematurity may be a risk factor. One study showed that macrolide antibiotics (both erythromycin and azithromycin) are associated with increased risk of IHPS, particularly when administered to infants younger than 2 weeks of age (Eberly, Eide, Thompson, & Nylund, 2015).

Symptoms

The classic presentation of pyloric stenosis is postprandial vomiting that is nonbilious and forceful (often described as "projectile" vomiting). The infant is often described as a "hungry vomiter," as they want to eat soon after vomiting. In premature infants, vomiting may be less forceful.

Focused PE Signs/Key Findings

Palpable "olive-shaped" mass at the lateral edge of the right upper quadrant (RUQ) of the abdomen. Patients were also described as being dehydrated (from repeated vomiting after feedings).

In addition, the history of vomiting in pyloric stenosis is typically forceful and non-bilious and tends to occur immediately after feeding compared with GERD, in which most episodes of vomiting are not forceful and may occur 10 minutes or more after a feeding.

The abdomen should also be evaluated for distension and bowel sounds. Abdominal distention or high-pitched bowel sounds suggest intestinal obstruction versus pyloric stenosis.

Lab Tests/Diagnostics

Patients with symptoms consistent with pyloric stenosis often have normal labs; however, in patients with prolonged vomiting, labs will show a hypochloremic, metabolic alkalosis due to the loss of large amounts of gastric acid. In addition, labs including prolonged vomiting indicate that the infant is at risk for hypokalemia as well. In addition, blood urea nitrogen and creatinine should be obtained to assess for dehydration and renal insufficiency. If obstruction is suspected, abdominal radiographs should be obtained. If pyloric stenosis is suspected, US is the procedure of choice for infants with a typical presentation.

Differentials

Malrotation, volvulus, or Hirschsprung's disease (HD) and other intestinal obstructions should be ruled out. GERD should also be ruled out. It is also important to consider cow's milk protein intolerance, adrenal crisis, and liver disease.

Don't Miss

The hypertrophied "olive" or pylorus can be palpated in up to 90% of cases.

Treatment

Surgical correction of the hypertrophied pylorus with a pyloromyotomy.

Follow-Up/Patient/Family Education

Mild regurgitation is common after a pyloromyotomy; however, this should not delay the initiation of feeding.

INFLAMMATORY BOWEL DISEASE

IBD is mainly comprised of two disorders: ulcerative colitis (UC) and Crohn's disease (CD). While some patients with IBD may present with nonspecific GI symptoms, making it difficult to distinguish between other GI disorders, the most common indicators of possible IBD in a child with abdominal pain are diarrhea, growth failure, pubertal delay, weight loss, rectal bleeding, pallor/fatigue, perianal skin tags (which can often be misdiagnosed as hemorrhoids), perianal fistulae or abscesses, a palpable abdominal mass, and a family history of IBD (Higuchi & Bousvaros, 2019; Table 6.5).

Table 6.5

Clinical Presentation and Differences Between Crohn Disease and Ulcerative Colitis

Type of IBD	CD	UC
	• Can involve any component of the GI tract from the oral cavity to the anus and is characterized by transmural inflammation	• Affects the colon and is inflammation of the mucosal layer
Epidemiology	20% of patients with CD present before the age of 20 years.	12% of patients with UC present before the age of 20 years.
Etiology/risk factors	IBD prevalence of 100–200/100,000 children in the United States.	
Symptoms	In addition, children with IBD often present with unique clinical features, including growth failure and delayed puberty.	
Focused PE signs/key findings	GI symptoms for IBD include loose stools or bloody diarrhea, abdominal pain, or tenesmus.	
	Growth: Growth failure (subnormal gains in height, weight, or weight loss) and/or delayed puberty.	
	PE: abdominal tenderness and/or mass (especially in the RLQ).	
	Extraintestinal manifestations include oral ulcerations (aphthous stomatitis), clubbing, rash (erythema nodosum or pyoderma gangrenous), eye inflammation (uveitis), jaundice, hepatomegaly, or arthritis. Other systemic symptoms can include fever and fatigue during flares of disease.	
Clinical features:		
Hematochezia	Common	Less common
Passage of mucus or puss	Rare	Common
Affects upper GI tract	Yes	No
Extraintestinal manifestations	Common	Common
Small bowel obstruction	Common	Rare
Fistulas and perianal disease	Common	No
Lab tests/diagnostics	Lab studies, radiographic studies, and endoscopy, including biopsies.	

(continued)

Chapter **6** Common Gastroenterologic Conditions Seen in Pediatric Primary Care

Table 6.5

Clinical Presentation and Differences Between Crohn Disease and Ulcerative Colitis (*continued*)

Differentials	Initial evaluation should include a comprehensive history and PE, including a family history. Establish extent of disease, disease activity. Consider/exclude infections such as giardia, CMV, Clostridium difficile, TB, HIV, and so on. If IBD is suspected based on initial evaluation, refer to GI specialist to establish IBD-like pathology by upper and lower GI endoscopy.
Don't Miss/Key Points:	
Treatment	Treat the underlying disease and its complications which usually includes drug therapy. Anti-inflammatory drugs are often the first step in the treatment of inflammatory bowel disease. They include corticosteroids such as prednisone and budesonide (Entocort EC), which can help reduce inflammation in your body. Biologics (such as infliximab and Humira) are often used when treatment escalates due to disease progression (i.e., worsening symptoms) **Biologics** Types of biologics used to treat CD include the following: • **Infliximab (Remicade), adalimumab (Humira), and golimumab (Simponi):** These drugs are called TNF inhibitors and work by neutralizing a protein produced by your immune system.	Treatment usually includes drug therapy and/or surgery. Therapy with 5-ASA is often the first step in the treatment of UC. Examples of this type of medication include sulfasalazine (Azulfidine), mesalamine (Asacol HD, Delzicol, others), balsalazide (Colazal), and olsalazine (Dipentum). Which one you should take and whether it is taken by mouth or as an enema or suppository depends on the area of your colon that is affected. Corticosteroids These drugs, which include prednisone and budesonide (Uceris), are generally reserved for moderate to severe UC. Due to the side effects, they are not usually given long term. Immunomodulator drugs These drugs also reduce inflammation, but they do so by suppressing the immune system response that starts the process of inflammation. Examples include the following: • **Azathioprine (Azasan, Imuran) and mercaptopurine (Purinethol, Purixan):** Taking these medications requires that you follow up closely with your doctor and have your blood checked regularly to look for side effects, including effects on the liver.

- **Cyclosporine (Gengraf, Neoral, Sandimmune):** This drug may be used for people who have not responded well to other medications and is not for long-term use.
- **Tofacitinib (Xeljanz):** This drug has recently been approved for treatment of conditions such as UC, rheumatoid arthritis, or psoriatic arthritis.

Biologics

Types of biologics used to treat UC include the following:

- **Infliximab (Remicade), adalimumab (Humira), and golimumab (Simponi):** These drugs are called TNF inhibitors and work by neutralizing a protein produced by your immune system.
- **Vedolizumab (Entyvio):** This gut-specific medication works by blocking inflammatory cells from getting to the site of inflammation.

Surgery can often eliminate UC. But that usually means removing your entire colon and rectum (proctocolectomy).

| Follow-up/patient/family education | Will be followed by a GI specialist. Important to monitor linear growth, skeletal development, and puberty |

5-ASA, 5-aminosalicylic acid; CD, Crohn's disease; CMV, cytomegalovirus; GI, gastrointestinal; IBD, inflammatory bowel disease; PE, physical exam; RLQ, right lower quadrant; TB, tuberculosis; TNF, tumor necrosis factor; UC, ulcerative colitis.

Chapter **6** Common Gastroenterologic Conditions Seen in Pediatric Primary Care

References

Benninga, M. A., Faure, C., Hyman, P. E., St. James, R., Schechter, N. L., & Nurko, S. (2016). Childhood functional gastrointestinal disorders: Neonate/Toddler. *Gastroenterology.* doi:10.1053/j.gastro.2016.02.016

Eberly, M. D., Eide, M. B., Thompson, J. L., & Nylund, C. M. (2015). Azithromycin in early infancy and pyloric stenosis. *Pediatrics, 135*(3), 483–488. doi:10.1542/peds.2014-2026

Higuchi, L. M., & Bousvaros, A. (2019). Clinical presentation and diagnosis of inflammatory bowel disease in children. *UpToDate.* Retrieved from https://www.uptodate.com/contents/clinical-presentation-and-diagnosis-of-inflammatory-bowel-disease-in-children

Kwon, H., Lee, J. H., Jeong, J. H., Yang, H. R., Kwak, Y. H., Kim, D. K., & Kim, K. (2019). A practice guideline for postreduction management of intussusception of children in the emergency department. *Pediatric Emergency Care, 35,* 533–538. doi:10.1097/PEC.0000000000001056

Lloyd, D. A., & Kenny, S. E. (2004). The surgical abdomen. In W. A. Walker, O. Goulet, & R. E. Kleinman (Eds.), *Pediatric gastrointestinal disease: Pathopsychology, diagnosis, management* (4th ed., p. 604). Hamilton, ON: BC Decker.

Matson, D. O., & O'Ryan, M. G. (2019). *Acute viral gastroenteritis in children in resource rich countries: Clinical features and diagnosis.* Retrieved from https://www.uptodate.com/contents/acute-viral-gastroenteritis-in-children-in-resource-rich-countries-clinical-features-and-diagnosis

Medscape. (2019). *Increased fracture risk in kids given early acid suppression therapy.* Retrieved from https://www.medscape.com

Pollock, B. H., Krischer, J. P., & Vietti, T. J. (1991). Interval between symptom onset and diagnosis of pediatric solid tumors. *Journal of Pediatrics, 119*(5), 725–732. doi:10.1016/s0022-3476(05)80287-2

Robin, S. G., Keller, C., Zwiener, R., Hyman, P. E., Nurko, S., Saps, M., . . . Van Tilburg, M. A. (2018). Prevalence of pediatric functional gastrointestinal disorders utilizing the Rome IV criteria. *Journal of Pediatrics, 195,* 134–139. doi:10.1016/j.jpeds.2017.12.012

Shalaby, M. S., Kuti, K., & Walker, G. (2013). Intestinal malrotation and volvulus in infants and children. *BMJ, 347,* f6949. doi:10.1136/bmj.f6949

Up to Date. (2019). *Pediatric gastroenterology.* Retrieved from https://www.uptodate.com/contents/table-of-contents/pediatrics/pediatric-gastroenterology

7

Common Neurologic Complaints Seen in Pediatric Primary Care

Michael S. Ruggiero

INTRODUCTION

Neurologic complaints in children are common; fortunately, the clear majority are not life-threatening, but clinicians need to know how to distinguish between those that are emergent and those that can be managed on an ambulatory outpatient basis. Most parents who bring their child to primary care want reassurance that the child's headaches are not cause for serious concern.

Despite most headaches being non–life-threatening, neurologic issues can have a significant impact on quality of life. The goal of this chapter is to review some of the more common neurologic complaints in children including headaches, dizziness, and concussions/head trauma.

OBJECTIVES

1. Identify common headaches that present in children.
2. List the most common cause of severe headache in children.
3. Describe what tests/neuroimaging must be performed prior to lumbar puncture (LP) in any patient who has a headache.
4. Understand the intervention and treatment for pediatric primary headaches.
5. Identify pediatric patients with headache who require emergent medical intervention.
6. Understand the workup and intervention for infectious causes of secondary headache in children including encephalitis.

HEADACHE

Headache is a common complaint in children and is responsible for an abundance of referrals to pediatric neurology departments; this complaint increases even more during the adolescent years.

Epidemiology

The prevalence of headaches is common in children with some study projections as high as 82% by age 15 (Merikangas, Kalaydjian, Khoromi, Knight, & Nelson, 2009). In addition, chronic or recurrent headaches occur in approximately 40% of children by 7 years of age. Most parents who seek help for a child who has headaches are looking for reassurance that the headache is not due to a serious cause. Boys are more frequently affected before puberty, and girls are more commonly affected after puberty. Headaches are a major cause of lost school and workdays and affects health-related quality of life in pediatric patients.

There are two main classifications of headaches: primary headaches and secondary headaches.

Primary headaches are commonly thought of as non–life-threatening, benign headaches that are not caused by an underlying illness, disease process, or structural abnormality. The three most common primary headaches are migraine, cluster, and tension. Despite their benign nature, primary headaches are the most common form of headache-related disability.

Secondary headaches are caused by an underlying illness, disease process, or structural abnormality such as infection, tumor, intracranial hemorrhage, or a vascular disorder. Most headaches in children are primary headaches or harmless secondary headaches, although less common secondary headaches are essential to identify when present as they can often be life-threatening or have long-term sequelae associated with them.

PRIMARY HEADACHES

■ CLUSTER HEADACHES

Etiology

Cluster headaches are the most common form of a group of headaches called trigeminal autonomic cephalalgias. Cluster headaches are the least common form of the primary headaches but are important to review as they are a source of severe pain and disability. Frequency of attacks can vary dramatically ranging from one every 2 days to eight in a day

Cluster headaches are more frequent among boys and men. Headaches tend to be short-lived but can vary in time between 15 minutes to 3 hours. The headache is described as unilateral involving with either the orbital, periorbital, or temporal region. These headaches are severe in nature.

Focused PE Findings

Examination will reveal a restless patient with autonomic findings that may include ipsilateral conjunctival injection, excessive lacrimation, swelling to the ipsilateral eyelid, pupil constriction, ptosis, and/or rhinorrhea/nasal congestion. There are not any findings during periods of remission or in between attacks.

The attacks are "clustered" in bouts lasting for weeks to months. There are two forms of cluster headaches: episodic and chronic. Episodic headaches are described as lasting from 7 days to 1 year, separated by pain-free periods lasting at least 3 months. Chronic cluster headaches are attacks that occur for more than 1 year without a remission period or a remission period that is less than 3 months.

Treatment/Prevention

Treatment is largely aimed at stopping the acute headache (see Box 7.1). Prophylaxis and prevention are more difficult given the unpredictable nature of cluster attacks. Abortive treatment is achieved with high flow 100% oxygen with a rebreather mask. Sumatriptan nasal spray has been shown to be effective but is not currently recommended by the manufacturer for pediatric use and would be off-label use. Corticosteroids, such as prednisone, have been a long-standing intervention for adults with cluster headaches, but research in children for cluster headaches is lacking. In adults, corticosteroids have been shown to be effective as an abortive treatment as well as prophylactic while waiting for some of the other preventive medications to be titrated up to effective doses.

Preventative medications such as verapamil 3 to 8 mg/kg/day in divided dosage q 8 hours and topiramate starting at 25 mg and titrating up over 4 weeks are commonly used in adults as effective preventative medications; however, the safety has not been established in children under 12 years old, despite being cited as preventative therapies in many texts. If verapamil is used in children as a preventative agent, cardiac exam and EKG need to be routinely monitored to detect atrioventricular block/PR interval prolongation.

■ MIGRAINE

Migraine headaches are the most common form of headache in children. Migraine headaches can be described as either migraine with aura or without aura.

- *Migraines without aura* are common signs and symptoms that are common of pediatric migraines. Migraine headaches last between 30 minutes and 72 hours with severity that is described as moderate to severe and tend to be aggravated by physical activity. The headache in children is most commonly frontotemporal and can be unilateral or bilateral. The headache is accompanied by nausea, vomiting, or photophobia.
- *Migraine with aura* has the aforementioned common symptoms and also include an aura for 5 to 60 minutes. The aura typically precedes the headache. An aura can be described as flashes, wavy, or squiggly lines that affect unilateral visual fields. This aura can be perceived with eye open or closed. This symptom is termed scintillating scotoma. It is important to note that this visual disturbance is completely reversible normally within an hour of onset, and prolonged continued visual changes should raise suspicion for another cause of headache and visual disturbance. Also common in migraine with aura is speech disturbance such as loss of speech precision and slowed speech.

Examination: The physical exam is normal except for the patient, who is visibly distressed or vomiting. There are no focal neurologic findings.

Triggers: There have been some well-documented triggers for migraine headaches: physical and emotional stress, sleep deprivation, chocolate, caffeine, monosodium glutamate, fragrances, and dehydration.

Workup for migraine: See under PE Workup for Primary Headaches.

Treatment: Treatment for primary headache consists of supportive and pharmacological intervention.

Sleep and rest in a quiet dark or dimly lit room with cool compress on the child's forehead is recommended.

BOX 7.1 FIRST-LINE PHARMACOLOGIC TREATMENT FOR PEDIATRIC HEADACHE

First-line OTC analgesics such as ibuprofen and/or acetaminophen.

Ibuprofen 10 mg/kg per dose repeated every 6 hours.

Acetaminophen 15 mg/kg/dose; not to exceed 1000 mg. Repeat as needed in 4 hours intervals with no more than three doses in 24 hours.

OTC, over the counter.

For patients with recurrent attacks, severe headache symptoms, or symptoms not improved by over-the-counter (OTC) analgesics, the second-line therapy includes the class of medications called triptans can be used in patients above the age of 5 years.

- Triptans come in several formulations, which is helpful for children who cannot swallow pills or if they are experiencing nausea and vomiting.
- Triptans come in tablets, dissolving tablets, and nasal spray depending on the manufacturers.
- Commonly use triptans for pediatric migraines are sumatriptan, rizatriptan, and zolmitriptan.

Treatment for the accompanying nausea and vomiting can be achieved with promethazine provided the children are 2 years or older. Oral dosing is fine for children who can take pills and for whom their vomiting does not interfere with taking the medication; otherwise, promethazine also comes in a rectal suppository.

Promethazine 0.25 to 0.5 mg/kg as needed at intervals of 4 to 6 hours.

When to Refer

- Patients with intractable migraine or status migrainosus (migraine longer than 72 hours) should be referred to the emergency department for management and possible admission.
- IV fluids, analgesics, and ergotamine (dihydroergotamine) treatment is usually successful in controlling the symptoms in the emergency department or inpatient ward.
- Any headache with neurologic findings should prompt immediate referral to an emergency medical center with imaging.
- Recurrent or chronic migraine, greater than 15 days of migraine per month, or ineffective treatment during attacks, warrants a neurologic consult.

Patient Education

Patients and/or parents/guardians should be encouraged to keep a migraine diary to help elicit more information of possible triggers and to establish days per month of migraine. This information can help in forming a prevention plan. Use of analgesics or triptans can lead to medication overuse headache. Using medication such as ibuprofen or acetaminophen for more than 14 days per month or triptans greater than 8 days a month has been associated with medication overuse headache. Chronic migraine that presents for more than 14 days per month would warrant a consult with a neurologist.

■ TENSION-TYPE HEADACHE/TENSION HEADACHE

Tension headaches are a common cause of headache in children and adolescents; unlike migraine headaches, the less prescriptive diagnostic criteria make true occurrence a little more difficult to estimate. Like migraine headaches, however, tension headaches are more prevalent as children age into adolescents and are a cause of disability in children. Tension headaches come in three separate subtypes (Do, Heldarskard, Kolding, Hvedstrup, & Schytz, 2018): Infrequent, which is less than one episode per month; frequent episodic, which is defined by one to 14 headaches per month; and chronic, which is 15 or more headaches per month.

Tension headaches are described as lasting from 30 minutes to 7 days. The typical presentation is a bilateral headache characterized as nonpulsating pressure or tightening sensation that is quantified as mild to moderate in severity. The headache is not made worse by physical activity. There is no nausea or vomiting associated with tension headaches. They can, in certain instances, have photophobia or phonophobia, but not both.

BOX 7.2 TREATMENT AND MANAGEMENT OF TENSION HEADACHES IN THE PEDIATRIC PATIENT

Acute management focuses on the appropriate use of OTC analgesics.

Ibuprofen 10 mg/kg per dose repeated every 6 hours.

Acetaminophen 15 mg/kg/dose; not to exceed 1000 mg. Repeat as needed in 4 hours intervals with no more than three doses in 24 hours.

For recurrent/episodic and chronic tension-type headache, there have been some studies that support the use of tricyclic antidepressants such as low-dose amitriptyline or nortriptyline.

Lifestyle modifications such as good sleep hygiene, physical activity, and balanced diet have also been recommended.

OTC, over the counter.

The diagnosis of tension headache is often given to headaches that do not entirely fulfill the required diagnostic criteria of migraine headaches.

Tension headaches do not have focal neurological findings, and the exam is benign but may reveal some myofascial trigger points upon palpation, specifically along the temporalis, suboccipital, sternocleidomastoid, and upper trapezius musculature.

■ PE WORKUP FOR PRIMARY HEADACHES

Seldom is workup necessary for primary headaches especially if they are of a recurrent or episodic nature and have persisted for more than 6 months. Any of the following would warrant neuroimaging and should have you reconsider a diagnosis of primary headache pattern: new onset of headache that is moderate or severe, headache in a child with preexisting neurologic anomaly or shunt, worst headache, associated focal neurological findings, signs or symptoms of increased intracranial pressure (ICP), associated seizure, altered mental status, or change in personality.

SECONDARY HEADACHES

Secondary headaches are most frequently caused by underlying illness. The most common causes are upper respiratory infections, sinus infections, and strep pharyngitis. A mild-to-moderate headache in conjunction with symptoms of a febrile upper respiratory infection, sinusitis, or pharyngitis tends to be a benign symptom of a self-limiting condition. There are, however, several types of secondary headaches that are life-threatening and require prompt identification.

■ ENCEPHALITIS

Etiology

Encephalitis results from inflammation of the brain parenchyma and may be caused by infections or autoimmune conditions, with viruses being the most common etiology.

Epidemiology

Encephalitis results in considerable morbidity and mortality. Its causes are like those of meningitis but involve the brain parenchyma as opposed to the meninges. Management of encephalitis, which can be fatal, requires understanding of a broad range of causative agents, pathophysiologic mechanisms, clinical syndromes, and outcomes.

Focused PE Findings

The signs and symptoms of encephalitis has commonality with meningitis such as headache and fever; however, it classically presents with altered mental status, behavior, and personality change and frequently includes difficulty with speech, ataxia, and seizure.

Workup

The workup of encephalitis is similar to that of meningitis. All cases of suspected encephalitis should undergo neuroimaging. Neuroimaging with MRI is preferred over CT scan if available and if the patient is stable enough for an MRI. Imaging should occur prior to LP.

LP is a critical part of the workup, but signs and symptoms of increased ICP need to be assessed prior to LP to help prevent cerebral herniation.

LP is used to assess the CSF for signs consistent with viral or bacterial infection and to isolate a pathogen. LP should be performed before the first dose of antibiotics.

CSF samples should be sent for analysis, gram stain, cultures, and viral studies that include enterovirus, HSV, arbovirus (arthropod-borne virus, i.e., West Nile virus, eastern equine encephalitis [EEE] virus, western equine encephalitis [WEE] virus, St. Louis encephalitis virus, etc.), and if clinically suspected, Rickettsiales. The CSF analysis is usually the quickest in turnaround giving information on distinguishing features of viral and bacterial infections (see Table 7.1).

Electroencephalography (EEG) should be performed as soon as feasible in patients who are suspected of having encephalitis.

Treatment

Children who are evaluated in the ambulatory setting and are suspected of having encephalitis need to be emergently transferred to an emergency medical center and preferably one with a pediatric ICU.

Treatment should be targeted at the causative pathogen that is isolated. However, treatment should not be delayed while waiting for results. Empiric treatment is typically aimed at covering likely bacterial and viral pathogens. Ceftriaxone and vancomycin plus acyclovir are most commonly used while awaiting cultures and lab results. If increased ICP or cerebral edema is suspected, then mannitol can be administered to help reduce ICP. Seizure related to the encephalitis can be treated with first-line medications lorazepam or midazolam.

Follow-Up

Children with encephalitis have a high incidence of long-term sequelae including learning difficulties, behavioral problems, hearing impairment, and motor deficits. Long-term follow-up is necessary for evaluation of the aforementioned sequelae. Developmental surveillance should continue throughout childhood, which may include neuropsychological testing

Don't Miss

Any patient who presents with severe headache, worst headache of their life, moderate-to-severe first headache, focal neurological findings, associated symptoms suggestive of increased ICP, seizure, significant trauma, altered mental status, or headache in the setting of preexisting structural neurological abnormality including shunts should be transferred to an emergency medical center.

■ MENINGITIS

Meningitis is an inflammatory process involving the meninges. Meningitis is caused most commonly by viruses and less frequently by bacteria.

Epidemiology

Viral meningitis has two peaks in children: first are neonates and second are children over 5 years old. Viral meningitis has its peaks in the fall and summer. The most common pathogens responsible for viral meningitis are enterovirus and to a lesser degree herpes simplex virus (HSV). Bacterial meningitis is most commonly caused by *Neisseria meningitides* and *Streptococcus pneumonia*.

Presentation

Viral and bacterial meningitis are similar and typically present with headache that is accompanied by fever, nausea, vomiting, stiff neck, and photophobia.

Examination is usually significant for fever, nuchal rigidity, and meningeal irritation as is seen in Brudzinski's and Kernig's signs. Petechial rash is also extremely common in patients presenting with *N. meningitides*. Newborns may present with fever, fussiness, and bulging fontanels.

Workup

Workup for meningitis is required to distinguish between the more benign viral meningitis and the life-threatening bacterial meningitis. The diagnostic test of choice for meningitis is an LP. Because of this, any patient who presents to an outpatient ambulatory practice with suspicion of meningitis should be transferred to an emergency medical center. Prompt LP and evaluation of cerebrospinal fluid (CSF) are required for a definitive diagnosis. However, due to the risk of cerebra herniation from increased ICP, a CT scan is often required prior to an LP. Some findings suggestive of increased risk of cerebral herniation from LP can be seen in Box 7.3.

LP is used to assess the CSF for signs consistent with viral or bacterial meningitis and to isolate a pathogen. LP should be performed before the first dose of antibiotics.

CSF samples should be sent for analysis, gram stain, cultures, and viral studies which include enterovirus, HSV, arbovirus (arthropod-borne virus, i.e., West Nile virus, eastern equine encephalitis [EEE] virus, western equine encephalitis [WEE] virus, St. Louis encephalitis virus, etc.). The CSF analysis is usually the quickest turnaround giving information on typical distinguishing features of viral and bacterial meningitis (see Table 7.1).

Serologic testing is used to rule in or out some of the specific causes of meningitis and is essential in guiding treatment, especially when empiric treatment is ineffective or if there is suspicion for some of the less common causes of meningitis.

BOX 7.3   INCREASED RISK OF CEREBRAL HERNIATION FROM LUMBAR PUNCTURE

Focal neurologic deficit
Papilledema
Seizure
Altered mental status
Immunocompromised
Respiratory compromise (tachypnea or depression)

Any history of neurosurgery
History or suspicion of space occupying lesion
Cerebrospinal fluid shunt
Signs or symptoms of meningeal infection

Table 7.1

CSF Analysis: Comparison of Viral and Bacterial Meningitis/Encephalitis		
	Viral	**Bacterial**
Appearance	Clear	Turbid
White blood cells	Less than 300 cells/mcg	Greater than 1,000 cells/mcg
Protein	Less than 200 mg/dl	Greater than 200 mg/dl
Glucose	Normal	Low

Some of the more common atypical causes on the differential are HSV, Lyme disease, syphilis, cytomegalovirus, Epstein–Barr, varicella measles, and mumps.

Treatment

- Treatment should not be withheld until cultures are back. If bacterial meningitis is suspected or cannot be ruled out, then IV ceftriaxone +/– vancomycin is the recommended treatment to cover bacterial meningitis and supportive care of IV hydration, cardiac, and respiratory monitoring.
- If HSV is high on the differential, IV acyclovir is also recommended.
- Treatment should be tailored to the offending organism once gram staining and cultures return.
- Viral meningitis is typically treated with supportive care such as IV hydration, fever, and pain management with acetaminophen.

Prognosis

Bacterial meningitis in the pediatric patient carries with it a 5% to 10% mortality rate and moderate rate of morbidity of which hearing loss is the most frequently encountered sequela (Mount & Boyle, 2017). Viral meningitis tends to resolve without any long-term sequelae or morbidity.

HEAD TRAUMA

Head trauma in children is a common injury and is responsible for an estimated 2 million medical visits per year. While most head trauma is mild and requires no intervention, the frequency of head trauma is great enough that there are real numbers of patients who require workup and intervention. This section will review intracranial hemorrhage and concussions.

Etiology

Most common injuries are due to sports injuries, bicycle accidents, falls, and motor vehicle accidents. Head injuries are more common in boys than girls.

Etiology tends to differ according to age of the patient. Adolescents sustain most head injuries in motor vehicle accidents, along with sports-related concussions and assaults. Preadolescents are getting more sports-related head trauma but more often as a pedestrian or while riding a bicycle.

Those under the age of 5 years are more prone to falls. Infants with head trauma need to be evaluated for abuse, as this is a particularly vulnerable group to abusive head trauma.

Concussion

Concussion is a disturbance of neurologic function and mental state resulting from trauma, occurring with or without actual loss of consciousness. Symptoms of concussion are typically self-limited, and concussion lacks any verifiable brain injury via neuroimaging. Concussion in children is most commonly seen in sports-related injury.

Epidemiology

There are an estimated 1.5 million concussions per year in child athletes. From 2007 to 2014, there was a 60% increase in concussion incidence, with a 143% increase in 10- to 14-year-olds and an 87% increase in 15- to 19-year-olds. Activities include but are not limited to football, soccer, wrestling, bicycling, hockey, lacrosse, field hockey, basketball, and playground injuries (Echemendia, 2017).

Clinical Presentation

Focused PE Signs

Symptoms of concussion have been well documented and have been increasingly studied over recent years given the millions of sports-related childhood concussions. Symptoms consist of headache, confusion or amnesia (ante- or retrograde), nausea or vomiting, and dizziness. Despite some older classifications requiring a loss of consciousness to diagnose concussion, this is no longer the case, and recent studies demonstrate that most concussions in children do not involve loss of consciousness.

There have been several tools over the years to help in the diagnosis of childhood concussion of which the most widely accepted has been one developed for sports-related concussions; the Sport Concussion Assessment Tool (SCAT5) and the Child-SCAT5 (Davis, Purcell, & Schneider, 2017) for children aged 5 to 12 years. The tool is a step-by-step approach to the evaluation of the child and includes "red flag" warnings that should prompt providers to transfer patients for emergency medical evaluation and neuroimaging.

These red flags are a combination of concern for cervical spine injury and increased ICP, severe or progressive headache, loss of consciousness, deteriorating conscious state, vomiting, double vision, seizure, neck pain, weakness, or paresthesia in arms or legs (Echemendia, 2017).

Management

- Signs and symptoms of concussion are self-limiting in most cases.
- Management of pediatric concussions is focused on symptom control and protecting the child from activities that may hinder their recovery.
- Cognitive, physical, and emotional rest is the recommendation.
- Patients must be instructed to avoid all activities that would place them at risk for additional head trauma during their recovery to avoid second impact syndrome.
- Light activity is encouraged, while taking caution to stay below their cognitive and physical symptom-exacerbation threshold. Rest for more than a few days may not hasten recovery and may lead to prolonged symptoms. Symptoms may be followed with a postconcussion symptom scale, with attention paid to the possible differentiation of clinical symptoms into separate clusters such as somatic/headache, cognitive, affective, cervical, vestibular, and/or oculomotor, which may assist in developing targeted rehabilitation.
- Concussed patients will often complain of increased symptoms with cognitive activities such as reading, video games, music, and texting. They often have difficulty attending school, focusing on schoolwork, and trying to keep up

with assignments. Initially, cognitive rest may include shortened school days, reduced workload, or even temporary leave of absence with gradual return to school.

- Medication may be considered in those with prolonged recovery and specific symptoms; however, there is no evidence-based pharmacologic treatment for a concussed athlete.
- Vestibular therapy consisting of balance and oculomotor exercises has shown results in combating dizziness and vertigo; an active rehabilitation program may facilitate recovery.
- On average children and adolescents require 2 to 4 weeks for a full recovery from a concussion, and this should be explained to the patient, parents, and stakeholders.
- While most patients will recover without incident, a small percentage of patients will develop persistent postconcussive symptoms such as headache, agitation, concentration difficulties, vestibular symptoms, and insomnia. Postconcussive symptoms or syndrome is when common concussive symptoms last more than 1 month. These patients should be referred to neurology for further evaluation and management of symptoms. Children who have protracted symptoms may also require interim adjustments at school or 504 accommodations.
- Any patient who presents with symptoms of intracranial bleed should be transferred to an emergency medical center for emergent neuroimaging and management.

BOX 7.4 SAMPLE OF CONSIDERATIONS FOR THE PEDIATRIC APC WHEN WRITING UP A POSTCONCUSSIVE RETURN TO SCHOOL MANAGEMENT PLAN

Management has been focused on activity modification and a gradual stepwise approach back to baseline cognitive and physical activity. An individualized plan should be developed by the pediatric APC for a return-to-school and return-to-athletics.

Rest should be encouraged for 1 to 2 days following the trauma and then implementing slow progression of cognitive and physical activity. Slow progression of school-like activities can begin after this period of rest and tends to involve activities of daily living, reading, and some homework, and if the child tolerates this, then returning to school for a half day and then progressing to a full day is a sound recommendation.

There is no conclusive evidence that medication hastens recovery.

Pharmacotherapy can be used for supportive or symptom control.
Children who are experiencing headache can usually be treated successfully with OTC acetaminophen or ibuprofen.
Ibuprofen 10mg/kg per dose repeated every 6 hours.
Acetaminophen 15mg/kg/dose; not to exceed 1000 mg. Repeat as needed in 4 hours intervals with no more than three doses in 24 hours.

Children and adolescents who are experiencing some vestibular symptoms such as vertigo and nausea may benefit from antihistamines such as diphenhydramine—oral: 5 mg/kg/day divided into three to four doses; usual dosing is 12.5 to 25 mg/dose (maximum daily dose: 300 mg/day). For children 12 years or older, oral: 25 to 100 mg/day in three or four divided doses. Caution should be used with analgesics as there is well-documented evidence that analgesia overuse is a common contributor to posttraumatic headache (Evan, 2017).

APC, advanced practicing clinician; OTC, over-the-counter.
Source: Evan, R. (2017). Sequelae of mild traumatic brain injury. In J. Wilterdink (Ed.), UptoDate. Retrieved from https://www-uptodate-com.treadwell.idm.oclc.org/contents/sequelae-of-mild-traumatic-brain-injury

Don't Miss

Return to Sports

Children should not begin a progression for athletic activity until they are able to return to school activity and remain asymptomatic. Once they have returned to school without restriction, they can begin a graduated return to sport. The graduated return to sport guidelines progress from light aerobic exercise to sports-specific exercise (with no risk of head impact), sports-specific drill and resistance training that are both non-contact and then a return-to-normal training activities with final step being return to competition. It should be noted that each step in the progress to play model is a minimum of 24 hours, and any symptoms would lead to a regression to the previous stage of asymptomatic activity.

Patient/Family Education

Observation should be for at least 24 hours. Signs and symptoms to be watched for include deteriorating mental status, seizures, focal neurologic signs, and worsening headache, nausea, or vomiting. Posthead injury instructions should be verbally explained to the caregiver, who should also be provided with written instructions and a means of returning to medical care should deterioration occur.

Don't Miss

Second impact syndrome is a devasting process that occurs when a concussion patient sustains a second head injury while recovering from a concussion, causing diffuse cerebral swelling, brain herniation, and high incidence of death.

■ INTRACRANIAL HEMORRHAGE

Etiology

Intracranial hemorrhage is bleeding with the skull. Most common reason for intracranial bleeds in children is trauma. The most common forms of intracranial hemorrhage are subarachnoid hemorrhage, subdural hematoma, and epidural hematoma.

There are anatomical differences to these types of intracranial hemorrhage and some differences in their presentation, but from a clinical standpoint, there are some key features that if identified would raise suspicion for an intracranial bleed and warrant neuroimaging to confirm the diagnosis.

In the setting of head trauma, findings such as any patient having a Glasgow Coma Scale score of less than 15, altered mental status, focal neurological signs, suspected skull fracture, loss of consciousness, seizure, or vomiting have been identified as high and intermediate risk indicators for intracranial bleeding (see Box 7.5). Any patient who presents with any combination of these symptoms in the setting of head trauma needs to be transferred to an emergency medical center for emergent evaluation observation and possible neuroimaging and preferably a center with a pediatric intensive care unit.

BOX 7.5 INTERMEDIATE AND HIGH RISK INDICATORS FOR INTRACRANIAL BLEED

Glasgow Coma Scale score of less than 15	Loss of consciousness
Altered mental status	Seizure
Focal neurological signs	Tachypnea
Suspected skull fracture	Vomiting

References

Davis, G. A., Purcell, L., & Schneider, K. J. (2017). The Child Sport Concussion Assessment Tool 5th Edition (Child SCAT5): Background and rationale. *British Journal of Sports Medicine, 51,* 859–861.

Do, T. P., Heldarskard, G., Kolding, G., Hvedstrup, J., & Schytz, H. W. (2018). Myofascial trigger points in migraine and tension-type headache. *Journal for Headache Pain, 19*(1), 84. doi:10.1186/s10194-018-0913-8

Echemendia, R. J. (2017). The SCAT5 in the evaluation of concussion management. *British Journal of Sports Medicine, 51,* 851–858. doi:10.1136/bjsports-2017-097506SCAT5

Evan, R. (2017). Sequelae of mild traumatic brain injury. In J. Wilterdink (Ed.), *UptoDate.* Retrieved from https://www-uptodate-com.treadwell.idm.oclc.org/contents/sequelae-of-mild-traumatic-brain-injury

Merikangas, K., Kalaydjan, A., Khoromi, S., Knight, E., & Nelson, K. (2009). Headache in a national cohort: Prevalence. *Journal of Child Neurology, 7*(23), 536–543.

Mount, H. R., & Boyle, S. D. (2017). Aseptic and bacterial meningitis: Evaluation, treatment, and prevention. *American Family Physician, 96*(5), 314–322.

8

Common Musculoskeletal Complaints Seen in Pediatric Primary Care

Michael S. Ruggiero

INTRODUCTION

With an estimated 15 million children under the age of 15 seeking medical care for musculoskeletal complaints each year, these are one of the most common reasons for pediatric visits. Diagnoses in the musculoskeletal system are vast and are too comprehensive for this chapter. This chapter will look at musculoskeletal complaints in two different lights, traumatic and atraumatic. Providers will take a logical approach to chief complaints that involve the musculoskeletal system. This chapter will introduce the provider to both common causes of acute joint pain and the approach to these complaints and then will explore some of the most common causes of acute musculoskeletal pain in children.

OBJECTIVES

1. Give pediatric advanced practice clinicians a thoughtful and reasonable approach to the management of children with common musculoskeletal complaints.
2. Understand an approach to work up the chief complaints that involve the musculoskeletal system.
3. Explain common causes of acute joint pain and the approach to these complaints
4. Explore some of the most common causes of acute musculoskeletal pain in children.

APPROACH TO TRAUMATIC MUSCULOSKELETAL COMPLAINTS

Musculoskeletal injuries are a common reason for office visits. Either due to accidental trauma, overuse, or sports-related injuries, having a quick guide to the management of these injuries is invaluable.

The easiest way to view these clinical problems is categorizing the injury into three groups: emergent, meaning the injury is life-threatening and limb-threatening and is capable of causing severe impairment; urgent, meaning the patient needs to be seen by a pediatric orthopedic specialist in the near future, as the treatment may involve specialized immobilization, reduction, and/or surgery; and routine, meaning something that primary care providers and nonorthopedic specialty providers can manage.

Next in the assessment of a musculoskeletal injury, one should try to make a judgment on whether the injury is a sprain/strain, fracture, or dislocation. The following section will help providers in the management of office orthopedics.

Common Principles

Traumatic musculoskeletal injuries are common in children and adolescents (Box 8.1). Despite the location of the pain or the specific diagnosis, the management of these is often similar.

BOX 8.1 TRAUMATIC MUSCULOSKELETAL INJURIES IN PEDIATRIC PATIENTS

Fractures:

- Fractures are less common in children than in adults, given the more pliable nature of the pediatric bone and the thick periosteum; however, they are still prevalent.
- Fractures should be suspected when there is a traumatic injury that results in any of the following: pain, limitation in function, deformity, swelling, ecchymosis, and point tenderness.
- Radiographs are indicated if a fracture is suspected.
- If an x-ray is to be performed, the provider must make sure that there at least two views performed and, at a minimum, they should be orthogonal to one another. In most cases, a good starting point is an AP view and a lateral view.
- Any pediatric fracture should be referred to a pediatric orthopedic specialist, especially if the joint and/or the epiphyseal growth plate is involved.
- The Salter Harris fracture classification is used to describe pediatric fractures that involve the epiphyseal plate/growth plate classified as I–V. See Figure 8.1.

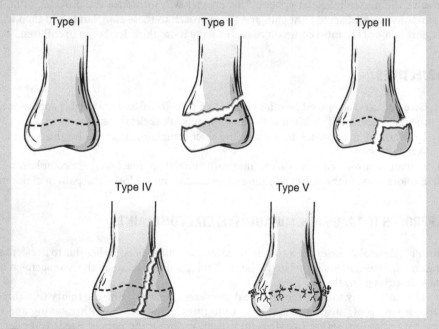

Figure 8.1 Salter Harris fracture classification.
Source: Reproduced from Fernandez, T., & Akerman, A. (2020). *The physician assistant student's guide to the clinical year: Pediatrics* (M. Knechtel, Ed.). New York, NY: Springer Publishing Company, p. 241.

BOX 8.1 TRAUMATIC MUSCULOSKELETAL INJURIES IN PEDIATRIC PATIENTS (*continued*)

- The most important aspects for a primary care provider in the diagnosis and management of a child with a fracture are to protect the injured area, assess for limb-threatening injuries, and prevent long-term dysfunction.
- All fractures should be assessed for concomitant neurovascular injures at the site and distally.
- Vascular injuries are an emergency and need to be addressed as such. An immediate referral to emergency medical center is required.
- Trauma-related compartment syndrome needs to be identified early and addressed immediately with a referral for emergency surgery. This also requires that parents/guardians are educated on the warning signs of compartment syndrome, as they often develop hours after the injury while at home.

Dislocations:
- Like fractures, dislocations require prompt attention and referral.
- Dislocations in children involving the large joints should be transferred to emergency medical centers for evaluation and reduction, as many of these children will need conscious sedation to reduce the dislocation.
- Dislocations of smaller joints, such as fingers and toes, can generally be reduced in an office setting with gentle traction and then splinted or buddy taped in extension. X-rays should be performed before and after reduction.
- Dislocations can also cause limb-threatening injuries due to vascular transection or more commonly compression.
- Any dislocation that is causing a pulseless limb should be emergently transferred to an emergency medical center.
- Attempts should be made by the primary care provider to reduce the joint and save the limb in the ambulatory setting if the child cannot be transferred to an emergency medical center within 4 hours.

Strains and sprains:
- A strain is an injury to a muscle or tendon. It usually occurs due to stretching or a strong muscular contraction. A sprain is an injury to a ligament usually due to force that puts "stretch" on the ligament.
- Both strains and sprains tend to be graded on a system of 1, 2, or 3 with increasing numbers reflecting higher amounts of damage to the structure.
- For example, type 1 strains or sprains have little structural damage to the tissue. Type 2 strains and sprains have mild to moderate tearing of the structure, which can adversely affect function. Type 3 strains are complete tear or ruptures of the structure leading to functional deficit and may require surgical intervention to repair. Type 3 sprains or tears to muscle and tendinous tissue are rare in children; but if they do occur, they are surgical urgencies to prevent long-term dysfunction.
- Examples of such tears would be of the Achilles tendon, distal bicep tendon, triceps tendon, or quadriceps or patella tendon.
- The urgency is related to the musculotendinous structure shortening and contracting, making successful surgical repair more difficult as time passes.
- As a general rule of thumb, orthopedic consultation should occur within a week of the injury.
- Sprains are a more common injury in children and are far more likely to be of the first- and second-degree variety. Type 3 sprains are increasing in prevalence as competitive sports and overuse injuries are occurring more as participation in year-round organized sports increases. Common type 3 ligament injuries are ACL tears, ulna collateral ligament tears (elbow), MCL/LCL tears, and anterior talofibular ligament tears (ankle).
- These injuries should be referred to orthopedic specialists as well; however, they tend not to be emergent as accessory musculature and other ligamentous structures help to preserve the joint stability and function.

ACL, anterior cruciate ligament; AP, anteroposterior; LCL, lateral collateral ligament; MCL, medial collateral ligament.

Most sprains and strains can be treated with the PRICE principle (protect, rest, ice, compression, elevation). Protect the area that has been injured via splinting and avoid weight bearing; rest the injured extremity; ice the injured region in the first 24 to 48 hours with careful attention not to develop a thermal injury; compress to help control swelling; and elevate to help control swelling and pain.

Most mild strains and sprains heal within 1 to 2 weeks and if moderate, within 3 to 4 weeks. It is important to have the child begin early, gentle range of motion (ROM) after the first 2 to 3 days of protection, which will help prevent a prolonged recovery from stiffness and pain. As stated in the aforementioned paragraphs, any complete tendinous or muscular tear should be referred expeditiously to orthopedic surgery. Any ligamentous injury or tear that renders a joint unstable should be referred to orthopedic surgery.

COMMON PEDIATRIC MUSCULOSKELETAL CONDITIONS

■ ELBOW

Elbow Fractures: Supracondylar Fractures

Epidemiology/Risk Factors

Elbow injuries are common in children of all ages. Most injuries are due to falls on an outstretched hand (FOOSH); these falls can lead to dislocations or fractures of the humerus, radius, or ulna. The most common form of fracture is a distal humerus fracture known as a supracondylar fracture.

Focused Physical Exam Signs/Findings

Due to the anatomy of neurovascular structures around the elbow, these particular fractures have a high incidence of disability and deformity due to neurovascular complications.

Any elbow fracture requires assessment of the brachial artery; median nerve, radial nerve, and ulnar nerve dysfunction can develop over time as hematoma formation or swelling increases.

Lab Tests/Diagnostics

X-ray is the imaging of choice in suspected elbow fractures. Images to order are an anteroposterior (AP) view of the elbow and a lateral elbow; an oblique view may also be beneficial. X-ray will help to classify the fracture according to the most widely used supracondylar classification system, the Gartland classification (see Figure 8.2; Gartland, 1959).

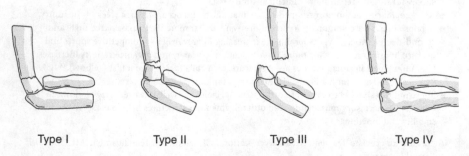

| Type I | Type II | Type III | Type IV |

Figure 8.2 Gartland classification of supracondylar fractures.

Management

Fractures of the elbow are common in childhood. Despite the exact diagnosis, it is generally accepted that all fractures about the elbow should have a referral to an orthopedist to help preserve normal ROM and function. It is also true that injuries commonly involve the neurovascular structure. All elbow injuries should raise suspicion for neurovascular injury that can lead to serious limb dysfunction, like a Volkmann contracture. Elbow fractures that have intra-articular extension can lead to difficulties with long-term ROM, especially extension.

In the setting of nondisplaced fractures with a normal neurovascular exam, it is generally agreed upon that splinting/casting in elbow flexion less than 90 degrees and sending to ortho for urgent follow-up is acceptable. Any signs of limb crisis or displaced fractures should be sent to the hospital for reduction and urgent orthopedic consult. Casts should not be circumferential without being split, as continued swelling can increase risk of compartment syndrome. Posterior splints are generally well-tolerated (see Figure 8.3a). Displaced fractures should be urgently reduced and splinted while awaiting surgery.

Patient Family Education/Follow-Up

Elevation is important to help prevent dependent swelling, which can be performed even in a posterior splint (see Figure 8.3b).

The parents must be educated on the signs of increased swelling and pressure.

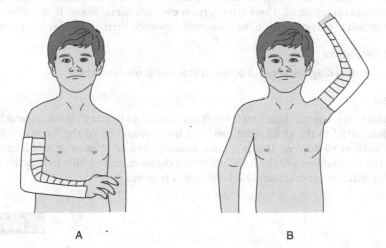

A	B

Figure 8.3 (A) Posterior arm splint. (B) Child able to elevate the arm for swelling control while arm is immobilized in posterior splint.

Don't Miss

Vigilance for clinical signs of a developing compartment syndrome is paramount. The earliest sign of compartment syndrome is pain out of proportion to the physical findings. Pain is the most reliable sign of compartment syndrome. Later findings are tense compartment. Less sensitive signs of compartment syndrome include pallor, paresthesia, and paralysis. Once these symptoms develop, there has typically been irreversible damage to the neuromuscular tissue.

(continued)

(continued)

Diagnosis may be supported by increased pain with passive tension of tendons and musculature that pass through the involved compartment, for example, passive extension of the fingers and wrist would increase pain in volar forearm compartment syndrome.

Nursemaid's Elbow

Etiology

A nursemaid's elbow occurs when the radial head annular ligament becomes interposed between the radial head and the capitellum. The mechanism of injury is due to longitudinal traction to the arm. The injury classically occurs from a *caretaker pulling or lifting a child by the wrist, hand, or forearm.*

Epidemiology/Risk Factors

Nursemaid's elbow is a common injury to children of toddler age (1–3 years old).

Focused Physical Exam Signs/Findings

The child refuses to use the involved limb and tends to hold the elbow in slight flexion with the forearm pronated. There is tenderness over the lateral elbow. ROM of the elbow in flexion and extension tends to be preserved; however, there is pain with supination.

Lab Tests/Diagnostics

This is a clinical diagnosis; x-rays do not reveal any acute findings.

Treatment

Reduction of the annular ligament is easily accomplished in an office setting and brings immediate relief to the child. First, perform hyperpronation of the forearm with the elbow flexed at 90 degrees. If that is unsuccessful, then an attempt should be made to reduce the annular ligament by fully supinating the forearm and fully flexing the elbow. No immobilization is necessary. No follow-up is required.

Don't Miss

Injuries to the elbow that raise suspicion for a fracture require an x-ray. X-ray findings can be subtle, and at times, no discernible fracture line can be seen. Providers must be on the lookout for subtle soft tissue findings suggestive of a fracture. A fat pad sign can alert providers to the presence of an elbow effusion due to a subtle fracture not yet visible on x-ray. It is generally accepted that a fat pad sign is pathognomonic for fracture in the setting of trauma.

■ HIP

Developmental Dysplasia of the Hip

Congenital hip dysplasia or developmental dysplasia of the hip (DDH) is a disorder of the hip(s) that causes excessive laxity of the femoral head within the acetabulum, leading to subluxation and dislocation of the hip.

Epidemiology

Estimations of DDH range greatly, but tend to be in the range of 10 in 1,000 births. Presentation can occur at different ages, however most cases are identified during the newborn period due to active screening.

Etiology/Risk Factors

The etiology of DDH is multifactorial; however, certain risk factors have been well-established for DDH. Risk factors include breech positioning in utero (20 times higher risk), female sex, being firstborn, and a positive family history.

Focused Physical Exam Findings

Screening during newborn physicals should include the Barlow and Ortolani physical examination maneuvers, testing for hip instability. These tests are less useful in older children. For the older infant and child, providers may find length discrepancy (Galeazzi sign), thigh fold asymmetry, and limited hip abduction. Children who are of walking age may have a Trendelenburg gait.

Lab Tests/Diagnostics

Imaging tests are used to aid in diagnosis for children with suspected DDH. Ultrasound is the preferred method of imaging in children under 6 months of age, given their largely cartilaginous structure. After 6 months, x-ray is the preferred imaging modality, as sufficient ossification has occurred at the femoral head. Imaging should be performed prior to discharge after birth in any child who has "risk factors" (i.e., a baby who was born breech) and subsequently in any child with positive findings on examination (such as positive Ortolani and Barlow maneuvers).

Treatment

Suspicion of, or diagnosis of, DDH in a child necessitates a referral to a pediatrician orthopedist. Treatment will consist of a Pavlik harness bracing by an orthopedic surgeon. The child must follow up every 1 to 2 weeks for adjustment of the brace, as the child is rapidly growing and usually imaging. The brace is generally worn full-time for 6 to 12 weeks (Yang, Zusman, Lieberman, & Goldstein, 2019). Failure of the Pavlik harness or late diagnosis (after 6 months) may require a more rigid orthosis or surgery.

Don't Miss

Children in Pavlik harness or DDH orthosis should be assessed for femoral nerve palsy due to compression. Parents may notice that the child does not actively try to extend the knee.

Legg–Calve–Perthes Disease

Legg–Calve–Perthes Disease (LCPD) is an avascular necrosis of the femoral head. The bone remodeling can lead to permanent deformity of the femoral head and early onset of hip arthritis and chronic pain. The condition tends to present acutely.

Epidemiology

LCPD affects approximately 5 in 100,000 children in the United States. The condition most commonly occurs during the ages of 4 and 9 years. Boys have a significantly higher incidence than females: 4:1. The disorder is most commonly unilateral, but in approximately 10%, both hips are affected.

Etiology/Risk Factors

Cause is thought to be multifactorial. There have been risk factors associated with LCPD. Risk factors include hip trauma, family history, secondhand smoke exposure, collagen disorders, and coagulopathy.

Focused Physical Exam Findings

Most children with LCPD present with caretaker who has noticed the child "limping." Children will complain of hip pain that may radiate to the anterior thigh or knee. Pain is better at rest and exacerbated with activity. Examination will often reveal a loss of abduction and internal rotation.

Lab Tests/Diagnostics

X-rays are the modality of choice for making the diagnosis of LCPD. Imaging should be an AP pelvis and a frog-leg lateral view. Findings may be subtle depending on the stage of disease. Findings can range from joint effusion with widening of the joint space to necrosis with flattening of the femoral head and widening of the femoral neck.

Treatment

Any patient suspected of having LCPD should be referred to a pediatric orthopedic surgeon. The goal of treatment is to maintain containment of the femoral head in the acetabulum. This containment is important to maintain a spherical shape to the femoral head (Georgiadis, Seeley, Yellin, & Sankar, 2015). Treatment depends on the age of the patient at presentation and the stage of disease. Treatment options range from symptomatic care with brief periods of bed rest, to adduction orthoses, to pelvic osteotomies.

Slipped Capital Femoral Epiphysis

Slipped capital femoral epiphysis (SCFE) is a hip disorder that occurs when there is displacement of the femoral head from the femoral neck through the physis. SCFE is the most common hip abnormality presenting in adolescence and is a primary cause of early-onset osteoarthritis.

Epidemiology

The incidence is estimated at approximately two per 100,000. It occurs more commonly in boys with a male-to-female ratio of 1.5:1. The age of onset is most common in adolescents. There is also a racial prevalence in Black, Pacific Islander, and Hispanic persons when compared with White persons. Risk factors include obesity, with approximately 80% of SCFE diagnoses occurring in obese children.

Presentation

The presenting complaint is usually groin or hip pain. Pain may be poorly localized referred to the anterior thigh or the knee. The patient will be of adolescent age and more likely overweight. Antalgic gait is present in most patients. The patients if standing still will often stand with the affected leg externally rotated. Examination reveals a limited internal rotation of the hip.

Workup

X-rays are the preferred imaging modality for SCFE diagnosis. Providers should order a bilateral AP pelvis and bilateral frog-leg lateral radiograph.

Treatment

SCFE treatment needs to begin immediately upon diagnosis. The primary care provider needs to prevent further slippage by placing a non–weight-bearing restriction on the patient, either by crutches or wheel chair, and an urgent referral to a pediatric orthopedist. Treatment is usually surgical via percutaneous screw fixation.

Special Considerations

Approximately 20% of patients have evidence of contralateral slip on initial presentation; the contralateral should be assessed and include x-ray evaluation, if deemed appropriate.

Transient Synovitis of the Hip

Transient synovitis (TS) of the hip or toxic synovitis of the hip is the most common cause of acute hip pain in children aged 3 to 10 years.

Epidemiology

TS is the most common cause of acute hip pain in children aged 4 to 10 years. It is more common in boys, with a male-to-female ratio of 2:1. It can affect adults but is most common in children.

Etiology/Risk Factors

While the exact etiology is unclear, there do appear to be well-documented risk factors. Risk factors are preceding viral upper respiratory infection, preceding bacterial infection, such as streptococcal infection, and trauma to the involved hip.

Focused Physical Exam Findings

TS presents most commonly with unilateral hip pain that is exacerbated with ambulation and manifests as an antalgic gait. Pain can be severe enough that the child refuses to weight bear. A recent history of an upper respiratory tract infection, or pharyngitis, or ear infection is often elicited. Examination reveals limited ROM in abduction and internal rotation. To ease discomfort, patients may rest with a flexed abducted and externally rotated hip.

Lab Tests/Diagnostics

There are no specific tests to diagnose TS. The most important job for a provider is to rule out a septic joint as TS, and septic joints present in a similar fashion and are difficult to differentiate. Inclusive workup is generally recommended as missing a septic joint can be devastating.

Providers should include temperature to check for fever, serum white blood cell (WBC) count, C-reactive protein (CRP), and erythrocyte sedimentation rate (ESR). The Kocher criteria are helpful in discerning between the two. The criteria include the increasing diagnostic probability in favor of a septic joint, yielding a 99.6% probability when all four criteria are met, and a 0.2% probability of septic joint if none are met.

Kocher criteria
WBC >12,000
Inability or refusal to weight bear
Febrile (>101.3°F or 38.5°C)
ESR >40 mm/hr

Treatment

Treatment of TS is largely supportive with symptoms improving within a couple of days and complete resolution on average within 2 weeks. Symptoms do not last. Nonsteroidal anti-inflammatory drugs (NSAIDs), such as ibuprofen, are generally sufficient in the management of TS pain. Consider admitting if pain control is difficult to achieve.

- **Ibuprofen** 10 mg/kg per dose repeated every 6 hours.

Don't Miss

The goal is to rule out a septic joint as opposed to confirming a diagnosis of TS. Much of the literature recommends ultrasound to check for an effusion. If there is an effusion present, then an ultrasound-guided joint aspiration is necessary.

■ KNEE

Anterior Cruciate Ligament Tear

Anterior cruciate ligament's (ACL's) primary function is to minimize anterior translation of the femur on the tibia. Complete tear or high-grade sprain can lead to instability of the knee. ACL tears are also a major cause of early-onset knee arthritis.

Epidemiology

There has been a growing rate of ACL injuries in children, as participation in competitive sports grows in children. Incidence of ACL tears in the pediatric community has varied significantly from study to study. In 2017, Beck, Lawrence, and Nordin et al. reviewed ACL tear patterns and trends over the past 20 years. The rate of ACL tears per 100,000 person years averaged 121 ± 19 (range 92–151). All trends increased. Overall, there was an annual increase of 2.3%. Females had significantly higher incidence except until ages of 17 to 18 years. Females peaked at the age of 16, and males at the age of 17, with rates of 392 ACL tears and 422 ACL tears per 100,000 person years, respectively (Beck et al., 2017).

Etiology/Risk Factors

ACL tears are due to traumatic events and tend to occur during sporting events. Injuries tend to be non-contact in nature but can occur due to contact, such as in a motor vehicle accident or blunt trauma to the leg. The typical mechanism is a hyperextension injury of the knee. The more common or classic description of the injury pattern is a non-contact injury in which a patient reports planting the ipsilateral foot and turning direction quickly.

Focused Physical Exam Signs/Findings

A patient presents with complaints of an acute knee injury. The knee is swollen typically with a large effusion. The patient will often report feeling a "pop" in the knee. If they are walking and weight bearing, they may report that the knee feels unstable. Estimation is often difficult in the acute phase, due to significant effusion and guarding. If effusion is large, contributing to pain and limitation in exam, then joint aspiration of the hemarthrosis is recommended. This often leads to significant improvement in symptoms. Examination test for integrity of the ACL will show laxity of the ACL when performing a Lachman's test or anterior drawer test.

Lab Tests/Diagnostics

Knee aspiration shows that hemarthrosis is consistent with an intra-articular injury. X-rays will not show the actual ACL disruption but may reveal bony changes or injury consistent with an ACL tear. X-rays should be performed to rule out a tibial plateau fracture or proximal tibial fracture but may show a Segond fracture that is an avulsion fracture of the anterolateral tibial plateau that is a common finding in ACL tears. Also, the site of ACL insertion of the tibial spine may show an avulsion, as, in some cases, the ACL injury is more of an avulsion fracture than a true ligament tear. ACL tears are a clinical diagnosis; however, given the fact the majority are repaired surgically, it is generally accepted that MRI should be performed to aid in diagnosis and to assess the injury further and detect concomitant structural damage.

Treatment

Complete tears of the ACL do not heal. All ACL injuries should be referred to orthopedic surgery where decisions will be made whether or not surgical reconstruction is necessary. Decisions are made based on the child's age, activity level, and severity of the injury. Reconstruction is the standard in treatment; however, bracing and strengthening with proprioception training may be appropriate in some patients. While awaiting orthopedic consultation, the child should use supportive bracing to help prevent instability and bulking of the knee, which can lead to further chondral injury. Partial weight bearing with crutches may be appropriate for children with pain and significant instability. Light, non–weight-bearing ROM of the knee should be encouraged while the child awaits orthopedic consult.

Osgood–Schlatter is one of the most common causes of anterior knee pain in young athletes, caused by repetitive microtrauma and subsequent traction apophysitis of the tibial tuberosity. It is commonly seen in 12- to 15-year-old boys or 8- to 12-year-old girls who participate in jumping activities. Patients present with anterior knee pain and swelling. Physical examination is usually diagnostic, with radiographs demonstrating soft tissue edema overlying the anterior tibial tuberosity, and some degree of fragmentation and irregularity of the tibial tubercle. MRI demonstrates edema in the tibial tuberosity and distal patellar tendon. Hoffa's fat pad may also show increased signal on fluid-sensitive sequences.

Patella Instability

Patellar instability (PI) is an umbrella term for patella problems ranging from patella tracking issues to subluxation to dislocation. The focus of this section will be on patella dislocation.

Epidemiology

PI accounts for the most predominant knee problems during growth. The overall incidence is around 50 in 100,000 children and adolescents per year, with a peak at 15 years old. Most patella instability and tracking issue occur laterally.

Etiology/Risk Factors

Obese patients, as well as female adolescent athletes, tend to have a higher predisposition as do patients with hypermobility disorders, such as Ehlers–Danlos syndrome. Mechanism of injury can be from direct trauma, but more frequently, it is a non-contact injury such as rapid deceleration and twisting of leg on a planted foot. However, dislocations can also coincide with traumatic events, such as direct impact to a partially flexed knee.

Focused Physical Exam Signs/Findings

Once dislocated, the patient will be holding the knee in a guarded position, with the knee in a slightly flexed position. The patient may state the knee is "locked" in that position. The patella is visibly laterally displaced. Patients tend to be in moderate pain and unable or unwilling to weight bear. Effusion is often present.

Lab Tests/Diagnostics

Prereduction x-rays are not necessary. However, x-rays should be obtained once reduction has occurred. AP, lateral, and sunrise views are recommended.

Treatment

Treatment consists of reducing the dislocation. Acute patella dislocation can often be achieved in an office setting. For lateral displacement, which is the vast majority of cases, reduction is achieved by placing the patient in the seated position and passively extending knee into slight hyperextension while applying gentle medial pressure to the lateral edge of the patella. Patient with medial dislocation would be similar just with lateral pressure applied to the medial edge of the patella. Unsuccessful attempt or patients who cannot tolerate the maneuver should be referred to an emergency medical center for conscious sedation, ultrasound-guided femoral nerve block, or analgesic prior to performing the same method. Once reduction is achieved, the patient should be fit for and educated on non–weight-bearing use of crutches. Knee immobilizer should be placed in the acute setting with orthopedic follow-up within a week (Hasler & Studer, 2017).

◼ SHOULDER

Clavicle Fracture

Etiology

The clavicle is the second most commonly broken bone in children. Most clavicle fractures in children heal uneventfully.

Epidemiology/Risk Factors

The mechanism of injury is a fall on an outstretched hand or a fall onto the shoulder.

Focused Physical Exam Signs/Findings

Children will present with cradling the affected arm, avoiding the use of the affected arm, and listing to the affected side. Due to the extreme pain, it can cause nausea and vomiting. Examination may show swelling and deformity at the fracture site and bruising, and it will be tender to palpation. *Note*: Distal neurovascular exam needs to be assessed. Check for subclavian hematoma.

Lab Tests/Diagnostics

Diagnosis of a clavicle fracture is confirmed by a clavicle x-ray.

Don't Miss

Displaced fractures may also compress the subclavian vessels or brachial plexus and produce vascular insufficiency, with diminution or absence of distal pulses, paresthesias, and paresis. Most fractures of the clavicle occur in the middle third of the clavicle and are seldom significantly displaced. Even with significant displacement, middle

(continued)

(continued)

third clavicle fractures in children tend to heal and remodel without functional deficit and without significant esthetic deformity. In the child with middle third clavicle fracture with no to mild displacement, treatment can consist of sling for comfort (or no sling for younger children who are not able to understand keeping their arm in a sling) and reassessment in 2-week intervals with the goal to resume normal activity after 4 weeks. Fractures that are of the distal third, proximal third, 100% displaced, or displaced and shortened should be referred to orthopedics for possible closed reduction and for follow-up.

Special considerations. Complications are rare; however, it is possible to injure the subclavian artery or vein. Suspicion for vascular injury should be raised if there is a large/increasing hematoma (Stepanyan, Gendelberg, & Hennrikus, 2018). Subclavian injuries are a surgical emergency, as they can cause morbidity and mortality. Children should be transferred immediately to an emergency medical center with vascular surgery service.

■ SPINE

Scoliosis

Epidemiology

This is a common disorder with a prevalence as high as 5% in some literature. Ninety percent of cases are idiopathic.

Etiology/Risk Factors

Scoliosis is a lateral curvature of the thoracolumbar spine measuring greater than 10 degrees. It is most commonly encountered during adolescence. Girls have a higher tendency and have a higher incidence of severe curvature than boys.

Focused Physical Exam Signs/Findings

Screening is often performed in schools and should be performed at each annual physical. Angles are calculated by performing a large plate spine x-ray with a Cobb angle calculation. Angles between 10 degrees and less than 20 degrees are managed with observation and core strengthening exercises, providers should consider a referral to a pediatric physical therapist to train the child and parent on a home exercise program.

Deformities with a curvature of greater than 20 degrees should be referred to an orthopedic pediatric spine specialist for management. Bracing is often utilized if curvature is greater than 20 degrees. Curvature less than 30 degrees at skeletal maturity rarely progresses; however, deformities of 50 degrees or greater tend to progress after skeletal maturity. Curvatures of 40 degrees or greater are likely to require surgery.

MUSCULOSKELETAL COMPLAINTS RELATED TO AUTOIMMUNE DISORDERS AND INFECTION

■ INFECTIOUS

Lyme Arthritis

Lyme disease is the most common tick-borne disease in North America. Most often, patients present with the pathognomonic erythema migrans rash; however, in many cases, the first sign of Lyme disease is not until weeks to months after the tick bite and manifests as acute arthritis. Lyme arthritis is most often a monoarthritis; however, in up to a one third of cases, patients will present with oligoarthritis.

Epidemiology

Lyme disease is caused by a group of spirochetal bacteria (genus *Borrelia*). Disease is transmitted by *Ixodes* ticks. It is prevalent in North America. Arthritis usually presents in children who do not receive antibiotics in the acute phase of Lyme disease if the tick bite or rash goes unnoticed. Prior to presentation with overt arthritis, children may report several weeks of nonspecific migratory arthralgias.

The knee is the most common joint involved—in some reports as high as 90% of the cases.

Presentation

There is joint swelling and effusion with loss of motion; pain is often described as mild to moderate. Patients may have low-grade fevers, headaches, or fatigue.

Presenting signs and symptoms are usually not as severe as SA. Weight bearing is maintained. Rash and other systemic signs of Lyme disease should be actively sought during the exam. History should be explicitly elicited concerning rashes and tick bites.

Workup

X-ray is seldom indicated. Arthrocentesis should be performed if there is an effusion present, generally to rule out a SA. Diagnosis is confirmed by serum ELISA IgM and IgG antibodies to *Borrelia burgdorferi* with a reflex Western blot to confirm positive tests.

Treatment

Children with Lyme arthritis are treated with doxycycline or amoxicillin. It is generally accepted that children who are less than 8 years old are treated with amoxicillin and those 8 years and older are treated with doxycycline. Treatment is for 4 weeks (28 days).

8 years or older: Doxycycline PO 2 to 4 mg/kg/day divided into two doses, up to adult dose of 100 mg twice a day.

Less than 8 years old: Amoxicillin PO 50 mg/kg/day divided into three doses, up to adult dose of 2 g/day (Cherry, Demmler-Harrison, Kaplan, Steinbach, & Hotez, 2019).

Septic Arthritis

Septic arthritis (SA) is a true pediatric orthopedic emergency. Diagnosis needs to occur efficiently to avoid destruction of the joint, prevent long-term morbidity, and prevent septicemia.

Epidemiology

Hematogenous infection is the most common; however, direct inoculation can occur from trauma or spread from an overlying skin infection. The incidence in developed countries is four to five cases per 100,000 children per year. Most commonly affected locations in the body are the large joints of the lower limb—hip, knee, and ankle joints. *Staphylococcus aureus* and respiratory pathogens are the most common causative agents.

Presentation

Presentation is classically an acutely swollen, red, painful joint with limited motion and fever. The child often refuses to weight bear on the affected limb. Neonates with a septic hip assume a characteristic position with the hip joint flexed and abducted in internal rotation.

Workup

SA is diagnosed clinically and supported by laboratory testing. The peripheral WBC count is frequently raised. Acute phase reactants, such as CRP and ESR, are often markedly raised. Joint aspirate and/or blood culture should be obtained before starting empiric antibiotic treatment and altered to treat the identified organism. The Kocher criteria are helpful in determining the likelihood of a diagnosis of SA. The criteria include the increasing diagnostic probability in favor of a septic joint, yielding a 99.6% probability when all four criteria are met and a 0.2% probability of septic joint if none are met.

The Kocher criteria include:

- WBC >12,000
- Inability or refusal to weight bear
- Febrile (>101.3°F or 38.5°C)
- ESR >40 mm/hr

Treatment

Patients should be admitted, and empiric treatment should begin immediately, following blood cultures and joint aspirate analysis. Treatment should be targeted to isolated organism(s). Empiric treatment should be started with vancomycin plus ceftriaxone plus oxacillin while awaiting the results of culture and joint aspirate. Patients generally are admitted for 2 to 4 days on parenteral antibiotics; if symptoms progress or fail to improve over the course of that time, then orthopedic arthroscopic lavage is largely indicated. Patients will be discharged on 2 to 4 weeks of oral antibiotics with close follow-up with orthopedics (Krogstad, 2019; Pääkkönen, 2017).

▪ RHEUMATIC DISORDERS

Autoimmunity and inflammation are the hallmarks of rheumatic disorder in children. Rheumatic disorders are autoimmune disorders in which the musculoskeletal system is most frequently targeted. The most prominent features of rheumatic disease tend to be atraumatic complaints of arthralgia, myalgia, and arthritis. Unlike adults of whom most cases of atraumatic joint discomfort tend to be degenerative conditions, atraumatic joint and muscle complaints in children have a higher incidence of being the manifestation of underlying rheumatic disease. The most common rheumatic conditions in children are juvenile rheumatoid arthritis/juvenile idiopathic arthritis (JIA), systemic lupus erythematosus, and dermatomyositis (Woo & Colbert, 2009).

Dermatomyositis/Juvenile Dermatomyositis (JDM)

Juvenile dermatomyositis (JDM) is an autoimmune-mediated inflammatory myopathy that presents with musculoskeletal complaints and dermatologic manifestations in children.

Epidemiology

Categorized as a rare disorder, it is still regarded as the most common inflammatory myopathy in children, accounting for more than 75% of the inflammatory myopathy diagnoses in children. Incidence is reported as 2.3 million children/year in the United States. The mean age of onset is 7 years, although about 25% of patients with JDM present under the age of 5 years. It is more common in females than males with a 2:1 ratio.

Clinical Manifestation

Children present with complaints of symmetrical proximal muscle weakness, such as difficulty combing hair, reaching above shoulder level, rising from a seated position, or climbing stairs. Most children will also present with some form of the dermatologic manifestations of the disease. Heliotropic rash that is a violet or bluish-purple rash that is most commonly found around the eyes and on the eyelids but is also frequently noted on the upper back, chest, and shoulders, known as the "shawl sign." Also considered pathognemonic for JDM are Gottron's papules that are violacious papules found most often on the dorsum of the hand over the metacarpal phalangeal joints but can also be seen on other extensor surfaces, such as elbows and knees. It is not uncommon for the dermatologic manifestations of the disease to present prior to myalgia and muscle weakness. Children during exam should have muscle strength testing performed and will often have notable weakness of the involved proximal muscle groups, and this deficit tends to be symmetric.

Workup

The workup for JDM begins with serum markers of which creatine phosphokinase (CPK) is the most sensitive. Elevations of greater than 1,000 IU/L are expected. The diagnosis is confirmed by muscle biopsy. Many centers are now recommending MRI prior to biopsy to help optimize the biopsy sensitivity. Biopsy of areas that display muscle edema on the MRI is likely to be more informative and has less risk of false negatives.

Treatment

A rheumatology referral or urgent consult is recommended once a diagnosis of dermatomyositis is suspected. Corticosteroids are the initial management choice for patients. Many specialists recommend admitting patients for 3 days of pulsed methylprednisolone and then discharging on oral prednisone. Continued treatment most commonly involves a combination of steroids and methotrexate.

Special Consideration

If JDM is considered, providers should work quickly to confirm the diagnosis and refer to appropriate specialists as delayed diagnosis has been shown to have higher rates of mortality. Also, symptoms of JDM without the dermatologic manifestations should raise suspicion for the less frequent childhood diagnosis of polymyositis.

Juvenile Idiopathic Arthritis

Epidemiology

JIA is the most common chronic rheumatic disease in children. The prevalence for JIA in North America is 113/100,000 children. Girls are more commonly affected than boys, and peaks of the illness manifest in toddlers. There are several different subtypes of JIA, and these subtypes range in variability among race and ethnicities. The most common subtypes as defined by the International league of Associations for Rheumatology (ILAR) are systemic arthritis, which accounts for 5% to 15% of children; pauciarticular or oligoarticular arthritis, which accounts for 50% to 80%; and polyarticular arthritis, which accounts for 15% to 25% of children.

Presentation

JIA is often symmetrical and polyarticular. Involved joints are swollen and can be painful but most often do not prevent weight bearing. They are generally not red or hot to touch. Boggy synovium can be palpated. Children may describe morning stiffness, with symptoms decreasing during the day as the joint is used. While joint manifestations are the hallmark of JIA, joint symptoms can be absent at onset and develop much later in the illness. Extra-articular manifestations that may occur prior to joint involvement are erythematous, salmon pink, evanescent macular rash that usually appears with fever duration of at least 6 weeks. Children should be examined for other common manifestations of the disorder as well such as hepatosplenomegaly, pericarditis, uveitis/iritis, and enthesitis.

Workup

No specific laboratory tests are available to confirm the diagnosis. The American College of Rheumatology established five criteria for the diagnosis of JIA: (a) age at onset younger than 16 years; (b) arthritis of one or more joints; (c) symptom duration of at least 6 weeks; (d) an onset type, after 6 months' observation, of the polyarticular form (five or more affected joints), the oligoarthritic form (fewer than five joints affected), or the systemic form with arthritis and characteristic fever; and (e) exclusion of other forms of arthritis. JIA is a clinical diagnosis. Thorough workup is required before making the diagnosis of JIA. Other emergent conditions that can cause arthritis and arthralgia must be ruled out. It should be mentioned that rheumatic conditions may be somewhat of a misnomer as the vast majority of children with JIA have a negative rheumatoid factor.

Note: Despite JIA often presenting as a multiple large joint arthritis, a subtype of pauciarticular JIA manifests as a low-grade inflammation of one or several joints in an otherwise well child. In approximately half of these patients, only one joint is involved. The knee is most often affected, with the ankle–subtalar and elbow joints next in frequency (Herring, 2014).

Treatment

Treatment involves a referral to a pediatric rheumatologist. Children should also be referred to an ophthalmologist for scheduled eye exams for possible ocular manifestations of the disorder. Treatment for symptoms of pain, stiffness, and swelling can begin in the primary care setting with NSAIDs Ibuprofen 10 mg/kg per dose repeated every 6 hours. Maximum dose is 3,200 mg/kg per dose.

Disease-modifying antirheumatic drugs are the mainstay of treatment for most cases of JIA. These are most often managed by a pediatric rheumatologist. The cornerstone of such treatment has been methotrexate. It is recommended that children have supplemental folic acid if on methotrexate.

Systemic corticosteroids are generally reserved for children with the systemic form of JIA who are presenting with high fever, pericarditis, or myorcarditis. Treatment has included high-dose pulse intravenous (IV) methylprednisolone or short courses of oral prednisone 1 to 2 mg/kg/day (maximum 60 mg/kg/day).

Rhabdomyolysis

Any child who presents with myalgia warrants an investigation of rhabdomyolysis. Rhabdomyolysis is a rapid dissolution of injured skeletal muscle. Disruption of skeletal muscle integrity releases intracellular muscle components, including myoglobin, creatine kinase, and electrolytes.

Etiology

Most cases of rhabdomyolysis are caused by direct trauma, strenuous activity, viral infections, and toxic effects of medications.

Presentation

Patients will present with myalgia and dark-colored urine due to myoglobinuria. Patients can develop life-threatening arrhythmias due to electrolyte abnormality. Up to 40% of children who present with rhabdomyolysis develop acute renal failure due to the nephrotoxic effects of myoglobin.

Workup

It will show a significantly elevated CPK. Labs to monitor renal function and electrolyte abnormalities should also be drawn.

Treatment

Focus of treatment is to remove offending agents if any are identified and to admit children for aggressive hydration with IV fluid to prevent acute renal failure and azotemia (Torres, Helmstetter, Kaye, & Kaye, 2015).

Systemic Lupus Erythematosus

Systemic lupus erythematosus (SLE) is an autoimmune disorder that can affect multiple organ systems in the body. Children often first present with vague complaints of muscle aches and joint pain.

Epidemiology

Childhood SLE (cSLE) is considered to be a rare disease; however, 20% of all cases of SLE begin in childhood. The incidence of cSLE is 0.3 to 0.9 per 100,000 children years. There is a higher frequency in Asian, Black, Hispanic, and Native Americans. Median age of onset of cSLE is 11 years. There is a higher rate of cSLE in females, with a female-to-male ratio of 8:1.

Clinical Manifestations

Because cSLE affects so many different organ systems, children can present with a host of different signs and symptoms. Most children will have musculoskeletal complaints, and specifically more than 80% of those diagnosed with cSLE will present with some degree of arthritis or arthralgia. The arthritis is polyarticular with effusions and often painful. Joints most commonly affected are those of the hand wrist, ankles, and knees. The joint pain and swelling are often symmetric. Other common manifestations of cSLE are constitutional symptoms, such as fever and malaise and cutaneous including the classic malar rash and temporal area alopecia (Levy & Kamphuis, 2012).

Workup

Serum markers of varying degree of sensitivity and specificity that are commonly used to help diagnose cSLE are antinuclear antibodies (ANAs), double-stranded DNA (dsDNA) antibodies, antibodies to the extractable nuclear antigens (ENAs), and antiphospholipid antibodies (aPLs). A negative ANA is generally considered exclusionary for a diagnosis of cSLE. If a child is suspected of having cSLE with a negative ANA, then another diagnosis needs to be considered, or a rare false-negative ANA may be explored with a repeat test. The American College of Rheumatology has developed a classification criteria to help aid in the diagnosis of SLE.

Treatment

All children suspected of having cSLE should be referred to a pediatric rheumatologist. Treatment usually begins with antimalarial drugs, such as hydroxychloroquine and prednisone, which should be tapered to the lowest effective dose.

Note: Children on hydroxychloroquine should be seen frequently by ophthalmology due to the ophthotoxic effects of the medication. Primary care should also be monitoring liver function, renal function, and CBC in patients diagnosed with cSLE (Okong'o, Esser, Wilmshurst, & Scott, 2016; Pachman & Khojah, 2018).

Don't Miss

All children with autoimmune disorders and specifically the aforementioned conditions are associated with a life-threatening condition known as macrophage activation syndrome (MAS). Symptoms and signs of MAS should be actively looked for in any child who presents with concerns for autoimmune disease. Fever in conjunction with any of the following should raise suspicion for MAS: ferritin >684 ng/mL, platelet count ≤181,000 microL, AST > 48 IU/L, triglycerides >156 mg/dL, or fibrinogen ≤360 mg/dL. A referral to an emergency medical center for prompt treatment with pulsed IV methylprednisolone is the typical treatment (Ravelli et al., 2016).

References

Beck, N. A., Lawrence, J. T. R., Nordin, J. D., DeFor, T. A., & Tompkins, M. (2017). ACL tears in school-aged children and adolescents over 20 years. *Pediatrics, 139*(3), e20161877. doi:10.1542/peds.2016-1877

Cherry, J., Demmler-Harrison, G. J., Kaplan, S. L., Steinbach, W. J., & Hotez, P. (2019). Lyme disease. In *Feigin and Cherry's textbook of pediatric infectious diseases* (8th ed., pp. 1246–1252. e2). Philadelphia, PA: Elsevier.

Fernandez, T., & Akerman, A. (2020). *The physician assistant student's guide to the clinical year: Pediatrics* (M. Knechtel, Ed.). New York, NY: Springer Publishing Company.

Gartland, J. (1959). Management of supracondylar fractures of the humerus in children. *Surgery Gynecology and Obstetrics, 109*(2), 145–159.

Georgiadis, A., Seeley, A. G., Yellin, M. A., & Sankar, W. N. (2015). The presentation of Legg-Calvé-Perthes disease in females. *Journal of Children's Orthopaedics, 9*(4), 243–247. doi:10.1007/s11832-015-0671-y

Hasler, C. C., & Studer, D. (2017). Patella instability in children and adolescents. *EFORT Open Reviews, 1*(5), 160–166. doi:10.1302/2058-5241.1.000018

Herring, J. A. (2014). Arthritis. In *Tachdjian's pediatric orthopaedics* (5th ed.). Philadelphia, PA: Elsevier.

Krogstad, P. (2019). Septic arthritis. In Cherry, J., Demmler-Harrison, G. J., Kaplan, S. L., Steinbach, W. J., & Hotez, P. (Eds.), *Feigin and Cherry's textbook of pediatric infectious diseases* (8th ed., pp. 529–534.e2). Philadelphia, PA: Elsevier.

Levy, D. M., & Kamphuis, S. (2012). Systemic lupus erythematosus in children and adolescents. *Pediatric Clinics of North America, 59*(2), 345–364. doi:10.1016/j.pcl.2012.03.007

Okong'o, L. O., Esser, M., Wilmshurst, J., & Scott, C. (2016). Characteristics and outcome of children with juvenile dermatomyositis in Cape Town: A cross-sectional study. *Pediatric Rheumatology Online Journal, 14*(1), 60. doi:10.1186/s12969-016-0118-0

Pääkkönen, M. (2017). Septic arthritis in children: Diagnosis and treatment. *Pediatric Health, Medicine and Therapeutics, 8*, 65–68. doi:10.2147/PHMT.S115429

Pachman, L. M., & Khojah, A. M. (2018). Advances in juvenile dermatomyositis: Myositis specific antibodies aid in understanding disease heterogeneity. *Journal of Pediatrics, 195*, 16–27. doi:10.1016/j.jpeds.2017.12.053

Ravelli, A., Minoia, F., Davì, S., Horne, A., Bovis, F., Pistorio, A., . . . Cron, R. Q. (2016). 2016 Classification criteria for macrophage activation syndrome complicating systemic juvenile idiopathic arthritis a European League against Rheumatism/American College of Rheumatology/Paediatric Rheumatology International Trials Organisation Collaborative Initiative. *Arthritis & Rheumatology, 68*(3), 566–576. doi:10.1002/ART.39332

Stepanyan, H., Gendelberg, D., & Hennrikus, W. L. (2018). Simple clavicle fractures, a primary care musculoskeletal injury. *Pediatrics, 141*, 204.

Torres, P. A., Helmstetter, J. A., Kaye, A. M., & Kaye, A. D. (2015). Rhabdomyolysis: Pathogenesis, diagnosis, and treatment. *The Ochsner Journal, 15*(1), 58–69.

Woo, P., & Colbert, R. A. (2009). An overview of genetics of pediatric rheumatic diseases. *Best Practice & Research. Clinical Rheumatology, 23*(5), 589–597. doi:10.1016/j.berh.2009.08.001

Yang, S., Zusman, N., Lieberman, E., & Goldstein, R. Y. (2019). Developmental dysplasia of the hip. *Pediatrics, 143*(1). doi:10.1542/peds.2018-1147

9

Dermatologic Abnormalities Commonly Seen in Pediatric Primary Care

Kristine M. Ruggiero

INTRODUCTION

Pediatric dermatologic conditions account for a large amount of pediatric primary care visits. A careful history and physical exam (PE) are key components to identifying and correctly managing a dermatologic condition; especially careful attention to lesion morphology, distribution, and color will allow ready identification of the nature of many common dermatologic conditions (many of them rashes). If the etiology of a rash is uncertain—especially in a child who appears ill, an immunocompromised child, or a neonate—prompt referral to a dermatologist is critical.

OBJECTIVES

1. Determine the extent and depth of a burn injury in a child and delineate how to evaluate a child who has an acute burn injury.
2. Understand how to differentiate between various dermatologic disorders in pediatric patients.
3. Discuss how to evaluate and manage various dermatologic disorders in a pediatric patient.

ASSESSMENT OF A CHILD WITH A DERMATOLOGIC CONDITION

The history and PE are important components when differentiating between various dermatologic conditions. One study showed the most common skin conditions seen in pediatrics are contact dermatitis and warts in younger children and acne vulgaris in teenagers (Özçelik, Kulaç, Yazıcı, & Öcal, 2018). It is important to ask the following: How long has the rash or lesion been present? Is it changing rapidly (over hours or days)? Do lesions come and go, or persist? Are there any systemic symptoms that appeared at the same time as the rash? Is the patient taking any medications (including over-the-counter [OTC] or herbal remedies)? Does this coincide with the onset of the rash? What are the skin symptoms? (Does the area of the rash itch or burn?) Does anyone else in the family have this particular rash?

Other important questions to ask is if the rash is scaly or not. Scaly rashes involve inflammation in the epidermis, and if the rash is diffuse, the most common diagnosis is a form of atopic dermatitis (AD; eczema). In general, eczematous eruptions are poorly marginated—that is, there are no areas within the region of the rash where the skin appears normal. It is this feature that helps to distinguish between eczema and lesions of tinea corporis or psoriasis, for example, which are characterized by distinct and discrete red, scaly lesions separated by normal skin. Non-scaly rashes result from injury to blood vessels in the dermis and usually are accompanied by some swelling. Dermal rashes are familiar to all primary care clinicians. Those seen most frequently are drug rashes and maculopapular eruptions that accompany viruses. Hives—also called urticaria, wheals, or welts—occur as the result of a vascular injury arising from immunologic or nonimmunologic mechanisms. Topical corticosteroids are not helpful and should not be used because these are effective only for epidermal inflammation that is clinically apparent as a scale. A viral exanthem may be clinically indistinguishable from a drug reaction; however, it should be noted in the child's chart if they had a rash while taking a drug.

BULLOUS LESION

Bullous Impetigo Versus Nonbullous Impetigo

Etiology

Bullous impetigo is a common cutaneous infection that primarily affects children between the ages of 2 and 5 years. It is caused almost exclusively by coagulase-positive *S. aureus*. It is a common manifestation of a staphylococcal toxin–mediated disease. Impetigo is caused by *Streptococcus* (strep) or *Staphylococcus* (staph) bacteria. Methicillin-resistant *S. aureus* (MRSA) is becoming a common cause. Bullous impetigo is less contagious than the nonbullous form (Mannschreck, Feig, Selph, & Cohen, 2020).

Focused PE Signs/Findings

Bullous impetigo presents as large blisters called bullae, usually in areas with skin folds, like the armpit, groin, between the fingers or toes, beneath the breast, and between the buttocks. In bullous impetigo, which usually affects children under the age of 2 years, fluid-filled blisters surrounded with red, itchy skin are present and tend to spread quickly over the body, eventually bursting and leaving a golden crust. They are usually found on the limbs and torso.

Nonbullous impetigo is usually a self-limited process that resolves within 2 weeks. Red sores are present, most commonly around the mouth and nose. These soon burst, oozing clear or pus-like fluid that goes on to form the "characteristic" golden crusts. Once the crusts dry out, reddish areas of skin are exposed. These usually heal without any scarring. It tends to affect the face, extremities, axillae, trunk, and perianal region of neonates, but older children can also be infected.

Lab Tests/Diagnostics

Generally, lab tests are not necessary, and the diagnosis can be made on the PE.

Differentials

Differentials can include ring worm, rashes, scabies, and chicken pox.

Don't Miss

Impetigo can spread to others. You can catch the infection from someone who has it if the fluid that oozes from their skin blisters touches an open area on your skin.

Treatment

Topical antibiotic ointment can be used as a first-line therapy for single lesions or non-bullous impetigo or small areas of involvement. Topical treatment includes topical antibiotics, such as mupirocin, retapamulin, and fusidic acid (Mannschreck et al., 2020). Oral antibiotic therapy can be used as first- or second-line therapy for a child with impetigo with large bullae or when topical therapy is impractical or unsuccessful. Oral antibiotics that are effective for treatment of impetigo are antistaphylococcal penicillins, amoxicillin/clavulanate, cephalosporins, and macrolides. In this situation, trimethoprim/sulfamethoxazole, clindamycin, or doxycycline in children older than 8 years can be used.

Prevention

Impetigo is a highly contagious disease. Impetigo is easily spread from person to person by direct contact with the lesions and/or indirectly by touching items (clothing, sheets, or toys) that have been used by individuals with impetigo.

Follow-Up/Patient/Family Education

A child diagnosed with impetigo can return to school 48 hours after antibiotic treatment is started, or when all sores have crusted and healed. At this point in time, the child will no longer be infectious.

Topical disinfectants, such as hydrogen peroxide, should not be used in the treatment of impetigo.

Impetigo is highly contagious; thus, avoid touching patches of impetigo, and stop other people touching them, too.

Hygiene is important: Always wash your hands after accidentally touching the area.

BURNS

As the largest organ of the body, the skin acts as a protective barrier to invading organisms, immune defenses, and fluid loss. When the skin is burned, it increases the risk of multiorgan injury and puts the patient at risk for systemic infections, such as sepsis, from invading organisms.

The criteria for outpatient management vary based on the center experience and resources. One such set of criteria in an experienced burn center includes burn affecting less than 15% total body surface area (TBSA), therefore not requiring fluid resuscitation; the ability to take in oral fluids, excluding serious perioral burns; no airway involvement or aspiration of hot liquid; no abuse; and dependable family able to transport the patient for clinic appointments. Once the child is ready to reenter school, the physician must discuss with the family and school staff any needs and expectations for the child, including wound care. Social reintegration can be difficult. Educating the teachers and staff of the child's appearance may help prepare the students.

Etiology

There can be various causes and various degrees of pediatric burns; some of the most serious types of burns are sustained in house fires. In addition, up to 20% of pediatric burns are a result of child abuse/neglect. The leading etiologies of pediatric burns seen in an outpatient pediatric setting are scald, thermal, and electrical injuries.

Epidemiology

The mortality rate increases dramatically if there is concomitant inhalation injury in addition to the burn injury.

Focused PE Signs/Findings

Assessment of a child with burn injury includes assessment of ABCs (airway, breathing, and circulation), followed by assessment of the extent of the burn (TBSA and depth of the burns). This is completed with a thorough head-to-toe examination. Using the Lund and Browder chart or the child's palm to represent 1% of the TBSA is more accurate in the pediatric patient than using the standard rule of nines for estimating the TBSA (Sheridan, 2018). Further evaluation of inhalation injury should also be assessed and is often used to risk-assess morbidity of severe burn patients.

A thorough history may involve obtaining information from people who witnessed the incident. Other basic elements, such as past medical history, surgical history, medications, allergies, and last tetanus immunization are critical.

It is also essential to establish the mechanism of the injury, including when and how the burn was sustained. Also, it is important to have a high level of suspicion for red flags for child abuse and neglect and use a detailed history and PE findings (such as pattern markings).

Blisters: These develop when damaged capillaries leak plasma into interstitial space (due to increased vascular permeability). This fluid contains plasma protein, inflammatory mediators, and cellular debris. The high osmolarity of this fluid can cause additional water absorption from underlying tissues, which can increase the local wound tissue pressure and can lead to more ischemia.

The American Burn Association (ABA) recommends that patients with burns >15% TBSA should be admitted and undergo fluid replacement therapy. IV fluid replacement therapy should be calculated in moderate to severe burns.

Lab Tests/Diagnostics

For minor burns (first-degree burns), no lab tests are indicated.

For major burns, transport to a hospital/emergency department (ED) is indicated. Patients should be placed on a cardiac monitor and pulse oximetry. Basic lab studies include a complete blood count (CBC) with differential and type and cross-match (in cases of trauma that may require a transfusion).

A chest x-ray may be indicated if smoke inhalation exposure occurred or is suspected.

Differentials

Burns should be distinguished from the following: pressure ulcers, cellulitis, and wound infections.

Don't Miss

First-degree burns are superficial, dry, and painful to touch and heal in less than 1 week. A second-degree burn is a partial-thickness injury. It presents with blistering of the involved skin and is typically pink or possibly mottled red, with potential weeping at the skin surface, and usually heals in 1 to 3 weeks (Sheridan, 2018). A third-degree burn is the most serious. It appears pearly white, charred, hard, or parchmentlike, and the dead skin (known as eschar) can be tan or black in color. Most burn injuries in children are scald injuries resulting from hot liquids, followed by electrical, chemical, and intentional burn injuries. Electrical burns are a common mechanism of injury in toddlers, as they tend to explore new things with their mouths and have the greatest potential to chew on live wires.

Treatment

Most superficial wounds and some partial-thickness wounds can be managed in a primary care setting. Outpatient management of burns can be divided into 6Cs: clothing, cooling, cleaning, chemoprophylaxis, covering, and comforting. Applying gauze soaked with cold water helps to stop the burn, relieve pain, and remove any chemicals or dirt from the wounds.

The initial management of burns involves assessment of burn depth and TBSA affected, a history, and PE. Calculation of percent of TBSA affected is an important determinant of the necessity for hospitalization versus outpatient management.

Superficial burns do not require any dressing, and patients should be instructed that if a blister forms, then return for further treatment. A skin lubricant, such as a thin layer of ointment, petroleum jelly, or aloe vera, can also be applied to the burn. The ointment does not need to be antibiotic.

Partial- and full-thickness burns should be covered with a sterile dressing after the wound is cleaned and a topical antibiotic is applied.

Electrical burns: Electrical injuries in children are common in children under the age of 2 years, as they often chew on live wires. A child with an oral burn should be irrigated, treated with topical antibiotics, and then referred to the ED for observation. Electrical injury from high voltages can cause arrhythmias.

Burns can be extremely painful. Pain management, which includes pharmacologic and nonpharmacologic approaches, is so important.

Topical treatments, which may provide relief of pruritus, include aloe vera, vaseline-based creams, cocoa butter, mineral oil, hydrogel sheets (e.g., Tegagel, Vigilon, FlexiGel), topical glucocorticoids, colloidal oatmeal in liquid paraffin and EMLA cream, and compression garments. Pain control can be achieved with weight-based dosing of ibuprofen or acetaminophen.

Follow-Up/Patient/Family Education

Teach parents the importance of having functioning smoke detectors, an important fire safety initiative that can prevent house fires and reduce the risk of death in fire by 60% (Sheridan, 2018).

Children should be instructed that in case of fire, hot doors should not be opened, and they should cover their mouth and stay low to avoid smoke inhalation.

PLAQUES

Psoriasis

Etiology

Up to 40% of people with psoriasis have symptoms before they are 16 years old, and 10% get it before they are 10 years old. A variety of clinical psoriasis types are seen in childhood, but plaque-type psoriasis is the most common form, followed by guttate. Other forms include erythrodermic, napkin, and nail-based disease. Like all autoimmune diseases, susceptibility is likely genetic, but environmental triggers are required to initiate disease activity. The most common trigger of childhood is an upper respiratory tract infection.

Epidemiology

There is limited epidemiological data regarding pediatric psoriasis. What is agreed upon is that about 3.5% of the general population is affected by psoriasis and approximately 1/3 of those cases began during childhood or adolescence.

Focused PE Signs/Findings

Psoriasis is a T cell–mediated chronic inflammatory disorder of the skin characterized by hyperproliferation of keratinocytes and consequent red, scaly skin plaques with lesions localized to the scalp, postauricular region, elbows, and knees (Eichenfield et al., 2018).

Erythroderma, pustular disease, including palmoplantar pustular psoriasis, and mucosal/glossitis can be observed as pediatric patterns of cutaneous psoriasis.

Diaper involvement is very common in infancy, but involvement of the groin is uncommon in older children.

Inverse psoriasis with involvement of the folds of the skin (axillae, inner thighs) represents a small minority of children.

Additionally, nail psoriasis can be noted in the setting of plaque-type psoriasis vulgaris, psoriatic arthritis, or isolated nail disease.

Involvement of joints with psoriatic arthritis is less prevalent in younger patients; however, it does occur in childhood disease and should be considered.

Lab Tests/Diagnostics

Biopsy can be helpful in differentiating psoriasis from these other illnesses.

Differentials

Differentials include pediatric arthritis, lichen planopilaris, psoriasiform ID reactions, nummular dermatitis, pityriasis rosea, and pityriasis rubra pilaris.

Don't Miss

Pharyngitis, stress, and trauma are often triggers for this autoimmune disease. Once disease has occurred, treatment is determined based on severity and presence of joint involvement.

Treatment

Topical therapies, including corticosteroids and calcipotriene, are the therapies of choice in the initial care of pediatric patients. Ultraviolet light, acitretin, and cyclosporine can clear skin symptoms, whereas methotrexate and etanercept can clear both cutaneous and joint diseases. Therapy should take into account several factors, including area of involvement, type and thickness of psoriasis, and age of the patient. In addition to topical steroids, other treatment options include phototherapy, calcineurin inhibitors, topical vitamin D analogues, tazarotene (off label), anthralin, methotrexate, and coal tar.

Despite the differences in pediatric psoriasis, the therapies used for pediatric psoriasis are essentially the same as those used in adulthood, with dosage and strength reductions calculated based on age, weight, and available formulations.

Prevention

While there are pharmacologic and nonpharmacologic things that can be done to control flare-ups, there is no cure for psoriasis.

Follow-Up/Patient/Family Education

Teach patients that while there is no cure, in addition to pharmacologic therapies, they can use moisturizing lotions, try to avoid dry or cold weather, use a humidifier, and get some sun, but not too much.

PRURITIS

Approach to a Child With Pruritis

Pruritus (itching) is a common symptom in pediatrics, rather than a specific disease. Pruritis may also be a presenting feature in other system disorders, specifically neurologic and psychiatric disorders. In addition, some drinks and foods can aggravate pruritus. These include caffeine-containing drinks, tomatoes, chocolate, and nuts.

Etiology

Dermatitis accounts for up to 90% of pruritus in childhood.

Epidemiology

The most common cause of itching in children is skin disease (rather than systemic illness). Pruritus is a common symptom that almost everyone experiences at some point in their lives. Sometimes in younger pediatric patients, it may be the only symptom. It is important to assess the patient with ongoing pruritus.

Symptoms

Itching

Focused PE Signs/Findings

See Table 9.1.

Lab Tests/Diagnostics

The initial evaluation should be made based on PE findings. While labs are not typically ordered, it is possible to rule out systemic disease with several labs including the following:

- CBC with differential to evaluate for iron deficiency and/or malignancy
- Serum bilirubin, transaminases, and alkaline phosphatase to look for liver disease
- Thyroid-stimulating hormone for thyroid disorders
- Blood urea nitrogen and creatinine for renal disease
- Chest radiograph for adenopathy

Differentials

Differentials for pruritus include infestations, such as scabies, pediculosis, and insect bites, or skin conditions such as AD, miliaria, contact dermatitis, and acute or chronic urticaria.

Prevention and Follow-Up/Patient Education

A detailed, careful history and thorough PE are important in the evaluation of a child with pruritus. In addition, identifying and avoiding the aggravating agent causing the pruritus is significant. If treatment is recommended, teach parents/children to closely follow treatment.

Pruritus that is limited to a specific area usually suggests a specific local cause. Systemic causes are usually associated with generalized pruritus. Timing is important to note in the history of pruritus. Pruritus from bedbugs and pinworm infestation usually occur at night. A recent onset suggests an infection, insect bite, drug reaction, urticaria, or contact dermatitis. Chronic pruritus is more common with AD or a chronic systemic illness.

Dry skin (xerosis), eczema (dermatitis), psoriasis, scabies, insect bites, and hives are some of the most common causes of pruritis in the pediatric patient.

Table 9.1

Common Pruritic Rashes in Pediatric Patients

Name	Etiology/Epidemiology	Symptoms/Other Clinical Manifestations	Treatment	Key Points
AD (aka atopic eczema)	Children with allergic rhinitis and asthma (the atopic triad) have a higher likelihood of developing AD.	Clinical features of AD include skin dryness, erythema, and crusting. Pruritus is a hallmark of the condition and is referred to as **the itch that scratches.** Scratching can lead to more inflammation and palpable thickening of affected skin (litchenification). Varying degrees of atopy: **Mild:** areas of dry skin, infrequent itching **Moderate:** areas of dry skin, frequent itching, redness (with or without excoriation and localized skin thickening) **Severe:** widespread areas of dry skin, incessant itching, redness (with or without excoriation, extensive skin thickening, bleeding, oozing, cracking, and alteration of pigmentation).	**Initial treatment:** Topically applied corticosteroids and emollients are the mainstay of therapy for AD. **Topical corticosteroids:** Treatment for **mild AD**: Low-potency corticosteroid cream (apply one to two times a day for 2–4 weeks (examples include desonide 0.05% or hydrocortisone 2.5%) Treatment for **moderate AD**: Medium- to high-potency corticosteroids (examples include fluocinolone 0.025% or betamethasone dipropionate 0.05%). Treatment for **severe AD**: Or in patients with an acute flare of AD, superhigh- or high-potency topical corticosteroids can be used (for 1–2 weeks) and then substituted with lower potency until the dermatitis resolves. **Second-line** therapy: Topical calcineurin inhibitors are generally recognized as being equal in strength to medium-potency topical steroids and should be considered a second-line therapy. Pimecrolimus 1% cream is a calcineurin inhibitor (inhibits cytokine production); it was developed specifically to treat inflammatory skin conditions.	Important considerations when prescribing high-dose topical steroids include adrenal suppression as a potential side effect in long-term dose. The face and skin folds are areas that are at high risk for atrophy with corticosteroids. Always examine the palms, soles, and mucous membranes of a pediatric patient with a rash. A rash limited to the trunk and extremities tends to be less serious than if the palms, soles, and mucous membranes are involved. Numbers are important in a rash because patients with tinea typically have only between one and five papulosquamous lesions. An annular plaque that looks like tinea is not tinea if there is no scale on the surface. Systemic symptoms, such as malaise, myalgias, photophobia, or joint swelling with a rash that appears to be eczematous, suggest an underlying systemic disease, such as lupus or dermatomyositis. Eczema is much more common than scabies, but scabies is likely if burrows are evident in the palms, if there is scaling between the fingers, and if the classic burrow lines appear on the wrists or ankles. Remember to rule out milk allergy in infantile eczema. Adverse side effects of calcineurin inhibitors include erythema, burning, and itching at the site.

| Contact dermatitis | Primary irritant contact dermatitis and allergic contact dermatitis are the two types. **Primary irritant contact dermatitis** is a nonallergic reaction to prolonged or repetitive contact with chemical irritants. | Type IV hypersensitivity reaction | |
| Urticaria | Urticaria is the result of dilation and increased capillary permeability and leads to edema of the upper corneum. **Type I** hypersensitivity to food, drugs, inhalants, and insect venoms is the most common mechanism, but **type II** (transfusion reaction) hypersensitivity or **type III** (serum sickness) hypersensitivity are also possible. Other types of urticaria include cold urticaria, solar urticaria, and pressure-induced urticaria. | Palpable, raised, and well-circumscribed wheals that blanch with pressure and typically resolve within a few hours. | Antihistamines are common first-line therapy to treat itch. Examples include diphenhydramine (Benadryl) or hydroxyzine (Atarax). | Remember if it is non-blanching when pressed, it is not urticaria. |

(continued)

Chapter **9**   Dermatologic Abnormalities Commonly Seen in Pediatric Primary Care

Table 9.1

Common Pruritic Rashes in Pediatric Patients (continued)

Name	Etiology/Epidemiology	Symptoms/Other Clinical Manifestations	Treatment	Key Points
Insect bites	Insect bites are especially a common cause of pruritis.			Papular urticaria is a delayed hypersensitivity reaction to an insect bite, is very itchy, and commonly presents to pediatric primary or urgent care.
Pediculosis capitis (aka head lice)	3% of school-aged children are affected with head lice. The louse infests only the human head; it sucks blood and secretes saliva, which results in an inflammatory reaction and itching.	Pediculosis capitis (head lice), pediculosis corporis (body lice), and pediculosis pubis (pubic lice aka crabs).		
Xerosis (aka dry skin)		Xerosis is the most common cause of itching in the absence of a rash.	Non–alcohol-based moisturizers, such as Aquaphor Baby Healing Ointment or Cetaphil Moisturizing Cream.	Teach parents to apply moisturizers while their child's skin is still a little wet to help trap in some moisture.

AD, atopic dermatitis.

RASH

■ POPULAR RASH

Warts and Molluscum Contagiosum

There are various types of warts (shown in Box 9.1), and they are caused by many different viruses. One more common group of viruses is the human papillomaviruses (HPVs) that infect epithelial tissues of skin and mucous membranes (American Academy of Dermatology Association, 2019). The most common clinical manifestations of HPV infection are warts (verrucae). There are various types of HPV. HPV type 1 commonly infects the soles of the feet and produces plantar warts, whereas HPV types 6 and 11 infect the anogenital area and cause anogenital warts (not covered here).

BOX 9.1 TYPES OF WARTS

Filiform warts often show up on areas such as the eyelids and around the mouth and nose and resemble skin tags.

Common warts are rough bumps on the skin. They can be anywhere but often seen on the hands. They may bleed if picked at.

Plantar warts appear as rough patches on the soles of the feet. They are often painful and can grow very large.

Flat warts look like very small flat, smooth bumps. They are often seen on the face.

Molluscum contagiosum is very common in children. It often has multiple papules with umbilicated center. It is highly contagious and often spread in daycare and other childcare centers and can be worsen in children with eczema.

Etiology

Warts, or verruca, are a very common skin infection caused by a virus. Children develop warts more often than adults. Warts are a benign growth of skin and less often mucosa. The human papillomavirus (HPV) is the virus responsible for causing warts. There are over 100 subtypes of HPV. The most common subtypes in warts are 2 and 4.

Epidemiology

Warts can occur at any age. They are unusual in infancy and early childhood. The incidence increases as children reach school age and prevalence among school-aged children is 10% to 20%. Prevalence peaks at 12 to 16 years.

Focused PE Signs/Findings

It is important to recognize the different types of warts (see Box 9.1).

Lab Tests/Diagnostics

Diagnosis is based on history and PE findings.

Differentials

The following are the differentials of rashes: common warts, filiform, plantar, flat, molluscum contagiosum, seborrheic warts.

Treatment

Most warts go away on their own after several months, so often treatment is not needed. While warts are a virus, and there is no treatment to "cure" warts, there are treatment options.

Initial treatment with topical salicylic acid (or other OTC medical irritants) and medical tape is usually recommended.

Salicylic Acid: Solutions of 17% salicylic acid are readily available OTC (such as compound W). Soak wart for 5 minutes in warm water; file down the wart by removing layers of dead skin with a callus file, emery board, or pumice stone; and then cover the wart with the salicylic acid and then medical or duct tape (both may also be purchased at a pharmacy/drug store). Repeat this process every 1 to 3 days until the wart is gone. Treatment may take several months.

Other treatments include the following:

- Freezing the wart with liquid nitrogen
- Applying an electrical current to the wart (electrocautery)
- Excising the wart
- Removing the wart with laser surgery

Don't Miss

Surgical excision and cautery are no longer recommended and often not covered by insurance plans, as they are often not curative and have been shown to increase the likelihood of localized spread.

Prevention

If treatment is recommended, teach parents and child to closely follow treatment for prescribed treatment period exactly as suggested. Encourage parents to teach children not to pick, bite, or scratch warts, as these can spread the virus.

Viral Exanthems

An exanthem is any skin rash that may be associated with fever or other systemic symptoms. Infections, in particular viral infections, are the most common causes of exanthems in children. Some exanthems have very specific patterns of eruption and other characteristics that help identify and manage them. For example, rashes caused by viral infections may cause reddish or pink spots over large parts of the body, such as the chest and back. Many viral rashes do not itch. Viral rashes are often seen on both the right and left sides of the body as opposed to one side. Table 9.2 reviews the most common pediatric viral exanthems. Perhaps 95% of pediatric rashes seen in primary care have an inflammatory component and, therefore, will be red; a rash that is not red is unusual and may require referral to a dermatologist for accurate identification (Arango & Jones, 2017).

SKIN ABSCESS, FOLLICULITIS, AND CELLULITIS

Clinical Manifestations

Common skin and soft tissue infections that pediatric patients may present with are skin abscesses, folliculitis, or cellulitis or any combination of these.

Skin Abscess

A skin abscess can be caused by more than one pathogen; the most common cause of skin abscess is *Staphylococcus aureus* (either methicillin-susceptible or methicillin-resistant *S. aureus*), which occurs in up to 75% of cases. Most abscesses are due to infection.

Table 9.2

The Most Common Pediatric Viral Exanthems

Name	Etiology	Focused PE Signs/Findings	Symptoms/Other Clinical Manifestations	Don't Miss/Key Points	Treatment
Erythema infectiosum (fifth disease)	Parovirus B19	Characteristic slapped cheek appearance, lacy rash	Erythematous rash; reticular extremities; rash may come and go over several weeks; aplastic crisis possible	Slapped cheek	Viral exanthems are self-limiting; supportive therapy includes acetaminophen for pain/discomfort; symptomatic treatment with resolution within several weeks
Measles (rubeola)	Measles virus	Begins at the hairline and spreads inferiorly (downward)	Erythematous macules and papules begin on the face; characteristic Kolpik spots, coryza and conjunctivitis, high fever	Kolpik spots	
Scarlet fever	Streptococcus pyogenes	Begins on the face and upper part of the trunk and spreads downward	Strawberry tongue, exudative pharyngitis, abdominal pain, rheumatic fever	Scarlatiniform rash	
Roseola (roseola infantum)	Human herpesvirus 6 and 7	Maculopapular rash; rose-pink appearance	Febrile seizures, lymphadenopathy	Rose-pink maculopapular rash	
Hand–foot–and–mouth disease	Coxsackie virus	Vesicles on an erythematous base	Vesicles on hands and feet and in the mouth (can be limited to just one area or all)	Highly contagious	
Varicella	Herpes zoster virus	Vesicles on an erythematous base that crust over; spreads from head and trunk proximodistal to extremities	Latent zoster infection; extreme pruritus	"Dew drop on a rose petal" rash	
Rubella	Rubvirus	Maculopapular rash; rose-pink appearance; spreads inferiorly	Forchheimer spots, lymphadenopathy, arthralgias	Forchheimer spots	

PE, physical exam.

Folliculitis

This is inflammation of one or more hair follicles. The diagnosis is often established clinically; rarely, Gram stain and culture or skin biopsy may be warranted to differentiate folliculitis from other conditions.

Cellulitis

This involves the deeper dermis layer of the skin and subcutaneous fat. It manifests as areas of skin erythema, edema, and warmth, resulting from a break in the skin barrier and entry of bacteria. Fever will likely be present. Lower extremities are the most common site of involvement.

Focused PE Findings/Symptoms

Purulence and localized lymphadenopathy, which may lead to an "orange peel" texture in the skin. Orbital cellulitis (shown as +EOMs) is a less common type of cellulitis around the eye orbit, but more serious and treated aggressively (patient should be admitted for intravenous [IV] antibiotics), as there is a risk for vision loss.

Lab Tests/Diagnostics

Not required.

Clinical Manifestations

Cellulitis = skin erythema, edema, and warmth

Skin abscess = painful erythematous nodule

Folliculitis = inflamed erythematous follicles.

Differential Diagnosis

Skin infections must be distinguished from the following infections: erythema migrans, septic arthritis, osteomyelitis, drug reaction, dermatitis, folliculitis, and abscess.

Treatment

Treatment usually includes oral antibiotic therapy. For more severe cases of cellulitis, IV antibiotics may be warranted. In addition, an incision and drainage (I&D) may be needed.

Don't Miss

Complications of cellulitis and skin abscess can include systemic spread of infection, leading to bacteremia, sepsis, and osteomyelitis, and complications of folliculitis include hair loss, skin scarring, or boils under the skin (furunculosis). Recurrent or spreading of the infection can be a complication of all of these skin infections.

References

American Academy of Dermatology Association. (2019). *Warts: Diagnosis and treatment.* Retrieved from https://www.aad.org/public/diseases/a-z/warts-treatment

Arango, C., & Jones, R. (2017). 8 viral exanthems of childhood. *Journal of Family Practice, 66*(10), 598–606.

Eichenfield, L., Paller, A., Tom, W. L., Sugarman, J., Hebert, A. A., Friedlander, S., . . . Cordoro, K. (2018). Pediatric psoriasis: Evolving perspectives. *Pediatric Dermatology, 35*(2), 170–181. doi:10.1111/pde.13382

Mannschreck, D., Feig, J., Selph, J., & Cohen, B. (2020). Disseminated bullous impetigo and atopic dermatitis: Case series and literature review. *Pediatric Dermatology, 37*(1), 103–108. doi:10.1111/pde.14032

Özçelik, S., Kulaç, İ., Yazıcı, M., & Öcal, E. (2018). Distribution of childhood skin diseases according to age and gender, a single institution experience. *Turk pediatri arsivi, 53*(2), 105–112. doi:10.5152/TurkPediatriArs.2018.6431

Sheridan, R. (2018). Burn care of children. *Pediatrics in Review, 39*(6), 273–296. doi:10.1542/pir.2016-0179

Common Pediatric Renal/Urologic Disorders Seen in Pediatric Primary Care

Michael S. Ruggiero

INTRODUCTION

Renal disease is a major cause of morbidity and mortality. Pediatric patients with renal disease, especially younger ones, may present with nonspecific signs and symptoms. Pediatric clinicians should be familiar with the modes of presentation of common renal disorders in the pediatric population. Pediatric patients may present with abnormal urinalysis, urinary tract infections (UTIs), or other signs and symptoms of a renal disorder. The role of the pediatric clinician and the approach to care of the child with common renal or urologic problems are presented in this chapter.

OBJECTIVES

1. Examine factors that contribute to the most common causes of dysuria, scrotal and penile pain, hematuria, and urethral and vaginal discharge in the pediatric population.
2. Identify common presenting clinical symptoms and clinical problems that are associated with dysuria, scrotal and penile pain, hematuria, and urethral and vaginal discharge.
3. Determine appropriate treatment options for these clinical problems.

DYSURIA

Dysuria is defined as painful urination. Painful urination in children manifests in different ways. The neonate and infant will present differently than the school-aged child and teenager. Dysuria can be broken down into two basic classifications: infectious and noninfectious. In this chapter, the focus will be on the most common cause of dysuria in children, which is infectious. The most common cause is a UTI. The following few pages will aim to guide the provider through identification, workup, and treatment of the pediatric patient with a UTI.

Urinary Tract Infection (UTI)

UTI is a common and important cause of illness, both febrile and afebrile, in infants and children, so much so that some estimates have UTIs accounting for up to 14% of pediatric ED visits. UTIs are infections that affect the bladder, known as cystitis, or the kidneys, known as pyelonephritis. Cystitis is known as a lower UTI, whereas pyelonephritis is known as an upper tract infection. Like many other pediatric disorders, presentation, workup, and treatment are specific to age. Most literature separates pediatric UTIs into age categories of neonates (both full and preterm): 2 months, 2 months to 2 years, and older than 2 years.

Etiology

Despite the age or sex of the child, *Escherichia coli* is the most common cause of UTIs, in both lower and upper tract infections. *E. coli* is the cause in greater than 80% of the UTIs and is due to ascending migration and, to a much lesser degree, homogenous spread. Less common organisms are *Klebsiella*, *Proteus*, and *Staphylococcus*. The exceptions to this are in the preterm neonate, children with indwelling catheters, and children who acquire their infection during or just after a hospital stay (nosocomial or hospital acquired). In these cases, approximately 50% are still due to *E. coli*, but there is significantly increased prevalence of *Candida* infections, *Klebsiella*, *Staphylococcus*, *Enterococcus*, and *Enterobacter* infections (Arshad & Seed, 2015).

Epidemiology

This is one of the most common bacterial infections in children. Prevalence depends on age. The highest rate for males is age less than 1 year and for females, less than 4 years. Females overall have four times greater a prevalence than boys. Uncircumcised boys have tenfold greater an incidence compared with circumcised boys. It is worth noting that in children less than 60 days old, uncircumcised males have the highest rate of UTIs of both sexes (Arshad & Seed, 2015).

Focused Physical Exam Signs, Symptoms, and Workup

The most common presenting symptoms of a child with a UTI less than 2 years of age is a fever. All neonates with fever of undetermined origin should have a urine sample sent for urinalysis and urine culture with sensitivity. Other signs/symptoms of UTI include blood in the urine, cloudy urine, foul-smelling or strong urine odor, frequent or urgent need to urinate, general ill feeling (malaise), pain or burning with urination, or enuresis after a period when the child has been toilet-trained. Physical exam (PE) may be normal but be sure to assess for any flank pain (with pyelonephritis) or any pressure or pain in the lower pelvis or lower back (UTI or pyelonephritis; see Table 10.1).

Lab Tests/Diagnostic Testing

Diagnostic testing is required to confirm the diagnosis of a UTI. Clinical manifestations help to determine who needs further workup for a UTI but will depend on urine sample to confirm the diagnosis and help determine treatment and follow up. Because collection of urine in young children is invasive, that is, catheterization or suprapubic aspiration, several organizations have developed guidelines and probability tools to help guide clinicians as to whether they should proceed with urine collection for children between the ages of 2 months and 2 years (Cherry, Demmler-Harrison, Kaplan, Steinbach, & Hotez, 2019). Any neonate with fever and no identifiable source of infection should have a urine sample collected, as should children with fever and no obvious source of infection. Any child with any of the following should prompt strong consideration for urine collection: urinary signs such as painful urination, foul-smelling urine, and hematuria and nonurinary signs such as poor feeding, jaundice, and vomiting (Balighian & Burke, 2018).

Table 10.1

Urinary Tract Infections: Age-Based Presentation, Workup, and Treatment			
	Neonate (< 2 months old)	**2–24 months old**	**Older than 2 years**
Symptoms	Occult/no subjective information	Occult/no subjective information Crying with urination may be noted	**Dysuria** **Increased frequency** of nausea Increased urgency Abdominal pain **Flank pain (pyelonephritis)**
Signs	**Fever** **Vomiting** **Poor feeding** **Irritability** **Foul-smelling urine** Apnea Tachypnea Jaundice Hematuria *Most diagnosed UTIs in neonates are of the upper tract (pyelonephritis)*	**Fever** **Vomiting** **Poor feeding** **Irritable** **Foul-smelling urine** Hematuria Jaundice	Fever Vomiting Suprapubic tenderness Hematuria CVA percussion tenderness (pyelonephritis)
Workup	Urinalysis **Urine culture and sensitivity (>10,000 CFU/mL)** *Catheterization Specimen* **Bacteremia workup** CBC Blood cultures LP if febrile Bilirubin if jaundice	Urinalysis **Urine culture and sensitivity (10,000–50,000 CFU/mL with pyuria)** Or **(>50,000 CFU/mL)** *Catheterization Specimen* **Bacteremia workup** CBC Blood cultures LP if febrile Bilirubin if jaundice **If well appearing and not febrile, no reason to do bacteremia workup**	Urine dip **(LE, nitrites, blood)** Urine culture and sensitivity **(>50,000 CFU/mL)** *Clean catch*
Empiric treatment (Treatment can be targeted once culture and sensitivity are back.)	**Admit** Empiric treatment with **ampicillin and gentamicin** **If nosocomial infection** is suspected, **treat with vancomycin and gentamicin.**	Can manage on outpatient basis unless high risk (outlined below) **Cefuroxime** 30 mg/kg per day by mouth in two divided doses for 10 days Or **Cefixime** 16 mg/kg by mouth on the first day, followed by 8 mg/kg once daily for 10 days	Can manage on outpatient basis unless high risk (see below) **Cefixime** 8 mg/kg every 24 hours or divided every 12 hours for 7 days for afebrile and 10 days for febrile

(continued)

Table 10.1

Urinary Tract Infections: Age-Based Presentation, Workup, and Treatment (*continued*)

	Neonate (< 2 months old)	2–24 months old	Older than 2 years
Follow-up and referral	**Renal US and VCUG:** once treatment and infection cleared **Renal ultrasound:** any child not responding to treatment to rule out abscess A pediatric urology referral for structural abnormalities on imaging	**Renal US and VCUG:** once treatment and infection cleared **Renal ultrasound:** any child not responding to treatment to rule out abscess A pediatric urology referral for patients with recurrent UTI or abnormalities on imaging	**Renal US and VCUG:** ■ Boys with first UTI ■ Girls <3 years old with first UTI ■ Child with febrile UTI ■ First UTI and family history of renal disease ■ Renal US: any child not responding to antibiotics A pediatric urology referral for patients with recurrent UTI or abnormalities on imaging
Complications	At increased risk of bacteremia and meningitis Increased association with CAKUT At increased risk for renal scarring (Arshad & Seed, 2015)	Recurrent febrile UTIs may lead to renal scarring.	Recurrent febrile UTIs may lead to renal scarring.

CAKUT, congenital anomalies of the kidney and urinary tract; CBC, complete blood count; CVA, cerebrovascular accident; LE, leukocyte esterase; LP, lumbar puncture; US, ultrasound; UTI, urinary tract infection; VCUG, voiding cystourethrogram.
Source: Arshad, M., & Seed, P. (2015). Urinary tract infections in the infant. *Clinics in Perinatology, 42*(1), 17–22. doi:10.1016/j.clp.2014.10.003

Admitting Patients With Suspected UTI

Identifying patients at high risk for complications associated with UTI is vital. The following are some identifiers of high-risk patients: less than 2 months old, signs of urosepsis, toxic appearance, hypotension, decreased capillary perfusion, immunocompromised, vomiting, worsening despite outpatient treatment, and less than 2 years old with a fever.

Noninfectious Causes of Dysuria

Urethritis in nonsexually active children is a common cause of noninfectious dysuria. This is typically due to urethral irritation from chemical soaps and lotions. Bubble baths are a common cause of this irritation. The patient presents with localized urinary symptoms without fever and without systemic symptoms. Urinalysis is unremarkable.

Infectious urethritis is covered later in this chapter, under the "Urethral and Vaginal Discharge" section.

HEMATURIA

There are few symptoms that bring more worry to patients and parents than gross hematuria. This chapter will focus on the approach to gross hematuria, focusing on the workup and management and exploring some of the most common causes.

■ GROSS HEMATURIA

Gross hematuria is defined as urine that has a substantial enough number of red blood cells (RBCs) in it to be visible without microscopy. It often presents as brown, tea-colored, or red/pink.

Epidemiology

Macroscopic hematuria has an estimated incidence of 1.3 per 1,000 children. Glomeruli, renal tubules and interstitium, or urinary tract (including collecting systems, ureters, bladder, and urethra) are all sources for gross hematuria.

Lab Tests/Diagnosis

The first step in the diagnosis of gross hematuria is to see if it is truly hematuria, as opposed to pigmenturia, such as myoglobinuria and hemoglobinuria (as outlined in Tables 10.2 and 10.3). Office-based urine dip sticks and laboratory urinalysis with microscopy are helpful in differentiating this.

Microscopic urinalysis is used to help assess the source of the urinary tract bleed. Microscopic findings of RBCs and RBC casts are suggestive of a glomerular source.

A quick way to distinguish myoglobinuria/hemoglobinuria from true hematuria in the office setting is to centrifuge the urine. Centrifuging the urine will separate the RBCs from the urine in cases of true hematuria. In cases of myoglobinuria or hemoglobinuria, the urine will stay pink/red/brown without separation.

Using ammonium sulfate to precipitate hemoglobin in the urine and then centrifuging it will cause separation. In myoglobinuria, the sample will stay in the supernate.

Imaging can be used to identify renal stones and congenital abnormalities of the urinary system. CT scans have been the gold standard; however, with its high radiation, ultrasound (US) is being used more frequently and is, in most cases, a sound first option.

All cases of hematuria need a renal function assessment; a minimum of serum creatinine and BUN are necessary to assess for acute renal failure.

In cases of hematuria that are believed to be from a glomerulonephritis as outlined in Table 10.4, further investigation may be necessary with more specific blood work, such as ANA, C3 and C4 compliment, IgA nephropathy, ANCA, and ant streptolysin O.

Table 10.2

Differentiating Between Gross Hematuria and Pigmenturia

Urine Dipstick	Microscopic Urinalysis	Hematuria or Pigmenturia
Positive	Positive	True hematuria
Positive	Negative for red blood cells	Hemoglobinuria or myoglobinuria
Negative	Negative	Dye, pigment in food or drink, medication (rifampin)

Table 10.3

The Differential for Hematuria, Hemoglobinuria, and Myoglobinuria

Hematuria	Hemoglobinuria	Myoglobinuria
Urinary tract infection	Paroxysmal cold	Rhabdomyolysis
Nephrolithiasis	hemoglobinuria	Electrocution
Hypercalciuria	Paroxysmal nocturnal	
Trauma	hemoglobinuria	
Hemorrhagic cystitis	Hemolytic uremic syndrome	
Glomerular causes IgA nephropathy,		
poststrep glomerulonephritis, lupus		
nephritis, HSP, Alport syndrome		
Coagulopathies		
Sickle cell disease		
AVM		

AVM, arteriovenous malformation; HSP, Henoch–Schönlein purpura; IgA, Immunoglobulin A.

PENILE PAIN

■ PAINLESS SCROTAL SWELLING

Painless scrotal swelling can often be dramatic in presentation but tends most often not to be an emergency. Common causes of scrotal swelling will be reviewed (see Table 10.5).

Don't Miss

Scrotal swelling that is accompanied by purpuric or petechial rash should raise suspicion for underlying Henoch–Schönlein Purpura (HSP) or Kawasaki's disease (Chapter 13, Endocrine Abnormalities Commonly Seen in Pediatric Primary Care). Testicular cancer is always in the differential for scrotal complaints, and palpation of a testicular mass is grounds for referral for US and urology consultation.

■ PARAPHIMOSIS

Paraphimosis is seen in uncircumcised males and is the inability to return the retracted foreskin to the normal position. This leads to a tourniquet effects to the glans penis.

Epidemiology

In uncircumcised males, the foreskin is retracted by the patient, caretaker, or medical provider and not returned promptly to the normal position. This can happen during cleaning and self-care or after an examination. This condition can happen at any age.

Symptoms

Pain tends to be the primary complaint along with urinary tract obstruction or voiding symptoms.

Table 10.4

Common Causes of Hematuria and Pigmenturia (Red-Brown Urine)

	Definition	Etiology	Signs and Symptoms	Workup	Treatment/Referral	
UTI	Inflammation and infection of the bladder or kidney	Most common is *Escherichia coli* (see Table 10.1)	Dysuria, increased frequency and urgency, hematuria	See Workup in Table 10.1	See Empiric Treatment in Table 10.1	
HUS	Clinical syndrome characterized by the triad of thrombotic microangiopathy, thrombocytopenia, and acute kidney injury	Common causes of acute renal damage in children STEC is the most common cause of HUS, *E. coli* O157:H7. Responsible for 90% of childhood HUS cases It most commonly occurs in children aged 5–7 years.	Hematuria, abdominal pain, nausea, vomiting, diarrhea, decreased urine, increased proteinuria in serum creatinine	Hemolytic anemia, thrombocytopenia, and renal damage For a definite diagnosis, Shiga toxin present in stool cultures.	Hospitalize adjustment of fluid and electrolyte balance, control of blood pressure, possibly dialysis	*Pneumococcus*-related HUS: Patients affected have a history of pneumococcus pneumonia infection. The diagnosis is made definitively with growth of *Streptococcus pneumoniae* in blood, pleural fluid, or cerebrospinal fluid cultures.
Rhabdomyolysis	Rapid destruction of injured myocytes	Traumatic injury drugs or toxins infections, muscle ischemia exertion, prolonged bed rest, hypo/hyperthermia	Weakness, myalgia, swelling, myoglobinuria.	Urine pigmented. Urine dip is positive for blood. Microscopic urinalysis is negative for blood. Serum CPK elevated.	Hospitalization supportive care, IV hydration, electrolyte regulation, possible dialysis for renal failure.	Acute renal failure occurs in about one third of all patients.

(continued)

Chapter **10** Common Pediatric Renal/Urologic Disorders Seen in Pediatric Primary Care

Table 10.4

Common Causes of Hematuria and Pigmenturia (Red-Brown Urine) (continued)

	Definition	Etiology	Signs and Symptoms	Workup	Treatment/Referral
Nephrolithiasis	Mineral stone in the urinary system, originating from the kidney	Hypercalciuria (idiopathic, hyperparathyroid, hypo/hyperthyroid, adrenal insufficiency, milk alkaline syndrome, adrenocorticosteroid excess)	Abdominal pain, flank pain, groin pain, nausea, vomiting, hematuria	Urinalysis, renal ultrasound, +/– CT scan, stone analysis, urine culture, spot urine CA:creatinine ratio, serum chemistrypanel, including creatinine, 24-hour urine	Children should be transferred to the emergency department for pain control and imaging. Obstructing stone in the setting of a UTI can rapidly lead to sepsis.
Glomerulonephritis PSGN/IgA/lupus/ HSP	Inflammation of the glomeruli, impairing the kidneys filtering ability	Autoimmune.	Hematuria, proteinuria, HTN, edema periorbital or peripheral, HSP—purpuric rash, PSGN—recent history of sore throat/ strep throat, IgA nephropathy—recent history of URI or GI symptoms, lupus—history of myalgia/ arthralgia/rash/malar rash.	Urine dip hematuria and proteinuria Urinalysis with microscopy will show RBCs and RBC casts. Serum BUN/creatinine Further workup to identify specific causes, such as ANA, C3 and C4 compliment, IgA, ANCA, and antistreptolysin O	Acute renal failure requires hospitalization for supportive care and possible dialysis. Patients with stable renal function and urine output can be worked up as outpatients. An urgent referral to a nephrologist is recommended.

ANA, antinuclear antibody; ANCA, antineutrophil cytoplasmic antibody; BUN, blood urea nitrogen; CA, calcium; CPK, creatine phosphokinase; GI, gastrointestinal; HSP, Henoch–Schönlein purpura; HTN, hypertension; HUS, hemolytic uremic syndrome; IgA, Immunoglobulin A; IV, intravenous; PSGN, poststreptococcal glomerulonephritis; RBC, red blood cells; STEC, Shiga toxin-producing *Escherichia coli*; URI, upper respiratory infection; UTI, urinary tract infection.

Table 10.5

Common Causes of Scrotal Swelling

	Varicocele	Hydrocele	Inguinal Hernia
Definition	Dilation of pampiniform plexus in the scrotum	Accumulation of peritoneal fluid into the scrotum through a patent processes vaginalis	Congenital or acquired defect of the processus vaginalis, allowing bowel into the inguinal canal and scrotum
Epidemiology	15% of adolescent males; Rare in patients under 10 years old 95% are left-sided.	Most common in newborns In older boys, hydrocele may develop because of testicular or epididymis inflammation.	Hernia is present in approximately 5% of all newborns. It is more common in boys than girls.
Exam	Exam performed in the standing position reveals scrotal swelling. Palpation reveals soft engorged vasculature around the spermatic cord often described as a "bag of worms" feeling. Valsalva maneuver may make the varicocele more prominent.	Painless scrotal swelling transilluminates on examination. Swelling tends to get worse with prolonged standing and crying and lessens with lying supine. Testicles are normal on examination.	Mass/bulge in the groin that is usually most prominent when there is increased abdominal pressure, that is, crying or straining. Scrotal swelling occurs with bowel in the scrotum. Bowel sound and peristalsis may sometimes be present.
Diagnosis	Clinical diagnosis	Clinical diagnosis	Clinical diagnosis
Treatment	No specific treatment for uncomplicated varicoceles.	Most hydroceles resolve by the second year of life. For persistent hydroceles, surgical intervention is recommended.	A surgical referral for repair is recommended.
Don't Miss	Right-sided varicoceles should raise suspicion for abdominal tumor and prompt abdominal imaging. Large varicoceles or varicoceles associated with testicular atrophy should be surgically referred to help preserve normal fertility.	Most hydroceles resolve by 1 to 2 years of age. Persistent hydroceles should be referred to urology. Hydroceles can be associated with testicular tumor, so it is imperative that full testicular exam is performed. If the hydrocele is hindering a complete and thorough testicular exam, then an ultrasound and urology referral is recommended.	Hernias that cannot be easily reduced should be sent for immediate surgical evaluation. Incarcerated and strangulated hernias are surgical emergencies.

Focused PE Signs

The glans penis is swollen due to venous and lymphatic congestions. The foreskin is seen proximal to the glans, with an inability to restore the foreskin to its normal resting position covering the head of the penis. Diagnostics are unnecessary, as this is a clinical diagnosis.

Treatment

Immediate manual reduction of the foreskin is recommended. If manual reduction cannot be performed, then an emergent referral to a medical center with surgical capabilities is required. Even if manual reduction is performed, the caregivers (if applicable) and patient should be instructed to avoid retraction of the foreskin for 1 week. Urology consultation should also be arranged, and discussion of preventative circumcision should be had.

Complications

Prolonged paraphimosis can lead to tissue necrosis and even possibly autoamputation.

Don't Miss

Penile pain can also be the result from a hair tourniquet. This occurs when hair or thread from clothing gets wrapped around the penis causing ischemia. Providers should perform a thorough inspection of the penis and scrotum to look for foreign bodies and hair/thread tourniquets.

SCROTAL AND PENILE PAIN

■ THE ACUTE SCROTUM

An acute scrotum is defined as testicular swelling with acute pain and can reflect multiple etiologies, including epididymitis, torsion of the spermatic cord, or torsion of the testicular appendages. Quick and accurate diagnosis of acute scrotum and its etiology are necessary because a delayed diagnosis of torsion for as little as 6 hours can cause irreparable testicular damage.

■ EPIDIDYMITIS

Inflammation of the epididymis is known as epididymitis. The epididymis is located along the posterior aspect of the testicle. Epididymitis can be acute, subacute, or chronic. Acute epididymitis will be the focus in this section. Identification of epididymitis is important, as early treatment can prevent long-term complications such as chronic pain. Several factors may predispose postpubertal boys to develop subacute epididymitis, including sexual activity, heavy physical exertion, and direct trauma (e.g., bicycle or motorcycle riding). Bacterial epididymitis in prepubertal boys is associated with structural anomalies of the urinary tract (McConaghy & Panchal, 2016).

Etiology

The etiologies include an ascending infection, viral causes, urinary reflux, and structural and functional anomalies of the urinary tract. Most cases of epididymitis in children are idiopathic without bacteriuria. Bacterial causes are likely to be from urine reflux and ascending infection from UTI; in these cases, *E. coli* is the most common bacterial infection. In teens who are sexually active, *Neisseria gonorrhoeae* and *Chlamydia trachomatis* are the most common causes of acute epididymitis.

Contributing factors of epididymitis include a history of UTIs or sexually transmitted infections (STIs), anatomic abnormalities, urinary tract surgeries or instrumentation, prolonged sitting, cycling, or trauma.

Epidemiology

Epididymitis occurs more frequently among late adolescents; however, it is not uncommon at any age. The annual incidence of acute epididymitis is approximately 1.2 per 1,000 boys of 2 to 13 years of age with one fourth of this group having recurrence within 5 years.

Symptoms

Patients with epididymitis may present with acute pain and swelling that gradually worsens over 24 hours. Pain tends to be isolated to the posterior epididymis. There are also times that inflammation may involve the ipsilateral testicle in a condition called epididymo-orchitis. Pain is reported as constant and not positional. Epididymitis related to ascending infection of the urinary tract may present with symptoms of UTI also, such as dysuria and fever.

In teens who are sexually active, urinary symptoms, such as urethral discharge and dysuria, may be present.

Signs

PE may reveal scrotal swelling. Testicular position and testicular lie are normal in epididymitis. Cremasteric reflex is preserved, and manual elevation of the testicles may relieve pain; this is known as a Prehn's sign. Palpation elicits pain over the posterior testicle. Focal swelling may be felt with palpation to the epididymis.

Diagnostics

A urinalysis and urine culture should be performed in patients presenting with epididymitis, to check for concomitant UTI; however, the majority of nonsexually active children and adolescents will have sterile urine with no evidence of pyuria or bacteriuria. Patients who have findings consistent with sexually transmitted epididymitis urethral discharge and dysuria should undergo STI testing for *C. trachomatis* and *N. gonorrhoeae*. Most labs now have the capability of performing nucleic acid amplification testing (NAAT) on urine samples.

Treatment

If there is an identified underlying infectious cause, then treat the underlying cause such as UTI or STI.

Most cases of epididymitis in children can be managed with analgesics/anti-inflammatories, scrotal elevation with supportive underwear, and a short course of bed rest if necessary. Any fever or systemic symptoms should prompt a thorough workup to investigate bacterial sources. Empiric treatment should be targeted toward most likely underlying infections (UTI for children and STI for sexually active teens).

■ ORCHITIS

Orchitis is inflammation of the testicle. This is most often caused by bacteria or viral infections. This is most commonly seen in prepubertal boys and related to mumps.

Men with epididymitis and orchitis typically present with a gradual onset of scrotal pain and symptoms of lower UTI, including fever. This presentation helps differentiate epididymitis and orchitis from testicular torsion, which is a surgical emergency.

Typical physical findings include a swollen, tender epididymis or testis located in the normal anatomic position with an intact ipsilateral cremasteric reflex. Laboratory studies, including urethral Gram stain, urinalysis and culture, and polymerase chain reaction assay for *C. trachomatis* and *N. gonorrhoeae*, help guide therapy. Initial outpatient therapy is empirical and targets the most common pathogens. When *C. trachomatis* and *N. gonorrhoeae* are suspected, ceftriaxone and doxycycline are recommended. When coliform bacteria are suspected, ofloxacin or levofloxacin is recommended.

Etiology

Orchitis is most commonly caused by infections. Infections are typically viral, the mumps virus being the most common. Despite a huge drop in mumps cases since vaccination became standard, there has been a steady increase in mumps infections since 2015. Approximately 30% of boys infected with mumps go on to develop orchitis; this tends to occur within 1 week of systemic and parotiditis findings. Other viruses have also been implicated in orchitis, such as coxsackie virus. Bacterial infections that cause orchitis in boys 2 to 14 years old are usually due to an extension of epididymitis from an *E. coli* infection, and in sexually active teens, orchitis is most commonly associated with STIs, such as *N. gonorrhoeae* and *C. trachomatis*.

Epidemiology

Males between 14 and 35 years of age are most often affected, and *C. trachomatis* and *N. gonorrhoeae* are the most common pathogens in this age group. In other age groups, coliform bacteria are the primary pathogens.

Symptoms

Gradual onset and worsening of unilateral or bilateral testicular pain and swelling are the symptoms of orchitis. Pain is not positional. It tends not to be associated with nausea or vomiting. Systemic symptoms are common and related to the underlying infectious cause.

Focused PE Signs

PE signs are testicular swelling, induration, and erythema of the scrotal skin. There may be fever, depending on the underling pathology. Normal lie of testicles and cremasteric reflex is preserved.

Diagnostics

A urinalysis and urine culture should be performed in patients presenting with orchitis, to check for underlying UTI. Patients who have findings consistent with sexually transmitted orchitis, urethral discharge, and dysuria should undergo STI testing for *C. trachomatis* and *N. gonorrhoeae*. If mumps is suspected in an unvaccinated patient, then an IgM antibody serum is recommended as soon as possible.

Treatment

Treatment for viral orchitis is supportive with bed rest; analgesics, such as acetaminophen or ibuprofen; and hot and cold packs as needed for analgesia. For suspected bacterial causes, antibiotics are used to treat the underlying cause. Children and adolescents with underlying bacterial epididymitis should be treated with antibiotics that have coverage for *E. coli*. For adolescent patients who are sexually active and have strong suspicion of STI, treatment should follow recommendations for STI treatment.

Don't Miss

Viral orchitis has been associated with testicular atrophy and subsequent subfertility. In rare cases, bilateral orchitis associated with mumps has led to infertility.

Any patient presenting with acute scrotal pain or scrotal swelling needs to have a complete exam of the scrotum. The provider should check for inguinal hernias to rule out hernia and incarcerated hernias. Also, although rare, the provider should check the scrotal skin for signs of Fournier gangrene. This is a rare complication associated with recent circumcision or insect bite to the scrotal tissue. This is a medical/surgical emergency and has a high rate of morbidity and mortality. Patients suspected of Fournier gangrene should be emergently transferred for multidisciplinary care, including surgical and intensive care.

■ TESTICULAR TORSION

Testicular torsion is the twisting of the testis on the spermatic cord. The spermatic cord contains the testicular artery, which is the blood supply perfusing the testicle. Twisting of the spermatic cord and vascular supply causes ischemia of the involved testicle, leading to necrosis. Testicular torsion is considered a surgical emergency. Any delay in diagnosis can lead to functional loss of the affected testis; therefore, radiologic assessment is frequently utilized in situations where testicular torsion is suspected to differentiate between torsion and similar conditions.

Epidemiology

Testicular torsion accounts for 10% to 15% of acute scrotal conditions in children. Testicular torsion occurs in 1 in 4,000 boys. Occurrence is bimodal with a peak in the neonatal period and, in most cases, teen years (ages 12–18 years). Testicular torsion is a surgical emergency, so it should be considered in children of any age presenting with testicular pain. There is some evidence to suggest that the risk of torsion can be inherited.

Symptoms

The following are the symptoms of testicular torsion: immediate onset of severe, unilateral scrotal pain, associated nausea/vomiting, and unrelenting and nonpositional pain, and abdominal pain

Focused PE Signs

The following are the PE signs: transverse testicular position, absent or diminished cremasteric reflex, high-riding testis palpation of the epididymis anteriorly, testicular tenderness, scrotal swelling, and erythema. The patient will likely be in distress due to intense scrotal pain.

Lab Tests/Diagnostics

Testicular torsion is a clinical diagnosis with time from diagnosis to intervention critical for successful outcome. Treatment and surgical evaluation should not be delayed waiting for imaging or diagnostic studies. The standard imaging historically has been Doppler ultrasound (US) with high sensitivity and specificity. Ultrasound has a 94% sensitivity and 96% specificity. Because of the time-sensitive nature of testicular torsion and a testicular salvage window time of 6 hours, unnecessary US can delay patients at high risk from getting appropriate surgical intervention and may be uneasy for patients at low risk. A clinical predicative tool has been developed, called Testicular Workup for Ischemia and Suspected Torsion (TWIST), for determining the risk of testicular torsion on clinical grounds. US is not recommended for patients with *high* clinical suspicion; instead, it is used in cases that tend to not be as clear. The TWIST scoring system is a clinical tool (Table 10.6) that assesses risk.

Patients with a score of 5 or higher are considered high risk. Scores between 2 and 4 are considered of an intermediate risk and tend to be the groups who require US confirmation to prevent unnecessary surgical exploration. Low-risk patients do not require US to rule out torsion, and high-risk patients can proceed directly to surgery.

Treatment

Surgery is the definitive treatment, and the goal of treatment is salvage of the involved testis and prevention of future torsion. This is accomplished through surgical correction and fixation. Testicular torsion is a surgical emergency, and time should not

Table 10.6

TWIST Predictive Clinical Tool		
Clinical Findings	**Degree of Risk**	**Intervention**
Hard testis (2 points)	Low risk: 0–1	Low probability of testicular torsion
Testis swelling (2 points) Absent cremasteric reflex (1 point)	Intermediate risk: 2–4	Intermediate risk of torsion: Emergent ultrasound or surgical exploration is recommended.
High riding testis (1 point) Nausea/vomiting (1 point)	High risk: 5 or more	High risk of torsion: Immediate surgical intervention is recommended.

TWIST, Testicular Workup for Ischemia and Suspected Torsion.
Source: Data from Sheth, K. R., Keays, M., Grimsby, G. M., Granberg, C. F., Menon, V. S., DaJusta, D. G., . . . Baker, L. A. (2016). Diagnosing testicular torsion before urological consultation and imaging: Validation of the TWIST score. *Journal of Urology, 195*(6), 1870–1876. doi:10.1016/j.juro.2016.01.101.

be delayed in diagnostic studies or periods of observation. Ambulatory practices should promptly refer patients to an emergency medical center with urology surgical services.

Attempts at correcting the torsion should be attempted in the office if presentation is less than 6 hours from onset of symptoms. Most torsion occurs medially, so detorsion would occur with lateral rotation. Right testis would be manually turned counterclockwise, whereas left would be turned clockwise. Detorsion is successful with the immediate relief of pain. Two to three rotations may be required, as torsion can be due to multiple rotations of the spermatic cord. If attempt is unsuccessful with lateral turning, then an attempt can be performed medially, as this may be a presentation of the uncommon lateral torsion. Even if manual detorsion is successful, surgical referral is still indicated to correct any residual perfusion abnormalities and to perform preventative testicular fixation.

URETHRAL AND VAGINAL DISCHARGE

It is uncommon in the nonsexually active pediatric population; however, genitourinary discharge is not uncommon in the sexually active adolescent population. The focus of the next few paragraphs is on urethral and vaginal discharge in the sexually active adolescent population.

■ PELVIC INFLAMMATORY DISEASE

Any female presenting with vaginal discharge, especially in the setting of abdominal pain, needs to be considered having an ascending infection from the vagina/cervix causing endometritis, salpingitis, tubo-ovarian abscess, or pelvic peritonitis.

Etiology

C. trachomatis and N. gonorrhoeae are the most common microorganisms associated with PID; however, other microorganisms may be involved.

Approximately 10% to 20% of women with chlamydial or gonorrheal infections may develop PID if not treated. Women with PID have a 20% chance of developing infertility from tubal scarring and have an increased risk of ectopic pregnancy.

Symptoms and Focused PE Signs

Presentation varies with the most common symptoms and signs being lower abdominal or pelvic pain, vaginal discharge, fever or chills, cramping, and dysuria. Some women also may have low back pain, nausea, and vomiting. PE produces one or more of the following: cervical motion, uterine, or adnexal tenderness.

Diagnosis

The diagnosis of PID is mostly clinical with confirmatory testing of underlying etiology via NAAT for C. trachomatis and N. gonorrhoeae. US may also be performed to check for free pelvic fluid or abscess.

Treatment

If mild to moderate illness, then outpatient treatment is acceptable. Standard treatment is ceftriaxone 250 mg intramuscularly one single dose in addition to doxycycline 100 mg twice a day (or every 12 hours) for 14 days. Consider adding metronidazole

500 mg every 12 hours for 14 days if trichomonas is suspected or if there has been recent instrumentation.

Patients should be hospitalized if they have severe illness, which manifests as any of the following: high fever, nausea, vomiting, severe abdominal pain, pelvic abscess, inability to take oral medications due to nausea and vomiting, pregnancy, or lack of response to oral medications after 24 hours of treatment (Curry, Williams, & Penny, 2019).

◼ URETHRITIS AND CERVICITIS/VAGINITIS

Urethral and cervical/vaginal discharge is most common among sexually active adolescents and is caused frequently by STIs. The most common STIs in this age group are trichomoniasis, chlamydia, and gonorrhea.

Etiology

The most common causes of sexually transmitted urethritis and cervicitis/vaginitis are infections with *N. gonorrhoeae*, *C. trachomatis*, and *Trichomonas vaginalis*. Most common non-STI causes of vaginitis are bacterial vaginosis and vulvovaginal candidiasis (see Table 10.7).

Epidemiology

Adolescents and young adults account for approximately half of all new STIs in the United States. There are approximately 6 million new cases a year of trichomonas, gonorrhea, and chlamydia reported each year. These numbers are likely underreported, as often infections are minimally symptomatic or asymptomatic.

Symptoms

The most common complaint of urethritis and cervicitis/vaginitis is discharge. The discharge can be scant or copious, depending on the underlying etiology. Voiding symptoms of dysuria may also be present. Patients may complain of itching or burning sensation at the distal urethra/meatus in males or vagina in females. Pelvic pain in females may accompany symptoms of cervicitis and vaginitis especially in the setting of pelvic inflammatory disease (PID). Males may experience testicular discomfort if there is an associated epididymitis. Systemic symptoms are rare.

Focused PE Signs

Signs can be subtle, depending on the cause (see Table 10.7). Discharge can be anything from scant and clear to copious and mucopurulent. Despite descriptions of discharge, there is no accurate way to diagnose cause based on appearance and amount of the discharge. There are seldom other findings on exam in the male experiencing urethritis, unless there is an ascending infection to the epididymis, in which case there would be palpation tenderness and swelling at the epididymis.

Females may also have a friable or erythematous cervix. Tenderness at the cervix should raise suspicion for an ascending infection and PID (Paladine, Urmi, & Desai, 2018).

Lab Tests/Diagnostics

NAAT is the lab testing of choice for gonorrhea and chlamydia infections. Samples can be taken from urine and endocervical and vaginal discharge. In males, urethral swabs

Table 10.7

Common STI Presentation, Testing, and Treatment

	Gonococcal urethritis or vaginitis	Chlamydia urethritis or vaginitis	Trichomoniasis	Bacterial vaginosis	Vulvovaginal candidiasis
Etiology	*Neisseria gonorrhoeae*	*Chlamydia trachomatis*	*Trichomonas vaginalis*	Increased pH Reduction of *lactobacilli* and increased *Gardnerella vaginalis*	*Candida albicans*
Presentation	Purulent discharge Dysuria Females are often asymptomatic carriers.	Thin urethral discharge Dysuria Females are often asymptomatic carriers.	Females Purulent discharge Malodorous Burning Cervical inflammation Strawberry cervix Males: most often asymptomatic and may have discharge and dysuria	Vaginal discharge Malodorous	Vaginal pruritis Vaginal irritation/ erythema White thick/curd-like discharge
Testing	NAAT Females: Urine or endocervical or vaginal swabs Males: Urine or urethral swab	NAAT Females: Urine or endocervical or vaginal swabs Males: Urine or urethral swab	NAAT Females: Urine or endocervical or vaginal swabs Males: Urine or urethral swab	Three of the following are positive on exam: Thin, gray-white discharge Vaginal pH >4.5 Positive whiff test Clue cells on wet mount	Microscopy reveals hyphae/pseudohyphae Culture
Treatment (adolescent)	**Ceftriaxone** 250 mg IM one dose Plus **Azithromycin** 1 g in a single PO dose	**Azithromycin** 1 g PO single dose (preferred) Or Doxycycline 100 mg BID for 7 days	**Metronidazole** 500 mg every 12 hours for 7 days	**Metronidazole** 500 mg every 12 hours for 7 days	**Fluconazole** 150 mg PO for one dose

(continued)

Chapter **10** Common Pediatric Renal/Urologic Disorders Seen in Pediatric Primary Care

Table 10.7

Common STI Presentation, Testing, and Treatment (continued)

	Gonococcal urethritis or vaginitis	Chlamydia urethritis or vaginitis	Trichomoniasis	Bacterial vaginosis	Vulvovaginal candidiasis
Don't Miss/Key Points	Untreated gonorrhea is a common cause of PID. Seldom causes disseminated disease, but it is the most common cause of infectious arthritis in young, sexually active patients. Patient is encouraged to inform sexual partner(s) to be tested/ treated. See individual state laws regarding expedited care of partners.	Common cause is reactive arthritis. Patient is encouraged to inform sexual partner(s) to be tested/treated. See individual state laws regarding expedited care of partners.	Increased risk of HIV transmission and other STIs; consider screening for other STIs, such as gonorrhea and chlamydia. Patient is encouraged to inform sexual partner(s) to be tested/ treated. See individual state laws regarding expedited care of partners.	Increased risk of HIV transmission and other STIs	Increased risk in patients with DM and recent antibiotic use

DM, diabetes mellitus; HIV, human immunodeficiency virus; NAAT, nucleic acid amplification testing; PID, pelvic inflammatory disease; STIs, sexually transmitted infections.

are also used. Self-swabbing in females is acceptable if there are no signs or symptoms of PID or any other compelling reason to perform a pelvic exam. Pelvic exam should be performed if there is concern for ascending infection. Concomitant infection is common in patients presenting with symptoms of an STI, so testing for gonorrhea and chlamydia at the time of testing is recommended.

Treatment

Treatment is outlined in Table 10.7.

Don't Miss

In patients presenting with continued symptoms of urethritis/vaginitis, despite negative screening for the aforementioned, consider urea plasma urealyticum or *Mycoplasma genitalium* infection.

References

Arshad, M., & Seed, P. (2015). Urinary tract infections in the infant. *Clinics in Perinatology, 42*(1), 17–22. doi:10.1016/j.clp.2014.10.003

Balighian, E., & Burke, M. (2018). Urinary tract infections in children. *Pediatrics in Review, 39*, 3–12. doi:10.1542/pir.2017-0007

Cherry, J., Demmler-Harrison, G. J., Kaplan, S. L., Steinbach, W. J., & Hotez, P. (2019). *Feigin and Cherry's textbook of pediatric infectious diseases* (8th ed.). Philadelphia, PA: Elsevier.

Curry, A., Williams, T., & Penny, M. L. (2019). Pelvic inflammatory disease: Diagnosis, management and prevention. *American Family Physician, 100*(6), 357–364.

McConaghy, J. R., & Panchal, B. (2016). Epididymitis: An overview. *American Family Physician, 94*(9), 723–726.

Paladine, H. L., Urmi, A., & Desai, A. (2019). Vaginitis: Diagnosis and treatment. *American Family Physician, 1*(97), 321–329.

Sheth, K. R., Keays, M., Grimsby, G. M., Granberg, C. F., Menon, V. S., DaJusta, D. G., . . . Baker, L. A. (2016). Diagnosing testicular torsion before urological consultation and imaging: Validation of the TWIST score. *Journal of Urology, 195*(6), 1870–1876. doi:10.1016/j.juro.2016.01.101

11

Common Neonatal Conditions Seen in Pediatric Primary Care

Meredith Scannell

INTRODUCTION

All advanced practicing clinicians (APCs) working in pediatrics should be skilled in newborn assessments. Newborn assessments are an essential tool to help identify any medical conditions, birth injuries, and anomalies. Newborn assessments should be conducted within 24 hours of birth, before discharge, and on the newborn (Scannell & Puka-Beals, 2019). Developing assessment skills is essential, as it aids in identifying normal deviations from those that may be life-threatening and those that require further evaluation, intervention or referral, and additional support.

When conducting the physical exam, all efforts should include the parents in the examination. For many newborns, the examination can be conducted in the crib in the room in which the parents are rooming. This allows for a more patient-centered approach and offers an opportunity for the parents to be involved by asking questions or discussing concerns they may have. It also gives an opportunity to ask parents questions that may be helpful in the examination such as family traits or other hereditary conditions.

OBJECTIVES

1. Identify normal variation in newborn assessment.
2. List common newborn conditions.
3. Describe common treatments for newborn complications.

APPROACH TO THE NORMAL NEWBORN

◼ APGAR SCORING

One of the very first assessments done after birth is Apgar scoring (Table 11.1). Apgar scoring gives a general assessment of the well-being of the newborn (American College of Obstetricians and Gynecologists, 2019). Apgar scoring is done at 1 minute of life

Table 11.1

Apgar Scoring for 1 minute and 5 minutes			
	0	1	2
Appearance	Completely cyanotic or pale/blue	Blue extremities (acrocyanosis), pink body (perfused face and trunk)	Completely perfused/pink body
Pulse	Absent	Less than 100 bpm	More than 100 bpm
Grimace	No response to stimulation	Grimace, weak, or slow response to stimulation	Cry is strong, prompt response to stimulation
Activity	Absent and flaccid	Some flexion of the arms and legs	Well-flexed arms and legs with active motion
Respiration	Absent	Weak, slow, or irregular cry	Vigorous cry

Source: American College of Obstetricians and Gynecologists. (2019). *The Apgar score (Committee opinion no. 644)*. Retrieved from https://www.acog.org/Clinical-Guidance-and-Publications/Committee-Opinions/Committee-on-Obstetric-Practice/The-Apgar-Score

and then 5 minutes of life. Scores of 7 or more indicate normal transition and scores less than 7 will require the newborn to be closely monitored with possible interventions, resuscitation, and typically admission to a neonatal intensive care unit, as scores below 6 are associated with neonatal morbidity and mortality and require emergent interventions.

MECONIUM ASPIRATION

Meconium aspiration syndrome (MAS) is a respiratory condition that occurs when the newborn aspirated meconium into the respiratory system. Aspiration often occurs in utero from an infant who has already passed meconium, or aspiration of meconium can happen during the birth process. The degree of severity of MAS ranges from mild to severe and life-threatening and is the leading cause of infant mortality and morbidity (Vain & Batton, 2017). Risk factors for MAS include a postmature infant, growth-restricted infant, and the presence of thick meconium-stained amniotic fluid at birth.

Symptoms

Newborns with MAS will have varying degrees of respiratory distress with nasal flaring and grunting. Other symptoms include cyanosis and tachycardia. Other findings include meconium staining of the skin, barrel chest due to hyperinflation, and rales or rhonchi on auscultation.

Diagnostics/Test

Diagnosis of MAS is often done at the birth of an infant who develops respiratory distress with a history of meconium-stained amniotic fluid (Vain & Batton, 2017). A diagnostic test for a newborn with MAS will often consist of chest x-rays showing diffuse, coarse, asymmetric patchy infiltrates, widespread consolidation, and areas of atelectasis and hyperinflation. It may also be necessary to obtain a blood gas sample to evaluate for hypoxia and acidosis.

Treatment

Treatment for MAS will depend on the degree of the condition. In some cases, suctioning will be required with oxygen therapy. In severe cases with significant respiratory distress, the newborn will require intubation with mechanical ventilation. For the newborn with significant respiratory distress, treatment with surfactant replacement of 100 to 150 mg/kg up to four doses is recommended. This is to aid the displacement of surfactant that occurs when meconium covers the alveolar surfaces and helps to prevent atelectasis.

Parent Follow-Up

For many parents, a child with MAS is a life-threatening condition. Parents will need to be educated on the seriousness of the condition and the various treatments.

NEWBORN DERMATOLOGICAL ASSESSMENTS

The newborn dermatological assessment is a critical aspect of the newborn assessment. Many dermatological conditions are present at birth and are often benign and will resolve spontaneously over time. The nurse practitioner/physician assistant must understand the common conditions, as they are often a significant concern for parents, and educating parents on the various dermatological conditions is essential (Martin & Rosenfeld, 2018).

Parent/Patient Follow-Up

Many newborn dermatological conditions are benign and will often resolve over time spontaneously. Parents need to be aware that although the condition may cause some concerns visually, there are often little to no treatments that will resolve dermatological conditions. Parents should avoid using over-the-counter creams or lotions, as these may irritate the skin more and worsen the condition.

For descriptions of common neonatal dermatologic conditions and their treatments and resolution periods, see Table 11.2.

NEWBORN HEAD AND FACE ABNORMALITIES

■ CAPUT SUCCEDANEUM

Caput succedaneum is the diffuse swelling of the newborn head due to a prolonged labor. The swelling can give the infant a "cone"-shaped head. This is seen immediately after birth and generally resolves within 24 hours of life.

Symptoms

The head of the newborn with caput succedaneum will often appear "cone" shaped. This is due to the pressure on the part of the head that was presenting into the birth canal. Other accompanying symptoms can be petechiae, ecchymosis, and purpura.

Focused Assessment

A focused assessment includes a close assessment of the swelling to ensure that there are no other injuries. Palpation can reveal pitting edema.

Table 11.2

Common Neonatal Dermatologic Conditions		
Common Skin Condition	**Description and Cause**	**Treatment and Resolution Period**
Erythema toxicum neonatorum	Benign rash that presents as small, irregular, flat red patches that are most commonly seen on the face, trunk, and extremities; onset is usually within the first 24–48 hours of life to 3 months of life.	No treatment is required. Most commonly appears within the first 14 days of life and can last up to 1 month of life.
Milia	Small epidermal or sebaceous cysts caused by immature sebaceous glands that commonly appear on the face and mucosa, less frequently found on the trunk of the newborn, and resemble white pimples.	Resolves spontaneously; treatment may include gentle cleaning with pumice stone, soap, or expression of content. Milia should resolve spontaneously 2–3 weeks after birth.
Congenital dermal melanocytosis (Mongolian spots)	Dark blue or gray patches of melanocytes that are most commonly found on the buttocks, flanks, or shoulders; can be mistaken for bruises.	No treatment required, and gradually fades over the first 3 years of life.
Seborrheic dermatitis (cradle cap)	Thick, yellowish crusty scaling lesions that usually appear on the scalp, face, head, and behind ears.	Treatment with daily shampoo to the head and corticosteroid cream to affected areas BID.
Transient neonatal pustular melanosis	Small pustules that begin as superficial pustules that are found most often on the chin, neck, and back at birth and can spread to the entire body, including palms and soles of the feet. Pustules begin as faint erythema and can progress to brown hyperpigmented macules.	Pustules typically present at birth and can last for months. No treatment is required as the pustules resolve spontaneously.
Acne neonatorum	Small reddish papules and pustules that are found on the chin, cheeks, and forehead around the third or fourth week of life.	Generally, no treatment is required; in severe cases, samples may need to be cultured. Resolves by the third or fourth month of life.

Source: Data from Martin, G. I., & Rosenfeld, W. (2018). *Common problems in the newborn nursery: An evidence and case-based guide.* Cham, Switzerland: Springer Nature Switzerland AG. doi:10.1007/978-3-319-95672-5; Scannell, M., & Puka-Beals, E. (2019). A guide to newborn assessment. *Nursing Made Incredibly Easy, 17*(4), 26–33.

Lab Test Diagnostics

There are no latest techniques; diagnosis is based on clinical findings.

Differentials

It is important for the healthcare provider to assess the newborn head for any trauma or cephalohematoma.

Treatment

There is no treatment for caput succedaneum, and swelling should resolve in 1 to 3 days (Venes, 2017).

Follow-Up/Patient/Parent Education

Parents should be instructed that the swelling will resolve over a few days, and the head will take on a more rounded appearance.

■ CEPHALOHEMATOMA

Cephalohematoma is a collection of blood over one of the skull plates located between the periosteum and the skull (Venes, 2017). Cephalohematoma often occurs due to trauma or pressure during a spontaneous birth or instrumental delivery, such as a vacuum-assisted or forceps-assisted birth (Lewis, 2014). Cephalohematoma does not cross the suture line and will be unilateral in appearance.

Etiology/Epidemiology

Cephalohematoma occurs between 1.5% and 2.5% of all deliveries (Venes, 2017).

Focused Assessment

Assessment of a cephalohematoma should be conducted to carefully examine the extent of the cephalohematoma and often occurs on one of the parietal bones or occipital bone, and in some cases, there can be two cephalohematomas and can occur on both parietal bones, with the suture line dividing the two cephalohematomas.

Diagnostics

Diagnosis is based on clinical assessment; however, a CAT scan or x-ray may be warranted to rule out skull fracture. Serial hematocrits may be necessary in some cases to determine the extent of blood loss and anemia. Aspiration is not recommended due to the risk of infection.

Don't Miss

Skull fractures are rare; however, they can occur and be present underneath the cephalohematoma. Infants with cephalohematoma should be evaluated for skull fracture especially if they develop neurological changes.

Treatment

Most cephalohematomas will resolve over 3 to 4 months (Lewis, 2014). Cephalohematomas require close monitoring, as they can worsen in the first 48 hours following birth (Lewis, 2014).

Follow-Up/Patient/Parent Education

Newborns with cephalohematoma are at risk for jaundice due to the breakdown of the red blood cells in the days/weeks following birth. Parents need to be educated on the risk of jaundice, and newborns need to be observed for clinical signs such as yellowish skin and scleral. In addition, these newborns are also at risk for infection, and thus, parents should be educated regarding early signs and symptoms of infections.

■ CLEFT LIP AND CLEFT PALATE

Cleft lip and cleft palate are the most common oral malformations in newborns. There are varying degrees and subtypes of a cleft lip and palate that occur when the facial bones do not fuse together completely, causing gaps. The different degrees can consist of complete or incomplete cleft lip/palate, and they can be unilateral or occur bilaterally. A cleft lip means that there will be a gap in tissues on the upper lip with partial or complete clefting. A cleft palate can occur in the absence of a cleft lip and can occur in the hard and soft palates.

Symptoms

- Split in the upper lip that appears as small-large notch
- Split palate
- Difficulty feeding
- Difficulty swallowing
- Chronic ear infections
- Dental problems
- Speech and language problems
- Hearing problems

Focused Assessment

Many cleft lips are visible and obvious when examining the newborn. Immediate assessment after the delivery focuses on oral airway and respiratory assessment, which can be compromised due to an inability to clear fluids effectively. The infant may also need supplemental oxygen if there is a respiratory compromise. A cleft palate may not be so obvious; the best approach to examine for a cleft palate is to insert a gloved finger into the newborn's mouth feeling the upper palate.

Don't Miss

Both a cleft lip and cleft palate can indicate other congenital malformations.

Treatment

Surgical repair is the primary treatment for cleft lip/palate; beginning at around 3 months of life, additional surgeries may be necessary depending on the degree of the cleft.

Follow-Up/Patient/Parent Education

- Often, these children will need to have surgeries and follow-up with a dentist who specializes in cleft lip/palates.
- Infants will also have feeding difficulties requiring early intervention with lactation consultant if breastfeeding is the preferred method of feeding.
- Parents and the newborn should also have a follow-up with a genetic counselor to review if the cleft lip/palate is indicative of a genetic condition.
- Mothers may need to be educated on the need for folic acid in the preconception period if they desire future pregnancies.

NEWBORN MUSCULOSKELETAL ABNORMALITIES

■ DEVELOPMENTAL DYSPLASIA OF THE HIP

Developmental dysplasia of the hip (DDH) occurs when the femoral head does not properly fit in the acetabulum, most commonly due to a flattened acetabulum.

Etiology/Epidemiology

DDH occurs in approximately 0.1% to 0.2% of births and can occur in both hips, but most commonly occurs in the left hip, and in infants who were in the breech position (especially frank breech) or born in the breech position (National Health Services, 2018b).

Symptoms

Symptoms of DDH include asymmetrical gluteal folds and leg lengths. Gluteal folds will also be asymmetrical, with an extra fold on the affected leg, or the gluteal folds may be asymmetrical with the folds uneven with a fold on one leg to be higher or lower than the fold on the other leg (International Hip Dysplasia Institute, 2018). Another symptom is asymmetrical leg length. The affected leg may appear shorter, which can indicate a dislocation (International Hip Dysplasia Institute, 2018).

Focused Assessment

Assessment should include inspection of the legs for symmetry in size as well as for symmetry in gluteal folds. The gluteal folds should be assessed in the prone and supine position. The Ortolani maneuver can be done in the supine position; the hips and knees are flexed in a circular motion while abducting and lifting the femurs (Venes, 2017). A palpable click or a clunking sound can indicate a subluxation or dislocation due to the femur slipping out of the acetabulum.

Lab Test Diagnostics

Ultrasound or an x-ray can confirm the diagnosis of DDH and should be performed if physical examination indicated DDH.

Don't Miss

Healthcare providers need to be aware that DDH may not have been diagnosed during the newborn examination, and assessing for DDH at a subsequent visit is an essential part of the infant examination.

Treatment

Treatment of DDH will depend on the degree of the condition. A Pavlik harness is a treatment that includes the use of a fabric harness that the infant is placed in so that the pelvis and legs remain in a stable position to allow for normal growth and development. It is used for several weeks without removal. Other treatments may include surgery and hard cast, especially if DDH was diagnosed after 6 months of age (National

Health Services, 2018b). Treatment for DDH is critical to prevent long-term sequelae of hip pain, ambulation problems, balance problems, and arthritis.

Follow-Up/Patient/Parent Education

The Pavlik harness must remain on at all times, and parents will need to be educated on the proper use of the Pavlik, how to change diapers and clothe without taking the Pavlik harness off, and how to clean the harness if it becomes soiled. Parents should be instructed to assess the skin daily around the harness for skin rubbing and irritation

◼ FRACTURED CLAVICLE

A fractured clavicle is one of the most common birth injuries of the newborn. This can occur during the birth process during a normal spontaneous delivery due to the infant squeezing through the birth canal, or it can be a result of an assisted delivery with instruments, and in some cases of emergency deliveries, the clavicle may be purposively fractured to assist in vaginal deliveries.

Symptoms

Symptoms of clavicle fractures include brachial plexus palsy, decreased movement, and asymmetric Moro reflex (Martin & Rosenfeld, 2018). Other signs include bruising, swelling, or discoloration of the affected arm and obvious discomfort when the affected arm is moved such as fussiness and/or crying (Martin & Rosenfeld, 2018).

Focused Assessment

The clavicles should be inspected by palpation to determine fracture. The clavicles should feel smooth and without any separations, irregularities, obvious cracks, unevenness, or breaks.

Lab Test Diagnostics

Diagnosis is confirmed with an x-ray, which can determine the degree of fracture.

Don't Miss

The surrounding skin should be palpated for crepitus, which will feel like Rice Krispies or small crackling that may indicate a punctured lung, which can occur from the fractured bone.

Treatment

There is no treatment for a fractured clavicle and healing will occur spontaneously. Pain analgesia may be prescribed as needed.

Follow-Up/Patient/Parent Education

Parents should be instructed to handle their infant gently and follow up with the pediatrician or healthcare provider within 2 weeks.

■ TALIPES EQUINOS (CLUBFOOT)

Talipes equinos, also known as clubfoot, is a congenital malformation of one or both feet. The foot will take on a C-shaped appearance, and the heel will point downward and inward, with the ankle inverted. A true talipes equinos is primarily due to genetics. Clubfoot can also occur due to mispositioning in utero, causing the foot to not grow or develop normally (National Health Services, 2018a).

Etiology/Epidemiology

The incidence of clubfoot occurs in approximately 1 in 1,000 live births. Parents with a history of clubfoot will have 30% chance of offspring developing clubfoot.

Focused Assessment

A clubfoot can be diagnosed on clinical assessment by obvious signs of the foot in a C-shape and heel pointed downward and inward. After this has been assessed, the healthcare practitioner needs to determine if the clubfoot is due to a congenital anomaly or due to malposition in utero.

Symptoms

An infant with clubfoot will have stiffness in the affected foot, absence of creases behind the heel of the affected foot, and an ankle that does not move properly. The foot will appear smaller in size, with a shortened Achilles tendon and wasting of the calf muscle.

Lab Test Diagnostics

X-rays of the legs should be done to determine the severity of the condition.

Differentials

Newborns with clubfoot may have other congenital anomalies. The healthcare provider needs to assess for other conditions seen with clubfoot such as spina bifida and amniotic band syndrome.

Treatment

Treatment is dependent on the degree of the condition. Nonsurgical manipulation often occurs shortly after birth. Some cases can be treated with physiotherapy with stretching of the ligaments and tendons into the correct alignment and position. Serial casting with long leg casts is another treatment option that consists of placing the affected foot in a cast after the foot is manipulated into position and requires resetting every few weeks. The Ponseti method is a well-known method involving stretching of the affected foot and the application of the Ponseti cast that is long leg cast. In some cases, a tendonectomy is required to strengthen the Achilles tendon.

Follow-Up/Patient/Parent Education

Parents will need follow-up visits with their healthcare provider, who is fitting and adjusting the cast, and pediatrician. Parents will need to be taught necessary cast care including how to assess for compromised circulation, pressure sores, skin problems, and neurovascular problems. As the infant grows, they may have ambulation difficulties and may need shoes of different sizes with one being smaller than the other. Parents may also need to follow up with a genetic counselor to determine underlying genetic conditions.

NEWBORN NEUROLOGICAL ABNORMALITITES

■ ERB'S PALSY

Erb's palsy is one form of brachial plexus injury that often thought to occur due to difficulty in birth such as shoulder dystocia, instrument-assisted delivery, or a large infant. The brachial plexus is a group of nerves that control sensation and movement in the arms and hands (American Academy of Orthopedic Surgeons, 2019). Damage to the upper aspect of the nerves in the brachial plexus will cause Erb's palsy. During birth, there can be pressure or damage to these nerves causing temporary or permanent nerve damage. It is easily identified at birth by a unilateral flaccid arm with little to no movement (Coroneos et al., 2017).

Etiology/Epidemiology

Erb's palsy is the most common brachial plexus injury occurring in 1 to 2 out of 1,000 live births (American Academy of Orthopedic Surgeons, 2019).

Symptoms

When Erb's palsy is present, one or both arms and hands are weak and have minimal movements; other accompanying symptoms can be a loss of feeling in the affected arm and total paralysis. Many infants will recover from Erb's palsy; however, those who do not can have long-term health consequences of arm weakness and a growth pattern that is uneven, resulting in uneven arms with the affected arm being smaller than the nonaffected arm (Coroneos et al., 2017).

Focused Assessment

All infants who have asymmetrical arm movements should be assessed for Erb's palsy.

Differentials

Differential diagnosis includes ruling out pseudo palsy that can occur due to a fractured clavicle and not Erb's palsy.

Don't Miss

Although Erb's palsy can be diagnosed at birth, the degree of the palsy can only be determined with serial examinations.

Treatment

Many infants with Erb's palsy will recover completely within a few days of birth (Coroneos et al., 2017). Treatment usually begins with a passive range of motion exercises to the affected arm. For severe cases, referral to specialized centers for extensive physical therapy treatment is necessary. Peripheral nerve graft may also be necessary in cases with ongoing paralysis.

Follow-Up/Patient/Parent Education

Parents will need to be educated on the importance of physiotherapy and adhering to all follow-up appointments. Parents need to follow a scheduled exercise program for the newborns; as newborns are unable to move their arm, parents will need to perform a range-of-motion exercises. Parents will need to be informed of the possibility of different growth patterns in the child's arm, which will become more noticeable as the child grows older.

References

American Academy of Orthopedic Surgeons. (2019). *Erb's palsy (brachial plexus birth palsy)*. Retrieved from https://orthoinfo.aaos.org/en/diseases--conditions/erbs-palsy-brachial-plexus-birth-palsy

American College of Obstetricians and Gynecologists. (2019). *The Apgar score (Committee opinion no. 644)*. Retrieved from https://www.acog.org/Clinical-Guidance-and-Publications/Committee-Opinions/Committee-on-Obstetric-Practice/The-Apgar-Score

Coroneos, C. J., Voineskos, S. H., Christakis, M. K., Thoma, A., Bain, J. R., & Brouwers, M. C. (2017). Obstetrical brachial plexus injury (OBPI): Canada's national clinical practice guideline. *BMJ Open, 7*(1), e014141. doi:10.1136/bmjopen-2016-014141

International Hip Dysplasia Institute. (2018). *Infant and child hip dysplasia*. Retrieved from https://hipdysplasia.org/developmental-dysplasia-of-the-hip/infant-signs-and-symptoms/asymmetry/

Lewis, M. L. (2014). A comprehensive newborn examination: Part I. general, head and neck, cardiopulmonary. *American Family Physician, 90*(5), 289–296.

Martin, G. I., & Rosenfeld, W. (2018). *Common problems in the newborn nursery: An evidence and case-based guide*. Cham, Switzerland: Springer Nature Switzerland AG. doi:10.1007/978-3-319-95672-5

National Health Services. (2018a). *Club foot*. Retrieved from https://www.nhs.uk/conditions/club-foot/

National Health Services. (2018b). *Developmental dysplasia of the hip*. Retrieved from https://www.nhs.uk/conditions/developmental-dysplasia-of-the-hip/

Scannell, M., & Puka-Beals, E. (2019). A guide to newborn assessment. *Nursing Made Incredibly Easy, 17*(4), 26–33.

Vain, N. E., & Batton, D. G. (2017). Meconium "aspiration" (or respiratory distress associated with meconium-stained amniotic fluid?). *Seminars in Fetal and Neonatal Medicine, 22*(4), 214–219. doi:10.1016/j.siny.2017.04.002

Venes, D. (2017). *Taber's cyclopedic medical dictionary*. Philadelphia, PA: F.A. Davis.

12

Infectious Diseases Commonly Seen in Pediatric Primary Care

Josh Merson and Kristine M. Ruggiero

INTRODUCTION

Although the incidence of serious infections has decreased after the introduction of conjugate vaccines, fever remains a major cause of laboratory investigation and hospital admissions. Clinical guidelines have been studied and vary widely; however, pediatric fever remains a chief complaint in many pediatric practices and urgent care settings. Therefore, the pediatric advanced practicing clinician (APC) should be knowledgeable about febrile conditions that occur in a variety of age groups in pediatrics. This review is to help the APC standardize their approach to care (separated by age of pediatric patient) for the most common causes of fever, to better help with the approach to caring for children with febrile illness.

Fever is a common complaint of children, accounting for approximately one-third of pediatric outpatient visits in the United States. A temperature of 38°C (100.4°F) or greater has generally been established as the definition of a fever requiring a workup. The most common etiology of fever differs between age groups, with infants younger than 3 months having unique risks for serious bacterial infections (SBIs); as such, their management is parsed out and discussed separately from that of older children in this chapter.

OBJECTIVES

1. Recognize fever and how to perform a fever workup in children of various ages:
   a. Fever in younger than 3 months
   b. Fever in 3 months to 36 months
   c. Fever in older than 36 months
2. Identify most common causes of fever by age.
3. Discern fever of unknown origin
   a. Serious bacterial infection (SBIs)

FEVER GUIDELINES

Epidemiology/risk factors: Children experienced around 14 infections during the first 3 years of life (Vissing, Chawes, Rasmussen, & Bisgard, 2018). Simply put, the younger the child, the higher the suspicion and workup should be for bacterial infection.

Etiology: Traditionally, a febrile neonate (temperature >100.4°F [>38°C]) undergoes a full sepsis workup, which includes a complete blood count (CBC), urinalysis, blood culture, urine culture, chest radiography, and diagnostic lumbar puncture (LP). The age group that is defined for this workup may vary and will be discussed later in this chapter.

Focused Physical Exam Signs/Finding: Fever

Lab Tests/Diagnostics: Vary by age and on the degree of suspicion of focal infection based on history and physical exam (PE) findings (see Tables 12.1 and 12.2).

Differentials: Vary by age (see Tables 12.1 and 12.2).

Don't Miss

- Fever work-up is divided by age groups: 0 to 28 days (neonates), 1–3 months, 3–36 months, over 3 years of age. Highest suspicion for SBI should be given to febrile neonates, and empiric treatment should be started immediately following a fever work-up. The standard treatment includes ampicillin plus either gentamicin or cefotaxime, which cover the bacterial organisms likely in this age group.
- Even though the height of the fever does not define the severity of illness by itself, there is an association with a greater likelihood of SBI for temperatures >39°C (especially in infants under 6 months).
- Temperatures above 41°C have also been associated with a higher risk of meningitis.
- However, children with SBI may also have a normal temperature or be hypothermic, especially in children with immune compromise (i.e., cancer patients, patients with immune deficiencies such as hypogammaglobulinemia or HIV infection).
- The most common cause of SBI in children continues to be UTI.

Key Points and Some Differences in Measuring Temperature

- The American Academy of Pediatrics suggests the following:
  - Rectal thermometry is used for children younger than 4 years of age.
  - In newborns, axillary temperature has been found to be as reliable as rectal temperature.
  - Oral thermometry is used in older children.
  - The gallium-in-glass thermometer has been suggested as an alternative for axillary thermometry, as it may be more accurate than digital thermometers; however, it has to be maintained in place for 5 minutes to assure correct measurement, and glass makes it unsuitable for young children.
  - Tympanic infrared thermometers represent a possible alternative, but their sensitivity is not optimal, and they are not accurate in children under 3 months of age.
  - Chemical forehead thermometers are unreliable.
  - Temporal artery thermometers and forehead noncontact infrared thermometers represent emerging techniques, but further studies are needed.
  - Parental report of tactile fever should never be dismissed!
- The National Institute for Health and Care Excellence (NICE) guidelines recommend measuring body temperature in the axilla, using an electronic thermometer for infants younger than 4 weeks of age and chemical dot or electronic thermometers in older children (Barbi, Marzuillo, Neri, Naviglio, & Krauss, 2017).

FEVER IN INFANTS LESS THAN 3 MONTHS

Rectal temperatures are the gold standard for obtaining a temperature in infants younger than 3 months of age, with a temperature of 38°C (100.4°F) or greater generally regarded as a fever.

Viral infections are the most common cause of fever in young infants, with human rhinovirus as most frequent, followed by respiratory syncytial virus (RSV), influenza, and parainfluenza.

The goal of evaluation of a febrile infant is to identify infants at risk for invasive bacterial infection (IBI; bacteremia and/or meningitis) requiring empiric antimicrobial therapy and hospitalization.

As standard practice, a full sepsis evaluation should occur on the following:

- Ill-appearing infants and neonates (infants younger than 28 days of life), including those with a diagnosed viral infection
- An infant with findings suggestive of HSV
- Infant 29 to 60 days of age with risk factors of invasive bacterial infection (including high temperature, congenital disease, technology dependent, or antibiotic use in the previous 7 days)
- Infants with a focal infection and abnormal CBC

In febrile infants up to 60 days of age, the combination of a normal urinalysis result, an absolute neutrophil count of less than 4,090 per mL (4.1×10^9 per L), and a serum procalcitonin level of less than 1.71 ng/mL is accurate at ruling out serious bacterial infections (Barry, 2019). Well-appearing infants 29 to 60 days of life who do not have a focal bacterial infection, clinical findings for HSV, and other risk factors for IBI and who have a rectal temperature <38.6°C (101.5°F) should undergo the following evaluation:

- CBC with differential
- Procalcitonin (PCT)
- C-reactive protein (CRP)
- Blood culture
- Urinalysis
- Urine culture
- Chest radiograph
- In addition, an LP should occur with any one of the following results:
  - White blood cell (WBC) count ≤5000/microL, ≥15,000/mcroL
  - Immature-to-mature neutrophil ratio >0.2
    - PCT >0.5 ng/mL
    - CRP >20 mg/L (2 mg/dL)
    - Findings of pneumonia on chest radiograph

A similar evaluation should occur for well-appearing febrile infants 29 to 90 days of life with a recognizable or testable viral infection.

Well-appearing infants 61 to 90 days of life with temperature ≤38.6°C without focal bacterial infection should undergo urinalysis and urine culture.

Other causes of infant ill-appearance may include the following:

- Congenital heart disease
- Adrenal hyperplasia
- Inborn errors of metabolism
- Malrotation with volvulus

FEVER IN CHILDREN 3 MONTHS TO 3 YEARS

A rectal temperature of ≥39°C (102.2°F) requires evaluation for a source of occult infection with no other identified source present on PE. Temperatures lower than this may also have an SBI requiring a careful assessment. Most children presenting to an outpatient evaluation will have an identified bacterial or viral infection on PE, and a majority of these will have acute otitis media. A small percentage of patients will have a recognizable viral illness including croup, bronchiolitis, influenza, varicella, or roseola.

SBIs in this age group may include meningitis, sepsis, pneumonia, septic arthritis, or cellulitis. Immunization reactions remain the most common source of noninfectious fever in this age group. Other noninfectious etiologies are uncommon but may include drug fever, malignancy, chronic inflammatory conditions, or Kawasaki disease. Bacterial infections that may not be clinically apparent even with a careful PE consist of urinary tract infections (UTIs), bacteremia, and pneumonia.

UTIs account for 8% to 10% of young children presenting with fever and remain the most common occult bacterial infection among febrile infants and young children. Fever is the most common clinical presentation of UTI in children younger than 2 years of age and should be on the differential even if not suggestive based on PE findings.

Symptoms: Symptoms include fever, urinary symptoms (frequency, urgency, dysuria, and incontinence), abdominal/suprapubic pain, vomiting, and back pain.

Physical exam: Examine temperature, suprapubic and/or costovertebral angle tenderness, and external genitalia for anatomic abnormalities.

Lab tests/diagnostics: Urinalysis catheterization or suprapubic aspiration preferred in non–toilet-trained children or clean-voided in toilet-trained children. UTI is defined as bacteriuria of a uropathogen in a symptomatic patient. Pyuria is present in most cases. For the diagnosis of UTI in children, pyuria is defined as positive leukocyte esterase on dipstick analysis or ≥5 WBC/hpf with standardized/automated microscopy.

10% to 20% of patients may not have pyuria. The definition of bacteriuria is defined as follows:

Clean-voided sample: Growth of ≥100,000 colony-forming units (CFU)/mL of a single uropathogen and <50,000 CFU/mL of a second uropathogen. This is the same standard definition as adults.

Catheter sample: Growth of ≥50,000 CFU/mL of a single uropathogen or ≥50,000 CFU/mL or one uropathogen and <10,000 CFU/mL of a second uropathogen.

Suprapubic sample: Growth of ≥1,000 CFU/mL of an uropathogen.

Treatment: Refer to local resistance patterns for antibiotic of choice.

Occult bacteremia is defined as the isolation of a bacterial pathogen in a blood culture taken from a febrile child with an otherwise normal exam. Bacteremia that occurs in a seriously ill patient with a focal infection including meningitis, septic arthritis, or cellulitis is usually readily identified. The risk of occult bacteremia is determined by immunization status. The risk of occult bacteremia in a completely immunized child who has a fever is <1%.

Lab tests/diagnostics: Blood cultures should be obtained prior to initiation of antimicrobial therapy for any patient in whom there is suspicion of bacteremia.

Treatment: Refer to local resistance patterns for antibiotic of choice.

Most children with fever and pneumonia have associated cough, tachypnea, abnormal lung sounds, hypoxia, retractions, nasal flaring, and/or any combination of the above.

Lab Tests/diagnostics: Chest radiographs are not necessary to confirm the diagnosis of pneumonia if the diagnosis of community-acquired pneumonia is suspected based on clinical findings, and patients are well enough to be treated as outpatients.

Treatment: Refer to local resistance patterns for antibiotic of choice.

FEVER IN CHILDREN OLDER THAN 3 YEARS

Many infectious and noninfectious diseases may cause a fever in children older than 3 years with generalized or local infection being the most common etiology including upper respiratory infections (URIs), otitis media, croup, bronchiolitis, and UTIs (Table 12.1).

Table 12.1

Most Common Causes of Fever in Children Over 3 Years of Age			
Disease	History	Examination	Diagnostics
URI/viral	Nasal congestion Rhinorrhea	Clear or colored nasal discharge Fever	RSV/influenza swab
Otitis media	Ear pain	Bulging tympanic membrane TM erythema Fever Middle ear effusion	Clinical
UTI	Frequency Urgency Dysuria Hematuria Abdominal pain	Suprapubic tenderness Costovertebral angle tenderness	Bacteriuria Pyuria Hematuria Positive urine culture
Gastroenteritis	Exposures Nausea Vomiting Diarrhea Abdominal pain	Abdominal pain	Clinical

RSV, respiratory syncytial virus; TM, tympanic membrane; URI, upper respiratory infection; UTI, urinary tract infection.

FEVER OF UNKNOWN ORIGIN/FEVER WITHOUT A FOCUS

The term *fever of unknown origin* (FUO) is generally applied to children with fever >38.3°C (101°F) that lasts 8 or more days in duration, in whom no diagnosis is apparent after initial outpatient or inpatient evaluation. FUO is usually caused by a common pediatric infection with an atypically prolonged time course.

Differential Diagnosis

There is an extensive number of infectious and noninfectious etiologies of FUO usually caused by common disorders with an unusual presentation. The most common etiologies are presented in decreasing order in Table 12.2 and include infectious diseases, connective tissue disorders/disease, and neoplastic disease. However, in many cases, a diagnosis is never established and the fever resolves.

History and PE Findings

Obtaining a detailed history of exposures with a careful repeated history, PE, and interpretation of laboratory testing may be critical in making a diagnosis. The age and gender of the pediatric patient narrows the differential diagnosis. Inflammatory bowel disease and connective tissue disorders are uncommon in younger children. Autoimmune disorders occur more frequently in females. Sexual history, travel, current medications, exposure to animals, tick bites, antecedent illness, trauma, and family history are all important areas to ask about in the history of present illness. A thorough history and PE will often reveal the diagnosis in more than half of all cases of children with a fever as a chief complaint.

Physical Examination

Findings on a PE that may suggest/identify a specific cause of a fever and direct further evaluation include the following:

- Conjunctivitis
- Absence of tears, dry mucous membranes
- Rashes
- Lymphadenopathy
- Joint tenderness
- Oral ulcers
- Thrush
- Heart murmurs
- Cutaneous manifestations (rash, hyperpigmentation)
- Mental status changes

In addition, red flags for SBI include the following:

- Skin: pallor, mottled appearance, ashen or blue skin color
- General: reduced activity (exhibited by poor feeding, no smile, decreased response to stimuli, lethargy, weak high-pitched cry)
- Respiratory: tachypnea
- Cards: tachycardia, capillary refill time >3 s
- Genitourinary: reduced urine output

Table.12.2

The Most Common Etiologies of Fever of Unknown Origin				
		Common	**Less Common**	**Rare**
Infectious	**Generalized**	Cat scratch disease	Brucellosis	Enterovirus
		Salmonella	Leptospirosis	Fungal
		Malaria	Toxoplasmosis	Hepatitis viruses
		Tuberculosis	Tularemia	HIV
		Viral		Psittacosis
	Local	Infective endocarditis		
		Intra-abdominal abscess		
		Liver infection		
		Osteomyelitis		
		URI		
		UTI		
Rheumatologic		Juvenile idiopathic arthritis		
		Systemic lupus erythematosus		
		Vasculitis		
		Common	**Less Common**	
Malignancies		Leukemia	Atrial myxoma	
		Lymphoma	Hepatoma	
			Neuroblastoma	
			Sarcoma	

URI, upper respiratory infection; UTI, urinary tract infection.

Don't Miss

Fever in children is a common concern for parents and one of the most frequent presenting complaints in pediatric primary care and urgent/emergent care.

Treatment

Varies and depends on source of infection.

Prevention

Follow-Up/Patient/Family Education

Encourage the child's caretaker/parent to keep their child with a fever hydrated by encouraging fluids or breastmilk if breastfeeding. Encourage parents to seek further evaluation if a child has a sunken or bulging fontanelle, has a dry mouth or sunken eyes, or is not producing tears. Antipyretics are the most common medications administered to children with fever, and weight- or age-based dosing with acetaminophen or ibuprofen should be written out and reviewed with parent/caretaker as misuse of over-the-counter (OTC) medications is common.

References

Barbi, E., Marzuillo, P., Neri, E., Naviglio, S., & Krauss, B. S. (2017). Fever in children: Pearls and Pitfalls. *Children, 4*(9), 81. doi:10.3390/children4090081

Barry, H. C. (2019). Laboratory-based prediction model can rule out serious bacterial infections in febrile infants. *American Family Physician, 100*(7), 440.

Vissing, N. H., Chawes, B. L., Rasmussen, M. A., & Bisgard, H. (2018). Epidemiology and risk factors of infection in early childhood. *Pediatrics, 141*(6). doi:10.1542/peds.2017-0933

13

Endocrine Abnormalities Commonly Seen in Pediatric Primary Care

Casey Sweeney and Kristine M. Ruggiero

INTRODUCTION

Endocrinopathies are categorized by the most common presenting symptoms seen in pediatric primary care including weight loss, weight gain, and short stature. This chapter reviews the approach to the most common endocrine disorders that present to pediatric primary care.

OBJECTIVES

1. Describe the pathogenesis of type 1 and type 2 diabetes.
2. Identify acute and chronic complications of type 1 and type 2 diabetes.
3. Discern management options and treatment goals for type 1 diabetes.
4. Recognize the most common causes of weight loss, weight gain, and short stature in the pediatric population.
5. Identify labs to order to work up common endocrinopathies commonly seen in pediatric primary care.

CONSTITUTIONAL DELAY OF GROWTH

Etiology

Most cases of short stature in the United States are due to normal growth variation, and very few children who are referred for evaluation are found to have underlying pathology.

Constitutional delay of growth (CDG), a normal growth variant, is the most common cause of delayed puberty. Those with CGD are normal size at birth, appropriate for gestational age, and then experience a decrease in linear growth velocity starting around 3 to 6 months of age, dropping in height percentile. Typically, these children will resume a normal growth rate but continue along the lower growth percentile, although parallel to the curve.

Ultimately, there is delayed skeletal maturity, delayed puberty onset, and delayed pubertal growth spurt. Commonly, it is during this delayed puberty and associated growth period that growth and developmental discrepancy from peers is concerning and thus triggers health provider consultation. However, catchup growth is expected with achievement of genetic height potential.

Epidemiology/Risk Factors

- Constitutional delay of growth is inherited from both parents and occurs often in families with a history of parental delayed puberty or "late bloomers." CDG is more often diagnosed in males, which may reflect a tendency to seek consult for short stature or growth discrepancies from their peers rather than an increased incidence.
- While there are many potential causes for short stature and delayed growth, family history, systemic illness, and genetic disorders are often implicated.
- Globally, malnutrition is a significant cause of short stature.

Focused PE Signs/Findings

- The assessment of short stature should include a detailed health history including pregnancy and birth history, dietary history, school performance, medications, and a review of systems.
- Parental puberty onset and height should be recorded. A normal prepubertal PE is expected in CGD. Tanner staging should be examined as well in cases presenting with delayed puberty.
- A measured height greater than two standard deviations below the mean for age is considered short stature.

Lab Tests/Diagnostics

- **Radiographs:** Left hand and wrist radiographs are indicated to assess bone age. The bones of the hand and wrist have a predictable pattern of ossification allowing comparative measurement of biological and structural maturity.
- *Bone age less than chronological age is consistent with delayed skeletal maturity associated in CGD.*
- While otherwise asymptomatic short stature consistent with CGD may not indicate laboratory testing, many studies can help evaluate potential etiologies and may include complete blood cell count (CBC), complete metabolic panel, thyroid studies, celiac studies, insulin-like growth factor-1, and urinalysis. Low follicle-stimulating hormone, luteinizing hormone, testosterone, and estradiol may be found with puberty delay in CGD.

Differentials

Potential differential diagnoses for short stature or constitutional delay in growth and puberty include, but are not limited to, the following:

- Familial short stature
- Intrauterine growth restriction
- Autoimmune disease
- Endocrine disturbance
- Chronic systemic disease
- Genetic syndromes
- Occult malignancy.

Treatment

Treatment is rarely indicated in constitutional delay of growth and puberty except for those experiencing psychosocial distress.

Hormone therapy can be used to induce puberty but will not affect adult height achievement. Growth should be monitored at frequent intervals to observe growth trajectory and development.

Patient/Family Education

Patients and families should be well informed that constitutional delay of growth and puberty is a nonpathological normal variant of growth and development.

Patients are expected to achieve normal sexual development and genetic height potential.

Delayed puberty onset can cause patients and families distress and can benefit from multidisciplinary support and reassurance. Short courses of hormone therapy can be used to induce puberty with little adverse effect but are not expected to increase height achievement.

CUSHING SYNDROME

Etiology

Cushing's syndrome (CS) is caused by prolonged glucocorticoid excess and can be of exogenous or endogenous etiology. The most common cause of pediatric CS is exogenous due to corticosteroid therapy. Endogenous CS in the pediatric population is rare and accounts for only 10% of new cases annually. In older children, the most common cause of endogenous CS is pituitary adenoma (Cushing's disease), whereas infants and toddlers are more likely to have adrenal etiology. Ectopic (adrenocorticotrophic hormone [ACTH]) releasing tumors are very infrequent among pediatrics, accounting for only 1% of cases (National Institutes of Health, U.S. National Library of Medicine, Genetics Home Reference, 2019). Majority of pediatric CS cases present with decreasing growth velocity and weight gain. The presentation of these symptoms can be insidious and is often mistaken for other pathologies delaying appropriate diagnosis of CS. CS can have significant consequences and thus should be considered in all pediatric cases presenting with delayed growth velocity and weight gain.

Most cases of CS are sporadic without familial inheritance although some syndromes that manifest CS can be inherited. CS is slightly more common in females than males during adolescence, but otherwise there is no confirmed sex predominance in pediatrics.

Risk Factors

Asthma and ectopic dermatitis are conditions commonly treated with prolonged corticosteroid therapy and thus pose a risk for the development of CS. Other risk factors include ACTH for the treatment of seizure disorder, obesity, type 2 diabetes mellitus, hypertension, and adrenal or pituitary tumors.

Focused PE Signs/Findings

As discussed earlier, the assessment of pediatric growth variation should include pregnancy and birth history, dietary history, school performance, medications, and review of systems. Since CS is associated with psychiatric and psychological symptoms, which should be considered during assessment, Tanner staging should be examined for delayed pubertal development. The most common presentation of pediatric CS is decreased height percentile with obesity. Excess glucocorticoids lead to adiposity particularly on the face (moon facies), neck, and trunk with dorsocervical fat pad. Other PE findings can include truncal adiposity and obesity with thin extremities, muscle wasting, and weakness; easy bruising and purple striae; delayed puberty; or reported irregular menses. Hirsutism, acne, and virilization may be noted upon PE related to excess androgen exposure. Younger children are unlikely to present with many of the most classic symptoms. Excess mineralocorticoid exposure can lead to hypertension and abnormal metabolic laboratory results.

Lab Tests/Diagnostics

Initial laboratory evaluation for CS is to examine for hypercortisolism. No single screening test has perfect diagnostic accuracy, and two different abnormal test results are required to confirm diagnosis. Cortisol has a circadian pattern, and therefore, random serum cortisol levels are not a part of the diagnostic process. The three accepted screening tests are urinary free cortisol testing via 24-hour urine collection, midnight salivary cortisol testing, and dexamethasone suppression testing. Once hypercortisolism has been confirmed, ACTH dependency must be determined and is measured with a midnight plasma ACTH. Results indicating ACTH dependency are consistent with pituitary or extrapituitary (ectopic) etiology, and MRI is indicated. Results indicating ACTH independency are consistent with adrenal etiology, and CT is indicated. Other laboratory findings associated with CS include hypokalemia, hypernatremia, glucose intolerance, glycosuria, polymorphonuclear leukocytosis, lymphopenia, eosinophilia, and polycythemia.

Differentials

Potential differential diagnoses for pediatric CS include but are not limited to constitutional growth delay, familial short stature, growth hormone deficiency (GHD), metabolic syndrome, obesity, polycystic ovarian syndrome, or other endocrine disorders.

Treatment

- In cases of pediatric CS due to exogenous glucocorticoid therapy, treatment dose should be titrated to the minimum dose required to achieve enough treatment effect, and growth should be continuously monitored. Transsphenoidal surgery (TSS) is indicated in all cases of CS due to pituitary adenoma, with a first surgery 90% cure rate.
- GHD is common following TSS, which should be monitored for and treated to improved height achievement. Single adrenalectomy is indicated in cases of unilateral adrenal masses and yields a nearly 100% cure rate.
- Bilateral adrenal disease requires bilateral adrenalectomy and subsequent lifetime replacement of glucocorticoids and mineralocorticoids. Postoperative transient adrenal insufficiency requires initial replacement with glucocorticoid stress dosing regimen to avoid adrenal crisis.
- Medical therapy with adrenal inhibitors is available as an adjunct therapy in cases of surgical failure or when ectopic ACTH secretion cannot be localized.

Patient/Family Education

Most immediately, patients and families should be well informed of the expected surgical management outcomes as well as potential postoperative complications, which are rare but can include transient DI, syndrome of inappropriate antidiuretic hormone secretion, hypothyroidism, GHD, bleeding, and infection.

The diagnosis and management of pediatric CS is multidisciplinary and requires long-term follow-up. Patients and families should be well informed of the posttreatment expectations and goals in optimizing height potential, normalization of body composition, and management of potentially persistent pathology including adiposity, insulin resistance, hypertension, and osteoporosis. The role of healthy lifestyle practice in improving outcomes should be emphasized as a part of initial and ongoing management.

Key Points

- Inhaled corticosteroids (ICS) play an important role in the prevention of severe asthma exacerbation. The potential effect of *chronic ICS use during childhood on pediatric growth velocity and adult height is controversial and unclear.*
- While research has not yet consistently demonstrated an effect, some suggests that there may be a risk of minimally decreased adult height among children treated with ICS over time. In the absence of definitive data, potential risks should be weighed against the known benefits of ICS in asthma management.
- Recommendations include using the use of lowest dose for therapeutic effect, not using in conjunction with other corticosteroids (oral, nasal, topical), and close monitoring of pediatric growth and development.

GROWTH HORMONE DEFICIENCY

Etiology

Congenital GHD is thought to be present at birth but often has delayed diagnosis until later in childhood when short stature is recognized. Most cases of pediatric GHD are idiopathic. GHD is a relatively rare cause of short stature in children. The most common known etiologies are intracranial lesions or radiation treatment.

Epidemiology/Risk Factors

- Pediatric onset GHD can be congenital or acquired and affects approximately 1 in 3,500.
- In congenital GHD, newborns are typically of normal size or appropriate for gestational age at birth but may have jaundice, periods of hypoglycemia, microphallus, or midline craniofacial abnormalities such as cleft palate. Pediatric-onset GHD ultimately manifests as a decrease in growth velocity and failure to achieve expected growth increments over the course of development. Delayed skeletal maturation, specifically delayed lengthening of long bones, is observable as short stature. Weight is often appropriate for age but appears out of proportion to height.
- While GHD may occasionally run in families, it is most often isolated rather than inherited. Like other pediatric cases of short stature, GHD is more often diagnosed in males; however, this may be somewhat attributable to an increased tendency to seek consult rather than increased incidence.
- Acquired pediatric GHD can be caused by central nervous system infection, central nervous system or head and neck radiation, pituitary or hypothalamus tumors, head trauma, or birth trauma.

Focused PE Signs/Findings

As discussed earlier, the assessment of short stature should include detailed health history including pregnancy and birth history, dietary history, school performance, medications, and a review of systems. Tanner staging should be examined for delayed pubertal development. Parental developmental history, as well as calculation of midparental height, should be taken. In addition to decreased growth velocity and short stature, PE findings may include delayed closure of fontanels, delayed dental development, fine hair, and poor nail growth. Truncal adiposity may be noted since growth hormone (GH) promotes lipolysis.

Bones should be assessed using left hand and wrist radiographs. The bones of the hand and wrist have a predictable pattern of ossification allowing comparative measurement of biological and structural maturity. Bone age less than chronological age is consistent with delayed skeletal maturity of GHD.

Lab Tests/Diagnostics

The potential laboratory assessment of delayed growth velocity and short stature can include the following:

- Labs: CBC, complete metabolic panel, thyroid studies, and celiac studies.
- GHD may coexist with another pituitary hormone deficiency, and this should be considered when planning laboratory evaluation.
- Interpretation of GH laboratory measurements is complex since GH has pulsatile secretion, is most often present in very low or undetectable levels, and may also be affected by nutritional status or systemic disease. Thus, single measurements are insufficient for diagnosis alone.
- The common first step in measurement of GH sufficiency is insulin-like growth factor 1 (IGF-1) and may be found low or normal levels in GHD. Insulin-like growth factor–binding protein 3 (IGFBP-3) is a less sensitive marker of GHD but also often included as it is less affected by nutritional status than IGF-1.
- GH provocation testing has limitations but often follows IGF-1 and IGFBP-3 screening in suspected cases. GH provocation testing (aka GH stimulation testing) is meant to stimulate the pituitary to secrete GH also allowing for interval measurement. Stimulating agents may include insulin, arginine, levodopa, clonidine, or glucagon, and the test is both administered and interpreted by specialized pediatric endocrinology.
- Since some patients with GHD also often have tumors or other anomalies of the pituitary gland and hypothalamus, MRI may also be indicated.

Differentials

Potential differential diagnoses for pediatric GHD include but are not limited to constitutional delay in growth and puberty, familial short stature, hypopituitarism, intrauterine growth restriction, autoimmune disease, endocrine disturbance, chronic systemic disease, genetic syndromes, and occult malignancy.

Treatment

- Treatment with recombinant growth hormone (rhGH) is indicated in all cases of pediatric hormone deficiency and is USFDA approved.
- The dose is typically increased during puberty and discontinued at completion of skeletal maturity.

- rhGH therapy increases height velocity, and it is expected that with rhGH therapy, children will achieve their height potential with the predicted midparental height range.
- Treatment should be monitored with height measurement at regular intervals throughout and should include periodic bone age studies.

Patient/Family Education

Patients and families should be informed of the expectation to achieve normal or near-normal potential height with rhGH therapy. Treatment includes daily dosing and frequent follow-up to monitor growth. Side effects of rhGH therapy are rare, with the most common side effects being headaches and pain at the injection site. Other less common side effects include intracranial hypertension or pseudotumor cerebri, slipped capital femoral epiphysis (SCFE), and peripheral edema (Polack et al., 2017; Sperling, 2014).

PRIMARY ADRENAL INSUFFICIENCY (CONGENITAL ADRENAL HYPERPLASIA, ADDISON DISEASE)

Etiology

Adrenal insufficiency (AI) can be congenital or acquired and is characterized by a disorder of the adrenal cortex (primary), insufficient production of ACTH by the pituitary (secondary), or insufficient cortisol-releasing hormone (CRH) by the hypothalamus (tertiary).

Ultimately, primary adrenal insufficiency manifests in deficiency of glucocorticoids with or without mineralocorticoid deficiency and abnormal adrenal androgens.

AI can have variable presentation from acute crisis to more insidious and nonspecific symptoms, sometimes making diagnosis challenging, but timely diagnosis and treatment is essential in preventing associated morbidity and mortality (Auron & Raissouni, 2015).

Epidemiology/Risk Factors

- The most common cause of pediatric primary AI is congenital adrenal hyperplasia (CAH), accounting for 70% of cases.
- CAH is an inherited autosomal recessive disorder of impaired enzyme activity in adrenal steroidogenesis and present in approximately 1 in 14,000 live births.
- The classic manifestation includes aldosterone deficiency with salt wasting and most commonly presents in the newborn period. Since neonatal salt wasting is difficult to diagnose and is potentially fatal, CAH is part of mandated newborn screening in the United States and many other countries as well.
- Autoimmune adrenalitis (Addison's disease), caused by autoimmune destruction of the adrenal cortex, accounts for approximately 15% of pediatric primary AI cases. The clinical presentation may include autoimmune destruction of other endocrine glands as well.
- Overall, adrenal insufficiency has female sex predominance. The development of CAH is inherited and may be more common in those with Ashkenazi Jewish lineage.
- Genetic, immune, and environmental factors can play a role in the development of PI, but it is often associated with the presence of eventual development of other autoimmune diseases. Addison's disease has been associated with hypoparathyroidism, hypothyroidism, hypogonadism, pernicious anemia, and diabetes mellitus of polyglandular autoimmune syndromes.

Focused PE Signs/Findings

- **Infants:** Primary adrenal insufficiency in infants can present at birth, and in cases of CAH, female newborns may present with ambiguous genitalia. During the newborn period, there may be prolonged jaundice and periods of hypoglycemia. Infants can experience poor weight gain or weight loss, lethargy, or irritability. The neonatal period carries risk for adrenal crisis.
- **Older children and adolescence:** Symptom manifestation can include fatigue, muscle weakness, anorexia, headache, nausea, vomiting, diarrhea, and abdominal pain. In aldosterone deficiency, salt craving is a common presenting symptom.
- Growth and development manifestations in childhood and adolescents can include hirsutism, weight loss, slow growth, or growth acceleration including premature adrenarche or precocious puberty. Adolescents can report decreased libido, loss of pubic, and axillary hair.
- Hyperpigmentation is classic finding present in over 90% of cases of AI and is generalized or observable at oral mucosa, skin creases, scars, areola, and genitalia.
- Hypotension or orthostatic hypotension may be measured upon exam. Laboratory findings of PI will be variable dependent upon aldosterone deficiency or excess and can include hyponatremia, hyperkalemia, hypoglycemia, ketomenia, and ketonuria.

Acute adrenal crisis can progress quickly and be fatal. Symptoms include hypotension, tachycardia, diaphoresis, dizziness, nausea, vomiting, confusion, hyponatremic dehydration, metabolic acidosis, and coma.

Lab Tests/Diagnostics

Testing for primary AI starts with a morning measurement of serum cortisol with expected low levels. Concurrent increased ACTH is expected in primary AI as well. Other dynamic laboratory evaluation of primary AI in cases of clinical uncertainty can include ACTH stimulation testing to measure cortisol and aldosterone levels following a dose of intravenous ACTH. Adrenal autoantibody testing establishes autoimmune origin.

Differentials

Differential diagnoses for PI due to CAH or autoimmune Addison's disease include but are not limited to other endocrine syndromes, other autoimmune syndromes, other disorders of growth and development, muscular disorders, nephritis, anorexia, depression, gastroenteritis, infection, and secondary or tertiary adrenal insufficiency.

Treatment

The multisystem complexity of both acute adrenal crisis and primary adrenal insufficiency necessitates pediatric specialty care. Acute adrenal crisis is life-threatening, which requires acute emergency treatment with the initial goal of hemodynamic stabilization. Chronic adrenal insufficiency in pediatrics requires glucocorticoid replacement. Oral hydrocortisone is preferred to minimize growth suppression. Those with salt-wasting CAH require mineralocorticoid and sodium chloride supplementation therapy.

Patient/Family Education

Patients and families should be well informed of the expected growth and development as well as the importance of treatment adherence and need for routine follow-up. The associated risk of adrenal collapse with surgery or other acute stress circumstances will require stress dosing of glucocorticoids during these episodes. When managed appropriately, pediatric patients are ultimately expected to lead normal lives.

WEIGHT GAIN

■ PEDIATRIC HYPOTHYROIDISM (HASHIMOTO THYROIDITIS)

Etiology

Hypothyroidism is a common endocrine disorder and in pediatrics may be congenital or acquired. Globally, iodine deficiency is the most common cause of hypothyroidism but is rare in the United States.

Epidemiology/Risk Factors

Congenital hypothyroidism affects 1 in 3,000 or 4,000 infants and is most typically due to thyroid gland dysgenesis. Congenital hypothyroidism causes significant but preventable consequences including developmental cognitive delay and intellectual disability and is therefore part of routine newborn screening in the United States and many other countries.

Acquired hypothyroidism in the United States is most commonly caused by autoimmune thyroiditis (Hashimoto thyroiditis). Other less frequent causes of hypothyroidism may be attributed to radiation exposure for cancer treatment of secondary drug effects. Symptoms typically present in late childhood or adolescence and affect 1 in 1,250 children in the United States. Hashimoto is more common in females, and symptoms typically present in late childhood or adolescence.

Risk Factors

Congenital hypothyroidism is most commonly sporadic but can be inherited. Hashimoto thyroiditis is frequently associated with a family history of autoimmune thyroiditis and is more common in those with other autoimmune diseases or syndromes.

Symptoms

Hashimoto thyroiditis can have an insidious onset but most often presents with asymptomatic goiter or possibly associated symptoms such as dysphagia, hoarseness, or sleep disturbance due to obstructive sleep apnea. Other symptoms can include fatigue, lethargy, constipation, decreased appetite, and cold intolerance. Of note, some pediatric cases of Hashimoto may initially present with hyperthyroid symptoms of the initial transient thyrotoxic phase and then manifest as hypothyroid (Hanley, Lord, & Bauer, 2016).

Weight gain can be associated with Hashimoto although skeletal maturation is more affected, and thus, these children may appear overweight for their height. The disruption in linear growth velocity can manifest in short stature and delayed dental eruption. Parents may also present with concerns of pubertal delay and menstrual irregularities, or less often precocious sexual development such as testicular enlargement, breast development, galactorrhea, and vaginal bleeding in cases of prolonged, untreated hypothyroidism.

Focused PE Signs/Findings

Goiter is the most common PE finding in pediatric Hashimoto. Palpation typically reveals a nontender, firm, diffusely enlarged thyroid and possibly nodules or pseudonodules. Other exam findings may include bradycardia, paroxysmal muscle weakness, abnormal deep tendon reflexes, myxedema, short stature, delayed fontanel closure, and delayed dental eruption.

Lab Tests/Diagnostics

- Following history and PE, the evaluation of Hashimoto thyroiditis requires serum thyroid function tests.
  - T3 and total T4 are not considered helpful in examining suspected hypothyroid.
  - *TSH is expected to be high with a low level of free serum thyroxine.*
- Elevated TSH with normal free T4 is subclinical.
- Elevated TSH with low free T4 is suggestive of central hypothyroidism and requires further investigation with imaging to assess the pituitary gland.
- The thyroid antibodies antithyroglobulin and antithyroid peroxidase are expected to be elevated in autoimmune cases but are not crucial to diagnosis.
- *Thyroid uptake scans are not considered* helpful in diagnosis of Hashimoto, and surgical or needle biopsy, while diagnostic, is rarely indicated.
- Skeletal studies may demonstrate delayed bone age or delayed epiphyseal development.

Differentials

Potential differential diagnoses for pediatric Hashimoto include, but are not limited to, the following:

- Constipation
- Malabsorption syndromes
- Genetic syndromes
- Constitutional growth delay
- Growth hormone deficiency (GHD)
- Depression
- Short stature

Treatment

The treatment for Hashimoto thyroiditis is levothyroxine, synthetic T4, once daily. Age- and weight-based dosing of levothyroxine is often initiated at low levels and titrated to achieve euthyroid state, observed through repeat thyroid testing.

Long-term monitoring of thyroid function is essential in the management of pediatric hypothyroid to ensure appropriate growth and development through adolescence.

Patient/Family Education

- Patients and families should be well informed that the goals of hypothyroid treatment are to restore normal thyroid function, reduce symptoms, reduce goiter size, and protect growth and development.
- Levothyroxine should not be taken concurrently with iron, calcium, or soy, as they decrease thyroid hormone absorption.

TYPE 2 DIABETES

Etiology

Type 2 diabetes mellitus is characterized by two underlying defects. The earliest abnormality in an individual who develops type 2 diabetes mellitus is insulin resistance, which initially is compensated with an increase in insulin secretion.

Type 2 diabetes mellitus then develops due to a defect in insulin secretion; the amount of insulin production cannot keep up the demand (increased requirements needed) from matching the increased requirements imposed by the insulin-resistant state.

Epidemiology/Risk Factors

The percentage of cases of diabetes in children and adolescents caused by type 2 diabetes has risen in the past one to two decades.

Because of the early age of onset and longer diabetes duration, children with type 1 or 2 diabetes are at risk for developing diabetes-related complications at a younger age. This can significantly affect their quality of life and shorten their life expectancy.

Focused PE Signs/Findings

PE findings may be within normal limits, with greater tendency for patients being over-weight or obese. In addition, patients may often have signs of insulin resistance, such as hypertension, PCOS (polycystic ovarian syndrome), or acanthosis nigricans.

Lab Tests/Diagnostics

The American Diabetes Association (ADA) criteria for the diagnosis of diabetes are any of the following (ADA, 2010):

- an HbA1c level of 6.5% or higher; the test should be performed in a laboratory using a method that is certified by the National Glycohemoglobin Standardization Program (NGSP) and standardized or traceable to the Diabetes Control and Complications Trial (DCCT) reference assay, or
- a fasting plasma glucose level of 126 mg/dL (7.0 mmol/L) or higher; fasting is defined as no caloric intake for at least 8 hours, or
- a 2-hour plasma glucose level of 200 mg/dL (11.1 mmol/L) or higher during a 75-g oral glucose tolerance test, or
- a random plasma glucose of 200 mg/dL (11.1 mmol/L) or higher in a patient with classic symptoms of hyperglycemia (i.e., polyuria, polydipsia, polyphagia, weight loss) or hyperglycemic crisis

Differentials

See "Differentials" under "Type 1 Diabetes" section.

Treatments

Some children diagnosed with type 2 diabetes can achieve their target blood sugar levels with diet and exercise alone. Others may require diabetes medications or insulin therapy.

Examples of possible treatments for type 2 diabetes include metformin (Glucophage, Glumetza). In addition, the USFDA recently approved Victoza (liraglutide) injections for treatment of pediatric patients 10 years or older with type 2 diabetes. Victoza is the first noninsulin drug approved to treat type 2 diabetes in pediatric patients since metformin was approved for pediatric use in 2000 (USFDA, 2019).

Patient/Family Education

The working group on type 2 diabetes care in children recommended guidelines that healthcare professionals should offer children and young people with type 2 diabetes and their family. The group specifically recommended that the program includes the following core topics (National Collaborating Centre for Women's and Children's Health, 2015a, 2015b):

- HbA1c monitoring and targets
- The effects of diet, physical activity, body weight, and intercurrent illness on blood glucose control

■ The aims of metformin therapy and possible adverse effects

■ The complications of type 2 diabetes and how to prevent them

WEIGHT LOSS

■ PEDIATRIC HYPERTHYROIDISM (GRAVES' DISEASE)

Etiology

While hyperthyroidism is a relatively rare childhood disorder, it has potentially significant effects and thus requires prompt diagnosis and referral. Pediatric hyperthyroidism is most commonly (>90%) due to autoimmune etiology, Graves' disease, with an incidence of 1 per 10,000 children in the United States. Graves' disease is more common in females and most often occurs between 10 and 15 years of age. Other, less frequent causes of hyperthyroidism can be attributed to autonomously functioning thyroid nodules, thyroid-stimulating hormone (TSH)–producing tumors, adverse drug effects, infection, and iodine exposure (Rivkees & Bauer, 2019).

Epidemiology/Risk Factors

The development of Graves' disease appears to be multifactorial involving genetic, immune, and environmental factors. Research has demonstrated clustering of Graves' in families and an association with risk for development of other autoimmune disorders.

Symptoms

Hyperthyroidism may have an insidious presentation and can be cyclic in nature with periods of remission and exacerbation. Common symptoms include weight loss, increased appetite, insomnia, heat intolerance, diaphoresis, heart palpitations, diarrhea, polyuria, and irregular menses. The presentation of hyperactivity, nervousness, poor concentration, emotional liability, or moodiness may erroneously be attributed to other behavioral diagnoses. Changes in behavior and decreased school performance should prompt consideration of hyperthyroidism.

Differentials

Potential differential diagnoses for pediatric Graves' include, but are not limited, to the following:

a. Hypermetabolic conditions
b. Excessive exogenous thyroid hormone
c. McCune–Albright syndrome
d. Early-phase Hashimoto's thyroiditis
e. Pituitary adenoma
f. Attention deficit hyperactivity disorder
g. Anxiety disorders
h. Anorexia

Focused PE Signs/Findings

Common PE findings include warm moist skin, tremors, paroxysmal muscle weakness, tachycardia, systolic hypertension, and increased pulse pressure.

Examination of the neck is expected to reveal a diffusely enlarged, nonnodular goiter with or without thyroid bruit upon auscultation.

Children and adolescents may also present with ophthalmic findings such as eyelid retraction, eyelid lag, periorbital edema, erythema, conjunctivitis, and exophthalmos.

While the clinical manifestations of pediatric hyperthyroidism are like those of adults, hyperthyroidism can affect childhood growth and development including premature craniosynostosis, early bone growth acceleration, advanced bone age, and delayed puberty.

Don't Miss

Thyroid storm is a rare but severe complication in pediatric hyperthyroidism and should not be missed. Symptoms include tachycardia, hyperthermia, hypertension, congestive heart failure, and delirium that can quickly progress to coma and death.

Lab Tests/Diagnostics

- Following history and PE, the evaluation of suspected hyperthyroidism requires serum thyroid function tests.
- TSH will be suppressed with elevated free thyroxine (T4) and triiodothyronine (T3).
- Following the laboratory diagnosis of hyperthyroidism, Graves' etiology can be confirmed by the presence of thyroid-stimulating immunoglobulin (TSI). TSH receptor-binding antibodies are also often elevated.
- Other diagnostic evaluations of hyperthyroidism can include thyroid ultrasound, CT scan, fine-needle aspiration for biopsy, and radionuclide scanning particularly considered in cases of negative antibody testing, thyroid gland asymmetry, or nodular thyroid.

Treatment

- The antithyroid medication methimazole is considered first-line treatment for pediatric Graves' disease.
- Age- and weight-based dosing is initiated to normalized FT4 or T4, followed by maintenance dosing to achieve remission.
- Thyroid function studies are evaluated every 2 weeks until values normalized and then every 3 to 4 months to monitor.
- Remission is typically assessed following 2 years of therapy by a reduction in medication dose or discontinuation.
- The use of methimazole and the pathology of Graves' itself also requires baseline measurement and observation of absolute neutrophil count and liver function over the course of treatment.
- Common minor drug side effects can include nausea, rash, myalgia, and arthralgia.
- Major drug adverse effects are uncommon but include agranulocytosis, vasculitis, or hepatitis and require treatment discontinuation.
- Beta-adrenergic blockers are indicated in cases with severe tachycardia and hypertension but also offer symptomatic relief from nervousness, palpitations, tremor, and so on.

Don't Miss

Propylthiouracil (PTU) is an alternative thionamide more commonly used in adults but carries a U.S. Food and Drug Administration (USFDA) black-box warning due to severe pediatric hepatotoxicity. PTU is thus avoided except for unique circumstances

(continued)

(continued)

such methimazole hypersensitivity or adverse effect requiring drug discontinuation, pregnancy, or cases of contraindicated radioactive iodine or surgical management. Iodine therapy and radioactive iodine ablation are infrequent approaches reserved for antithyroid treatment failure or extreme thyrotoxicity. Subtotal or total thyroidectomy is rarely indicated in pediatric Graves' cases, but there are exceptions.

Patient/Family Education

Families should be well informed that the goal of methimazole treatment is to achieve a state of remission. Remission rates are variable, and some may experience exacerbations, but prolonged remission is achieved in up to two-thirds of children. Thus, the initial and long-term management of pediatric Graves' requires routine follow-up to monitor thyroid stabilization, maintenance dosing, and remission. Families must also be vigilant in observing for side effects and potential adverse drug effects requiring dose reduction or discontinuation.

■ TYPE 1 DIABETES (INSULIN-DEPENDENT DIABETES MELLITUS)

Etiology

Although the exact cause/etiology of insulin-dependent diabetes mellitus (IDDM) is unknown, genetic, autoimmune, and environmental factors have all been linked to the cause of type 1 diabetes. Diabetes is a chronic metabolic disorder characterized by hyperglycemia and abnormal energy metabolism due to absent or diminished insulin secretion. Type 1 diabetes mellitus (T1DM) results from the lack of insulin production in the beta cells of the pancreas.

After 90% of the beta cell function has been destroyed, loss of insulin secretion becomes clinically significant. The lack of insulin prevents glucose from entering the cell, and hyperglycemia results.

The production of ketoacids is brought about in this increased catabolic state. When blood glucose levels exceed 180 mg/dL, glycosuria results in an osmotic diuresis and polyuria ensues. If insulin deficiency is severe, ketones are produced in large quantities leading to diabetic ketoacidosis (DKA).

Epidemiology/Risk Factors

T1DM, one of the most common chronic diseases in childhood, is caused by insulin deficiency following the destruction of the insulin-producing pancreatic beta cells. It most commonly presents in childhood.

Symptoms

As shown in Box 13.1, a history of new-onset weight loss, polydipsia, polyphagia, and polyuria is consistent with T1DM.

Differentials

- Type 2 DM
- MODY (maturity onset diabetes in the young), several hereditary forms of DM that carry a strong family history
- Psychogenic polydipsia

BOX 13.1 THE MOST COMMON CLINICAL MANIFESTATIONS OF TYPE 1 DIABETES MELLITUS

"The 3 P's" (Polyuria, Polydipsia, Polyphagia)

Weight loss

Increased thirst and frequent urination (due to excess sugar building up in child's bloodstream that pulls fluid from tissues)

Extreme hunger

Fatigue

Irritability or behavior changes

Fruity-smelling breath

Blurred vision

Yeast infection

- Nephrogenic diabetes insipidus (DI)
- High-output renal failure
- Transient hyperglycemia with illness and other stress
- Steroid therapy

Focused Physical Exam Signs/Findings

A physical exam (PE) is usually within normal limits in a child with T1DM, unless DKA is present (see Box 13.2).

Treatment

Treatment of IDDM is through insulin replacement. Usually, 0.5 to 1.0 unit/kg of insulin per day is the daily diabetic requirement. This is divided into two to three insulin

BOX 13.2 DON'T MISS/FAIL TO SPOT THE SIGNS AND SYMPTOMS OF DIABETIC KETOACIDOSIS AND HYPOGLYCEMIA IN A DIABETIC PATIENT

DKA: The child with DKA will present as acutely ill-appearing and significantly dehydrated. Symptoms can include polyuria, polydipsia, fatigue, headache, nausea, emesis, and abdominal pain. The child may have altered mental status (confused to comatose), and on PE, tachycardia will be present with hyperpnea (Kussmaul respirations) are often present. From the ketosis, a fruity odor may be present on their breath. Intravascular volume depletion can lead to hypovolemia, and while cerebral edema is a rare very late finding, it is often fatal. Signs of changing mental status, unequal pupils, or decorticate or decerebrate posturing and/or seizure indicate cerebral edema. Early ID and management are the keys to improving outcomes.

Hypoglycemia: Signs of hypoglycemia can include trembling, diaphoresis, flushing, tachycardia, sleepiness, confusion, mood changes, seizure, and coma. A blood glucose level should be checked on any patient with known type 1 or type 2 DM who presents to primary care for a sick visit, as illness can affect blood sugar levels. During times of stress, additional insulin may be needed. Treatment of hypoglycemia includes eating a carbohydrate snack to increase serum glucose concentration. If the child is vomiting, cake icing or Monogel instant glucose can be applied to the buccal mucosa to provide glucose.

DKA, diabetic ketoacidosis; DM, diabetes mellitus; ID, identification; PE, physical examination.

injections per day: two-thirds of the total daily dose before breakfast and one-third before dinner; in addition, insulin is divided between short-acting regular insulin and intermediate-acting NPH insulin (Rosner & Roman-Urrestarazu, 2019). Sometimes insulin pumps are used, which deliver a basal-bolus of insulin.

Hemoglobin A1C, a test measuring glycosylated hemoglobin, should be monitored every 3 months to assess average glycemic control. An A1C goal of <7.5% (58 mmol/mol) is recommended across all pediatric age groups.

Patient/Family Education

Patient and family education play a vital role in management of T1DM. A child with IDDM is treated through insulin replacement, diet, exercise, psychological support, and regular medical follow-up. Diabetes education in the pediatric patient varies depending on the age and developmental level of the child at diagnosis, and care should be taken to take this into account when providing education (i.e., a 3-year-old child may be able to pick which snack they want, versus a 10-year-old child should become familiar with checking their own blood sugars (BSs), versus an adolescent should be able to start becoming more autonomous in the chronic management of their diabetes; Rosner & Roman-Urrestarazu, 2019).

References

Auron, M., & Raissouni, N. (2015). Adrenal insufficiency. *Pediatrics in Review, 36*(3), 92–102. doi:10.1542/pir.36-3-92

Hanley, P., Lord, K., & Bauer, A. (2016). Thyroid disorders in children and adolescents: A review. *JAMA Pediatrics, 170*(10), 1008–1019. doi:10.1001/jamapediatrics.2016.0486

Marino, B. S., Cassedy, A., Drotar, D., & Wray, J. (2016). The impact of neurodevelopmental and psychosocial outcomes on health-related quality of life in survivors of congenital heart disease. *The Journal of Pediatrics, 174*, 11–22. doi:10.1016/j.jpeds.2016.03.071

National Collaborating Centre for Women's and Children's Health. (2015a). *Diabetes (type 1 and type 2) in children and young people: Diagnosis and management.* London: National Institute for Health and Care Excellence.

National Collaborating Centre for Women's and Children's Health. (2015b). *Education for children and young people with type 2 diabetes.* Retrieved from https://www.ncbi.nlm.nih.gov/books/NBK343400/

National Institutes of Health, U.S. National Library of Medicine, Genetics Home Reference. (2019). *Cushing disease.* Retrieved from https://ghr.nlm.nih.gov/condition/cushing-disease

Polak, M., Blair, J., Kotnik, P., Pournara, E., Pedersen, B. T., & Rohrer, T. R. (2017). Early growth hormone treatment start in childhood growth hormone deficiency improves near adult height: Analysis from NordiNet International Outcome Study. *European Journal of Endocrinology, 177*(5), 421–429. doi:10.1530/EJE-16-1024

Rivkees, S., & Bauer, A. (2019). Thyroid disorders: Manifestations, evaluations, and management in children and adolescents. *Contemporary Pediatrics.* Retrieved from https://www.contemporarypediatrics.com/endocrinology/thyroid-disorders-manifestations-evaluation-and-management-children-and-adolescents

Rosner, B., & Roman-Urrestarazu, A. (2019). Health-related quality of life in paediatric patients with Type 1 diabetes mellitus using insulin infusion systems. A systematic review and meta-analysis. *PLoS One, 14*(6), e0217655. doi:10.1371/journal.pone.0217655

Sperling, M. (2014). *Pediatric endocrinology* (4th ed.). Philadelphia, PA: Elsevier/Saunders.

U.S. Food and Drug Administration. (2019, July 17). Retrieved from https://www.fda.gov

14

Common Allergies and Immunodeficiencies Seen in Pediatric Primary Care

Laura Cline

INTRODUCTION

Allergies and infections are a common cause for pediatric urgent care visits. Often, an infant or child may have different types of allergies or recurrent infections that do not respond to first-line therapies, and it is important to understand the common presentations, approach to care, and various treatment modalities for children with allergies and immune disorders. This chapter will outline the approach to care of the child with allergies, anaphylaxis, and recurrent infections and common immunodeficiencies in pediatrics that would be seen in pediatric ambulatory care.

OBJECTIVES

1. Identify different types of allergy presentations and the various treatment modalities.
   - Understand the difference between intolerance and an allergic reaction.
2. Recognize signs and symptoms of anaphylaxis and be familiar with the treatment of anaphylaxis, including when to administer epinephrine.
3. Understand the management of the child with recurrent infections/immunodeficiency.
   - Recognize the clinical features suggestive of a primary immunodeficiency.
   - Review the lab studies to order to evaluate the immune system.

ALLERGY

Etiology

An allergy is a specific reaction to an exposure of a substance. Allergies can develop at any age. A child can become allergic to a food, medication, or other substance the first time they are exposed to it or after repeated exposures. Common environmental allergens include pollen, bees, animals (cats, dogs), grass, or dust. Common food allergies include milk, peanuts, fruits, seafood, or eggs.

Allergies are an allergy-specific IgE-mediated response within the body. Patients can be sensitized to antigens without having a reaction. Sensitization is the presence of an IgE-mediated response without clinical symptoms upon exposure. It is essential for healthcare providers to know and understand the difference between intolerance and an allergy when dealing with the pediatric population.

A food allergy is a specific immune response that occurs reproducibly upon subsequent exposures of certain offending foods. Food allergies are potentially life-threatening. A food intolerance is a specific ingredient in food (usually a protein) that elicits an immunological reaction to an allergen-specific immune cell. Food intolerances are not life-threatening (Boyce et al., 2010). Different allergies and intolerances are diagnosed with knowing previous reactions (what symptoms they presented with, how soon after exposure, how it was relieved), skin testing, blood testing, and potentially food or drug challenges.

There are multiple forms of allergen exposure. The following are the most common forms: ingestion, contact, or inhalation. For exposure by ingestion, the patient has been exposed orally to the substance. Ingestion can happen through eating the substance directly or through the saliva of someone who has eaten the substance. Exposure to an allergen by contact happens through the skin. Contact exposure often occurs by direct contact via skin with the allergen, which causes a rash or hives to develop. Inhalation exposure is when particles of the substance have been inhaled. Allergic reactions via inhalation exposure are very rare, although still possible. Early introduction to foods that cause allergies is highly recommended. The American Academy of Pediatrics recommends that early introduction of high-allergen foods not be delayed beyond the age of 6 months (National Academies of Sciences, Engineering, and Medicine, 2017).

ALLERGIC TRIAD

In pediatrics, it is important to look for the allergic triad, which consists of AR, AD, and asthma. These reactions often come hand in hand, and a child can present with one, two, or all three symptoms. Although asthma is typically followed and monitored by pulmonologists, it is important to note when discussing allergies in the pediatric population.

ALLERGIC RHINITIS

Allergic rhinitis (AR) is also known as hay fever. AR is almost always a genetic disease. There can be seasonal AR (typically caused by pollen and usually develops after the age of 6 years old) and perennial AR (present throughout the year and can be seen in any age group). The most common offenders are pollen, dust mites, mold, and animal dander.

Signs and symptoms of AR are as follows: sneezing, congestion, itchy nose, throat, eyes, and ears, clear rhinorrhea, allergic shiners, nosebleeds (from rubbing nose), swollen nostrils or boggy nasal turbinates, recurrent ear complaints (fluid in ears), snoring, mouth breathing, fatigue, and the allergic salute. Treatment for AR is as follows: avoid the allergen, over-the-counter (OTC) antihistamines (both long-acting and short-acting), anti-inflammatory nasal sprays, corticosteroid nasal sprays, decongestants, and allergic eye drops.

ALLERGY TESTING

Lab Tests

Skin or scratch testing is performed when a small amount of solution that contains different allergens is either injected under the skin or applied with a small scratch of the skin. When there is a positive, the skin test will present with both a wheal and a flare. A wheal is a bump that appears on the skin after an antigen has been applied, and a flare is the erythematous or inflamed area after an antigen has been applied. Blood testing or RAST testing, i.e., IgE blood testing, is also used to confirm allergies. The gold standard of testing once an allergen is confirmed is either a food or drug challenge, which is performed under the recommendation and supervision of a pediatric allergist (Sicherer et al., 2017).

ANAPHYLAXIS

Etiology

Anaphylaxis is an IgE-mediated immune response within the body that produces a sudden release of mast cells and basophil-derived mediators into circulation throughout the body.

Epidemiology/Risk Factors

An antigen triggers production of IgE-mediated antibodies by IgE binding to the surface of mast cells or basophils. These basophils are triggered with subsequent exposures to the antigen causing anaphylaxis. Anaphylaxis presents differently in each person, and subsequent reactions can even present differently in each patient.

Don't Miss

When discussing anaphylaxis, it is essential to remember that when two or more body systems are involved, epinephrine is always necessary to prevent further progression of the reaction. Children can exhibit anaphylaxis to any known or unknown allergen. The eight most common food allergens that induce anaphylaxis are tree nuts, soy, fish, peanuts, shellfish, eggs, wheat, and dairy (American Academy of Allergy, Asthma, and Immunology, 2015).

The signs and symptoms of anaphylaxis are triggered when the histamine is released either locally or systemically within the body. When it is released locally, it causes urticarial or hives. Systemic release of a histamine causes both hemodynamic and cardiovascular changes. Histamines bind to H1 and H2 receptors and lead to flushing, headaches, and hypotension. When histamines act on H1 receptors, the following symptoms can be produced: pruritus, vasodilation, tachycardia, bronchoconstriction, flushing, and headaches (O'Keefe et al., 2017).

Anaphylaxis incorporates three different potential reaction phases. The first or uniphasic phase is most commonly how anaphylaxis presents. Typically, the uniphasic phase develops within minutes to 1-hour postexposure. The symptoms resolve within hours of treatment, and there are no rebound symptoms. Next, we potentially see the biphasic phase; this is when symptoms reappear after resolution. The biphasic phase is typically seen within 8 to 10 hours postexposure. Finally, there is the protracted phase. The protracted phase is the rarest phase and happens when the anaphylactic reaction lasts for hours, days, and in some cases weeks (O'Keefe et al., 2017).

Focused PE Signs/Findings

The most common signs and symptoms of anaphylaxis by body system:

Skin: Urticaria, angioedema, pruritus, erythema, periorbital itching/erythema/edema

Respiratory: Upper airway: nasal congestion, sneezing, cough, hoarseness, oropharyngeal/laryngeal edema

Lower airway: bronchospasm, wheezing, chest tightness

Cardiovascular: dizziness, tachycardia, syncope, hypotension

Hypotension symptoms: fatigue, palpitations, clammy/cool/pale skin, rapid/shallow breathing, blurred vision, dizziness/lightheadedness

GI: abdominal pain, nausea, vomiting, diarrhea

Neuro: feelings of impending doom

Diagnostic Criteria for Anaphylaxis

Anaphylaxis is highly likely when any one of the following criteria is fulfilled:

- Acute onset of illness (minutes to less than 2 hours)
- Involvement of skin/mucosal tissue plus
  - Respiratory involvement
  - Hypotension (in infants and children, if there is a greater than 30% decrease in systolic BP; O'Keefe et al., 2017)

Treatment

The first line of treatment for anaphylaxis is always epinephrine.

Epinephrine Dosing
<25 kg: 0.15 mg every 5 minutes as needed.
≥25 kg: 0.3 mg every 5 minutes as needed.

Epinephrine can be given every 3 to 5 minutes in severe cases. Epinephrine is an alpha- and beta-agonist. It decreases the mediated mast cell release. The alpha component works on smooth muscle contraction, whereas the beta component increases the cardiac output. The onset of action of epinephrine is within 5 to 10 minutes. Epinephrine is given intra-muscularly (IM)/subcutaneously. Epinephrine has a very short half-life and is eliminated within 5 minutes. Epinephrine is metabolized in the liver and excreted through the urine.

The following are additional adjunct treatments that are used in combination with epinephrine for anaphylactic reactions in the outpatient or hospital setting: short-acting antihistamines such as diphenhydramine or hydroxyzine; long-acting antihistamines such as loratadine, cetirizine, levocetirizine, and fexofenadine; medications for GI upset such as ranitidine/famotidine/ondansetron, and albuterol for respiratory symptoms. Steroids are no longer recommended for treatment.

Follow-Up/Patient Family Education

Prevention of anaphylaxis is key. Pediatric patients with a severe allergy should wear an emergency alert bracelet or necklace and carry their auto-injector with them at all times. A child with a history of an anaphylactic allergy should be followed by an allergist as well. Remind parents that a child with any allergy is at risk for an anphylactic reaction; however, children at increased risk of anaphylaxis include children with a history of a previous anaphylactic reaction, any other history of a severe allergic reaction in the past, and/or a history of allergies and asthma.

■ ATOPIC DERMATITIS

Etiology

Atopic dermatitis (AD) is an inflammatory, allergic, noncontagious skin disorder. AD is the most common chronic childhood skin disorder. There is a strong family history component. AD presents as itchy, erythematous, scaly, and flaky skin. AD is diagnosed by physical examination (PE) of the skin, with having a family history of allergies or asthma and with the patient having a personal history of allergies or asthma.

Focused PE Signs/Findings

AD presents as itchy, scaly, bumpy, erythematous, and edematous skin. Skin can become thickened (lichenification) and harden over time due to scratching. AD presents on flexural and/or extensor surfaces of skin depending upon age. The most common areas AD presents are creases of arms, neck, knees, trunk, and extremities.

Key Points

There are certain triggers for AD and they are as follows: food allergies, environmental allergies, dry skin, infection, heat or sweating, stress, contact irritants (certain soaps, lotions, laundry detergent, shampoo, body wash), long hot baths/showers, wool clothing, dust, cigarette smoke exposure, and certain foods. If AD appears in infants, question whether there is a food allergy component. Most often when the offensive food is removed, there is a significant clearance in the skin.

Treatment

Bathing daily in a warm bath/shower is important. Avoid hot water and avoid drying with a towel, as the friction can irritate the skin; allow the child to drip-dry and apply lotion while skin is still moist to help lock in additional moisture. There are multiple treatment modalities for AD: Topical medications such as steroid creams or ointments are often used to help manage inflammation of the skin. Examples of these are hydrocortisone, triamcinolone, and mometasone.

Oral medications such as daily nondrowsy/drowsy antihistamines are helpful in managing AD. Examples of nondrowsy daily antihistamines appropriate for use in the pediatric setting are cetirizine, loratadine, levocetirizine, and fexofenadine and drowsy antihistamines are diphenhydramine and hydroxyzine. It is appropriate depending on the severity of symptoms to use both a nondrowsy longer-acting antihistamine and a drowsy shorter-acting antihistamine together simultaneously with good effect (Wolters Kluwer, 2019).

Patient/Family Education

Other treatment modalities are wearing a pair of wet pajamas/socks underneath a pair of dry pajamas/socks to help lock in moisture, wearing gloves to bed, and keeping fingernails short to avoid scratching, as open skin leaves them open and more susceptible to systemic infections.

Bleach baths are a recommendation that oftentimes concerns parents. They help rid the skin of germs that can cause infections and can help neutralize any irritants on the skin. Explain that bleach baths are not harmful to patients, and ask the parents if they allow their children to swim in chlorine-treated pools: It is exactly the same efficacy. This often calms their nerves, and they are more receptive to trialing them. Bleach baths should consist of the following: use one-fourth cup of bleach for a half-bathtub full of water. For infant baths, you can use 1 teaspoon of bleach per gallon of water. Avoid getting water in the child's eyes. Allow them to soak in the bathtub of lukewarm bleach water for 10 to 15 minutes, and then rinse thoroughly and drip-dry and apply lotion while still moist. Bleach baths can be used a few times a week (Tollefston & Bruckner, 2014).

Oral steroids are often the last resort and only used sparingly in children for severe AD flares. The concerns of frequent and consistent use of oral steroids are stunted growth, roid rage, and increased appetite. When needed, they can be beneficial; however, this typically is not first- or second-line therapy for AD flares (Tollefston & Bruckner, 2014).

Prevention

AD is not a curable disease; however, AD can be well controlled with proper treatment and medications, as well as avoiding known triggers. The weather and climate have significant impacts on skin health. For example, in New England, cold weather is often a trigger for AD, and in many southern states, heat and humidity play a large role. Knowing how to avoid triggers is key in helping to successfully manage AD.

■ FOOD PROTEIN–INDUCED ENTEROCOLITIS SYNDROME

Etiology

Food protein–induced enterocolitis syndrome (FPIES) is not clearly understood. FPIES is an uncommon allergic response. It is a non–IgE-mediated gastrointestinal (GI) food hypersensitivity. The allergen causes GI inflammation due to a T cell–mediated response, which causes a fluid shift in the abdomen. FPIES presents as acute, recurrent vomiting and diarrhea, typically 2 to 4 hours after consumption of the offensive allergen.

Epidemiology/Risk Factors

This reaction commonly presents in infancy and commonly is outgrown by 6 years of age. The most common irritants are milk, soy, rice, and oats (American Academy of Allergy, Asthma and Immunology, 2019).

Treatment

Since FPIES is non–IgE-mediated response, it will not respond to typical IgE-mediated treatment such as epinephrine. There is a risk of hypotension, dehydration, and hypotensive shock due to volume and fluid depletion with vomiting and diarrhea; therefore, it is typically treated with an intravenous (IV) fluid bolus, ondansetron (either IV or PO), and Prilosec/Zantac.

■ ORAL ALLERGY SYNDROME

Oral allergy syndrome (OAS) is a common form of allergy present in those allergic to pollen or weeds that presents as itching or swelling of the oral pharynx. Skins of fruits and certain foods contain the largest amount of pollen, which causes OAS symptoms when these foods are consumed. If the skins are removed or the foods are cooked, the pollen proteins are denatured, and people are able to eat them without issue. OAS is only present in plant-based foods. OAS is becoming more prevalent in the population, as the prevalence of AR is also rising, and both are responses to pollen sensitivity.

Focused PE Signs and Findings

These include pruritus, tingling in mouth, mild erythema, and mild angioedema of lips, oral mucosa, palate, and throat. Symptoms typically present within 5 to 10 minutes of consumption of the allergen and resolve quickly without treatment when acid and digestive enzymes in the saliva break down the protein. Typically, no further symptoms progress.

Diagnostic criteria for OAS are as follows: the patient has symptoms, there is a known allergy or evidence of an allergy to pollen (such as AR), and there is confirmation of pollen allergies by either skin prick testing or IgE testing.

IMMUNOLOGY

Etiology

Immune diseases are inherited conditions that often present in childhood. Immunological diseases affect the immune system, particularly the white blood cells (WBCs). Immunity is your body's way of fighting off infectious organisms. There are several different types of WBCs that make up the immune system. Neutrophils are the components of WBC that fight bacteria and fungi. Lymphocytes are the types of WBCs that fight viruses. T cells and B cells are both subsets of lymphocytes. T cells play a vital role in creating an immune response within the body and create cell-mediated immunity. T cells are produced in the bone marrow and originate from hematopoietic stem cells. T cells are also known as invader cells. When T cells are deficient, your body can be affected by intracellular pathogens. T cells are necessary for B cell activation. B cells play a vital role in creating an immunological response by creating antibodies. B cells are affected by extracellular pathogens (Dean, & Jim, 2017).

Epidemiology/Risk Factors

Immune system disorders cause abnormally low activity or overactivity of the immune system. In cases of immune system overactivity, the body attacks and damages its own tissues (autoimmune diseases). Immune deficiency diseases decrease the body's ability to fight invaders, causing vulnerability to infections. Anyone is at risk for these disorders, and immune deficiencies typically present in early childhood, whereas autoimmune diseases can present at any time in life in childhood or adulthood.

Labs/Diagnostics

When questioning an immune deficiency, the important labs to orders include complete blood count (CBC) with differential and an Ig panel (which includes IgG, IgA, IgM, IgD, and IgE).

■ PRIMARY IMMUNE DEFICIENCY DISEASE (PIDD)

Infections are a normal part of life; however, when these infections are recurrent or do not clear with long treatment durations, it is essential for healthcare providers to understand the underlying differential diagnosis. Clear record-keeping of infection types, frequency of infections, duration of infections, and treatment modalities are key in helping to identify immune deficiencies in the pediatric population.

Primary immune deficiency diseases (PIDDs) range from mild to severe. PIDD can be present at birth; however, some individuals do not develop symptoms until much later in life. PIDDs are not contagious and oftentimes are difficult to detect. PIDDs are often made up of a combination of B lymphocyte antibody deficiencies and T lymphocyte deficiencies. Immune deficiencies can be difficult to detect; therefore, it is important to work with healthcare providers to recommend seeing a pediatric immunologist for further workup and testing. PIDD is often diagnosed with a strong medical history, PE, laboratory testing, and prenatal and newborn testing (American Academy of Allergy, Asthma and Immunology, 2015).

Symptoms

The most common signs and symptoms of PIDD are frequent infections such as bronchitis, ear infections, sinusitis, or pneumonia. PIDD may be genetic in nature; therefore, if one child in a family has a PIDD, it is important to have other siblings worked up to see if they too have an immune deficiency.

BOX 14.1 EXAMPLES OF SOME OF THE MORE COMMONLY KNOWN PRIMARY IMMUNODEFICIENCY DISEASES

Agammaglobulinemia or hypogammaglobulinemia **is a disease that affects a child's immune system by producing a very low level of antibodies (B cells) in the blood to fight infections. Agammaglobulinemia is more common in males.**

XLA **is an inherited form of primary immune deficiency. XLA is caused by a lymphocyte gene mutation.**

Hyper IgM **disease is a type of PIDD caused by a T cell surface protein deficiency. The T cells are unable to communicate with B cells to switch them from making IgM.**

WA **disease causes issues with T cells, B cells, and platelets. Patients have a low platelet count in addition to their platelets being a smaller size. Patients with WA have an increased tendency to bleed, recurrent infections, and often present with eczema.**

DiGeorge syndrome **is a genetic defect of chromosome 22. Patients with DiGeorge are known to have the following issues: abnormal facies, hypothyroidism, heart defects, autoimmune disorders, learning difficulties, and developmental delays.**

PIDD, primary immune deficiency disease; WA, Wiskott–Aldrich; XLA, X-linked agammaglobulinemia.

Don't Miss

The following are warnings that a child may have a PIDD: four or more new infections in a year, infections that are resistant to oral antibiotics and require IV antibiotic treatment, recurrent or persistent thrush, and long-term use of oral antibiotics with little or no effect on the disease. Some common visible signs of PIDD are eczema, serious skin infections, lymphadenopathy, chronic diarrhea, cramping and abdominal pain, and failure to thrive.

Treatment

First-line treatments for PIDDs (shown in Box 14.1) include low doses of prophylactic antibiotics and other medications. If patients do not respond to that treatment, they are often treated with IgG replacement therapy, which is the standard treatment for PIDD. IgG replacement therapy is known as immunoglobulin treatment. The most common types of immunoglobulin treatment are IV immunoglobulin and subcutaneous immunoglobulin, given through infusions. For severe cases, hematopoietic stem cell transplants are considered.

■ COMBINED VARIABLE IMMUNODEFICIENCY

Combined variable immunodeficiency (CVID) presents like most other PIDDs with recurrent infections. Diagnosis criteria for CVID must have at least one of the following elements: increased susceptibility to infection, an autoimmune manifestation, a family member with an antibody deficiency, personal history of a granulomatous disease, poor antibody response to vaccines, low switched memory B cells, and low IgG or IgA with or without IgM (measured at least twice). Patients typically aged 4 or older are diagnosed with CVID; however, most are not diagnosed until their second or third decade of life. There must be no evidence that there is a T cell deficiency present, and all secondary causes must be ruled out (National Institute of Allergy and Infectious Disease, 2020).

■ SEVERE COMBINED IMMUNODEFICIENCY

Etiology

Severe combined immunodeficiency (SCID) is a rare genetic disorder that affects 50 to 100 children born in the United States annually. SCID testing is part of the newborn screen. SCID is also known as bubble boy disease.

Focused PE Signs/Findings

Patients with SCID are often noted to have failure to thrive as infants and to have recurrent infections. SCID presents when there are severe deficiencies in both T and B cell functioning. Children with SCID are unable to produce B cells, due to their T cells not working. These children are left with no immune system functioning and are left completely susceptible to infections. Even common viral illnesses that are nonthreatening for those with healthy immune systems have the potential for serious and severe side effects for a child with SCID.

There is a form of SCID called X-linked SCID, which is due to a defective gene on the X chromosome. X-linked SCID affects only males. Females can be carriers and pass on the trait to their sons. If one child has SCID, it does not mean that the disease will affect all siblings, but they should be tested. It is important for mothers of children diagnosed with SCID who are planning to breastfeed to discuss this with their child's healthcare provider, as some diseases are able to be transmitted through breast milk. Patients with SCID should not receive any vaccines since they are unable to produce antibodies to the diseases being introduced to their system from the vaccines. SCID patients often received immunoglobulin infusions until they are able to find a suitable donor for the stem cell or bone marrow transplant. A hematopoietic stem cell or bone marrow transplant is the cure for SCID, which allows the patients to begin producing WBCs and have functioning T and B cells.

References

American Academy of Allergy, Asthma and Immunology. (2019). *About AAAAI*. Retrieved from https://www.aaaai.org/

Boyce, J. A., Assa'ad, A., Burks, A. W., Jones, S. M., Sampson, H. A., Wood, R. A., Plaut, M., Cooper, S. F., Fenton, M. J., Arshad, S. H., Bahna, S. L., Beck, L. A., Byrd-Bredbenner, C., Camargo, C. A., Jr, Eichenfield, L., Furuta, G. T., Hanifin, J. M., Jones, C., Kraft, M., … Schwaninger, J. M. (2010). Guidelines for the diagnosis and management of food allergy in the United States: Report of the NIAID-sponsored expert panel. *The Journal of Allergy and Clinical Immunology, 126*(6, Suppl.), S1–S58. doi:10.1016/j.jaci.2010.10.007

Dean, P., & Jim, D. (2017). B cells: The antibody factories of the immune system. *Leaf Science*. Retrieved from https://www.leafscience.org/b-cells/

National Academies of Sciences, Engineering, and Medicine. (2017). *Finding a path to safety in food allergy: Assessment of global burden, causes, prevention, management, and public policy*. Washington, DC: The National Academies Press.

National Institute of Allergy and Infectious Disease. (2020). *Food allergy*. Retrieved from https://www.niaid.nih.gov/diseases-conditions/food-allergy

O'Keefe, A., Clarke, A., St. Pierre, Y., Mill, J., Asai, Y., Eisman, H., . . . Ben-Shoshan, M. (2017). The risk of recurrent anaphylaxis. *Journal of Pediatrics, 180*, 217–221. doi:10.1016/j.jpeds.2016.09.028

Sicherer, S. H., Allen, K., Lack, G., Taylor, S. L., Donovan, S., & Oria, M. (2017). Critical issues in food allergies: A national academies consensus report. *Pediatrics, 140*(2). doi:10.1542/peds .2017-0194

Tollefston, M. M., & Bruckner, A. L. (2014). Atopic dermatitis: Skin-directed management. *Pediatrics, 134*(6), e1735–e1744. doi:10.1542/peds.2014-2812

Wolters Kluwer. (2020). *Lexicomp*. Retrieved from https://www.wolterskluwercdi.com/lexicomp -online/

Disorders in Hematology and Oncology Commonly Seen in Pediatric Primary Care

Kristine M. Ruggiero

INTRODUCTION

Being tired or fatigued is a common complaint by children and often a reason for a pediatric primary care visit. Fatigue is a common nonspecific symptom that can be attributed to apparent problems such as not getting enough sleep or getting over a recent illness, but when children complain of fatigue all the time it can be a symptom of a more serious problem, especially if this nonspecific symptom is associated with other constitutional symptoms such as weight loss and fever. This chapter will focus on the common organic causes of fatigue seen in pediatric primary care as well as the less common but more serious causes of fatigue such as cancer.

OBJECTIVES

1. Determine the common causes of fatigue seen in pediatric primary care.
2. Discern between various types of anemia common in children.
3. Determine the approach to care for a child presenting with fatigue.
4. Discern between common causes and less common causes of fatigue, including leukemia presentation, in a child.

ANEMIA

Etiology

Anemia is an abnormally low hemoglobin, hematocrit, or red blood cell (RBC) count. It can be classified based on the appearance of RBCs on a peripheral blood smear and RBC parameters such as mean corpuscular volume (MCV) and mean corpuscular hemoglobin concentration (MCHC). Because RBC parameters vary by age, it is important to know the age of the child before determining if the child has anemia. Anemias can be classified in terms of decreased RBC production, RBC destruction, RBC sequestration, or blood loss.

Research supports that iron deficiency anemia (IDA) during infancy and childhood can have long-lasting negative effects on neurodevelopmental outcomes. Iron is essential for normal neurodevelopment, and it is known that iron is the world's most common single-nutrient deficiency. Therefore, pediatric primary care advanced practicing clinicians (APCs) should strive to eliminate iron deficiency and IDA. Appropriate iron intakes for infants and toddlers as well as methods for prevention of IDA are presented in this chapter.

Anemia is not a disease, but rather a symptom of another disorder. Anemia is defined by the World Health Organization (WHO) as a hemoglobin (Hgb) concentration 2 SDs below the mean Hgb concentration for a normal population of the same gender and age range.

Hematocrit (HCT) is defined as the fractional volume of whole blood sample occupied by RBCs, expressed as a percentage.

Hemoglobin (Hgb) is defined as a measure of the concentration of the RBC pigment hemoglobin in whole blood, expressed as grams per 100 ml (dL) of whole blood.

Disorders of RBCs can be classified as quantitative, qualitative, or both. Most encounters seen in pediatric hematology are quantitative disorders, which are due to problems with decreased production in blood cells or increased loss of blood cells from the circulation. In pediatrics, abnormally low counts (i.e., anemias) are more common than high counts (seen in thrombocytosis or polycythemia). Qualitative disorders are less common in pediatrics and are due to intrinsic abnormalities in the blood cells themselves, although qualitative disorders can lead to quantitative disorders (i.e., sickle cell anemia is a qualitative disorder that can lead to a hemolytic anemia which is a quantitative disorder).

For this chapter, we will provide a general overview of anemia but focus on one of the most common types of anemia seen in pediatric primary care, IDA.

Epidemiology/Risk Factors

Patient Characteristics

The normal values of anemia vary by age. Different causes of anemia present at different ages. In infants, it is important to differentiate between physiologic anemia and pathologic anemia: the most common cause of anemia in young infants is physiologic anemia that occurs at 6 to 9 weeks of age (and can include causes of blood loss and Rh incompatibility).

The fetus draws from the mother the iron it will need for the first 6 months of life; therefore, IDA due to nutritional deficiency is unlikely in infants less than 6 months of age. Infants who are at risk for anemia include preterm infants (called anemia of prematurity) and infants born to mothers with anemia.

In toddlers and older children, acquired causes of anemia are more likely, such as blood loss or from diet. Too much cow's milk (>24 ounces/day) can induce a microcytic anemia (by causing inflammation in the gastrointestinal tract and inhibiting absorption of iron). This is common in toddlers and preschoolers who can be picky eaters but who like to drink milk.

Symptoms

Fatigue is a common symptom of anemia, specifically IDA. Other symptoms of IDA in the pediatric patient can include growth delay, developmental delays in the younger infant/child, or poor academic performance on standardized tests in the school-age child or adolescent.

In addition, the APC should ask about any history of fatigue, easy bruising, fevers, weight loss, rash, jaundice, or cough. Asking about a detailed medication history is also important, as certain medications can cause bone marrow suppression or hemolysis. It is also important to ask about any signs or symptoms of occult bleeding including melena, hematochezia, hematuria, hematemesis, abnormal menses, or epistaxis. Dietary history is also important and a common cause of IDA. In addition, family members with jaundice, gallstones, and splenomegaly may suggest an inherited hemolytic anemia.

In the history, it is important to obtain the prenatal history, which may reveal a history of prematurity or a mother with anemia, which are risk factors for iron deficiency anemia in the infant. Other patient characteristics to include in the history of a child with anemia are as follows:

- In neonates, infection and hemolytic disease are the most common causes of anemia.
- Hemoglobinopathies are more common in children with anemia around 3 to 6 months of age.
- IDAs are more common in school-age children (usually due to diet or blood loss).
- Some causes of anemia are X-linked (including G6PD deficiency) and are more common in males.
- Inherited disorders (a history of prior occurrences of anemia) versus acquired disorders (a new incident of anemia with a previously documented normal complete blood count [CBC]).
- Developmental delay is associated with IDA, vitamin B12/folic acid deficiency, and Fanconi's anemia.
- Consideration must be given to the possibility of lead poisoning because iron deficiency is often seen in children who also have lead toxicity.

Focused Physical Exam Signs/Important Findings

Vital sign assessment may reveal tachycardia or postural changes in heart rate and blood pressure, which are seen in acute blood loss. Other findings suggestive of blood loss include positive guaiac stool.

Examine the patient to assess the severity of the anemia. This includes assessing for pallor (skin, conjunctivae, and mucous membranes). In addition, it is important to assess for other signs of anemia including scleral icterus, jaundice (seen in hemolytic anemias), hepatomegaly, and splenomegaly. Assess the skin for petechia and purpura (seen in pancytopenia).

Lab Tests/Diagnostics

The lab exam should begin with a CBC, including RBC indices, reticulocyte count, and review of the peripheral bloom smear.

A CBC with a low Hgb and/or HCT may indicate anemia. Additional tests may be ordered to evaluate the levels of serum ferritin, iron, total iron-binding capacity, and/or transferrin. In a child with anemia from iron deficiency, in addition to a low Hgb and HCT, other tests usually show a low mean corpuscular volume (MCV), low ferritin, low serum iron, high transferrin or total iron-binding capacity (TIBC), and low iron saturation.

The peripheral smear may show small, oval-shaped cells with pale centers. In severe iron deficiency, the WBCs may be low and the platelets may be either high or low.

Universal screening for anemia is recommended at 9 to 12 months of age.

Table 15.1

Common Causes of Anemia When Other Cell Abnormalities Are Present

Pancytopenia	Anemia and Low PLTs	Anemia and High PLTs	Anemia and High WBC
Leukemia	HUS	Iron deficiency	Leukemia infection
Myelosuppressive	Evans syndrome	infection	
drugs/toxins	DIC		
Aplastic anemia			
Infection			
Vitamin B12/folate			
deficiency			

DIC, disseminated intravascular coagulopathy; HUS, hemolytic uremic syndrome; PLTs, platelets; WBC, white blood cell.

Source: Adapted from Srugnara, C., Oski, F. A., & Nathan, D. G. (2015). Diagnostic approach to the anemic patient. InS. H. Orkin, D. G. Nathan, D. Ginsburg, A. T. Look, D. E. Fisher, & S. E. Lux (Eds.), *Nathan and Oski's hematology and oncology of infancy and childhood* (8th ed., pp. 293–307). Philadelphia, PA: WB Saunders, p. 293

Don't Miss

The APC should then identify if other cell lines are affected. Table 15.1 reviews the differential diagnoses to consider depending on which cell lines are affected in combination with anemia.

Treatment

Treatment of anemia first depends on identifying the underlying cause and severity of anemia. Iron replacement is the treatment if IDA is the diagnosis. Treatments for IDA may include iron supplements, procedures, surgery, and dietary changes. Severe IDA may require intravenous (IV) iron therapy or a blood transfusion.

Prevention

Prevention of anemia is vital. For formula-fed infants, formula is fortified with iron; in addition, the introduction of iron-containing foods should begin at 4 to 6 months of age, including iron-fortified cereals. For breastfed (BF) infants, human milk contains very little iron. Therefore, exclusively breastfed infants are at increasing risk of IDA after 4 months of age (time the infant uses up mother's iron stores). Consequently, beginning at 4 months of age, BF infants should be supplemented with 1 mg/kg per day of oral iron until appropriate dietary intake of iron-rich or iron-fortified foods are introduced (4 to 6 months of age) in the diet.

For partially BF infants, the proportion of human milk versus formula is uncertain; therefore, beginning at 4 months of age, partially BF infants (more than half of their daily feedings as human milk) who are not receiving iron-containing complementary foods should also receive 1 mg/kg per day of supplemental iron.

Toddlers 1 through 3 years of age should have an iron intake of 7 mg/day. For toddlers not receiving this iron intake, liquid supplements are suitable for children 12 to 36 months of age, and chewable multivitamins can be used for children 3 years and older. In addition, intake of iron through diet includes eating red meats, cereals fortified with iron, vegetables that contain iron, and fruits with vitamin C, which augments the absorption of iron.

Endocrine Causes of Anemia

Hypothyroidism (see Chapter 13, Endocrine Abnormalities Commonly Seen in Pediatric Primary Care).

Infectious Causes of Fatigue

Mononucleosis (see Chapter 12, Infectious Diseases Commonly Seen in Pediatric Primary Care).

ONCOLOGIC CAUSES OF FATIGUE

Childhood cancer may present with signs and symptoms that are shared by other childhood illnesses, such as fever, weight loss, and fatigue. These are nonspecific symptoms that may be found in children with cancer.

In the absence of infection, unresolving fever may reflect a neoplasm. Approximately two-thirds of children with leukemia had fever at time of diagnosis.

■ LEUKEMIA

Acute lymphoblastic leukemia (ALL)
Acute myelocytic leukemia (AML)

Etiology

Childhood cancer is often difficult to detect in its early stages especially because children often get many colds and infections during the winter and spring months. Children also present more with metastasis at the time of diagnosis than adults. While the exact cause of leukemia is not known, it is thought to involve a combination of genetic and environmental factors. Leukemia cells have acquired mutations in their DNA that cause them to grow abnormally and lose functions of typical white blood cells (WBCs) (Radhi et al., 2015).

Epidemiology/Risk Factors

While cancer is not hereditary, people can inherit genetic abnormalities that increase their risk of developing cancer. Children with certain syndromes are at increased risk of developing certain neoplasms. For example, children with trisomy 21 are at increased risk of developing ALL among other hematopoietic disorders.

ALL is the most common malignancy in children. Leukemia develops due to changes or mutations in the DNA of bone marrow. In most cases, these mutations happen for no apparent reason; however, research shows that certain factors such as exposure to chemicals (including benzene, gasoline, increased radiation due to CT scans, and chemotherapy) and lifestyle (smoking) contribute to genetic mutations as well.

Differential

The differential includes idiopathic thrombocytopenic purpura (ITP), aplastic anemia, Epstein–Barr virus infection, rheumatologic disorders, and other malignancies.

Focused Physical Exam/Important Findings

Nonspecific symptoms may be uncovered in the **history** and include fatigue, malaise, and anorexia. Approximately 25% of patients complain of bone pain or arthralgias.

Progressive bone marrow failure can lead to fractures, pallor, ecchymoses, petechiae, and fever. Neurologic symptoms such as headache and papilledema can be found if there is central nervous system (CNS) involvement.

On physical exam (PE), lymphadenopathy may be present. The child may appear pale and tired. Examination of the skin may reveal petechiae or purpura.

Lab Tests/Diagnostics

Anemia, leukopenia, and thrombocytopenia often occur either as isolated findings or in combination in tumors that involve the bone marrow. Acute leukemias are the most common bone marrow tumors. Approximately 90% of children with leukemia have anemia and thrombocytopenia at diagnosis. In addition, leukemia can also present with elevation in WBC count or leukemoid reaction (increase in leukocyte concentration).

In the presence of positive constitution symptoms (fatigue, weight loss, fever), or other findings concerning for malignancy on a careful PE (such as supraclavicular lymphadenopathy) in the absence of a known source or cause of infection, a CBC with differential, a peripheral blood smear, blood culture, and chest x-ray should be performed. Additional studies may be indicated based on other signs and symptoms, and an infectious cause should always be explored in an abnormal peripheral blood smear.

Immature WBCs, normally only present in the bone marrow, may be observed in the peripheral blood in a variety of disorders including infection, erythropoietic stimulation caused by hemolysis or hemorrhage, rheumatoid arthritis, or septicemia.

The presence of circulating blasts, aka immature WBCs, or profound neutropenia or thrombocytopenia can suggest leukemia. Immature WBCs normally only present in the bone marrow may be observed in the peripheral blood in a variety of other disorders including infection, erythropoietic stimulation caused by hemolysis or hemorrhage, rheumatoid arthritis, or septicemia. A bone marrow aspirate and biopsy can confirm or exclude malignant disease involving the bone marrow. Conversely, the presence of atypical lymphocytes in a peripheral smear (can be seen in mononucleosis or other viral illnesses) can differentiate between other illnesses and cancer.

Treatment/Prevention

The APC should have a high level of suspicion and early referral to a pediatric oncologist when cancer is suspected, as early treatment may reduce morbidity and mortality.

The treatment strategy in leukemia is to treat the leukemia and manage complications of treatment.

ALL is the most common pediatric neoplasm and accounts for 80% of all cases of childhood acute leukemia. The prognosis for AML is worse than that for ALL. Standard-risk ALL has an 80% cure rate, whereas the prognoses for AML vary widely among subtypes.

References

Radhi, M., Fulbright, J. M., Ginn, K. F., & Guest, E. M. (2015). Childhood cancer for the primary care physician. *Primary Care, 42*(1), 43–55. doi:10.1016/j.pop.2014.09.006

Srugnara, C., Oski, F. A., & Nathan, D. G. (2015). Diagnostic approach to the anemic patient. In S. H. Orkin, D. G. Nathan, D. Ginsburg, A. T. Look, D. E. Fisher, & S. E. Lux (Eds.), *Nathan and Oski's hematology and oncology of infancy and childhood* (8th ed., pp. 293–307). Philadelphia, PA: WB Saunders.

16

Common Behavioral/Mental Health Complaints in Pediatric Primary Care

Kristine M. Ruggiero, Rebecca Sarvendram, and Elizabeth Maloney

INTRODUCTION

Despite the need for mental health services, current treatments are far from widely embraced by families. In one U.S. study, more than half of parents of children with emotional, behavioral, or developmental concerns did not discuss them with their child's pediatric provider (Wissow, Van Ginneken, Chandna, & Rahman, 2016). In addition, parents often differ significantly in their attitudes toward treatment options for mental health problems in the pediatric population. This chapter will focus on identification and management of the top three presenting symptoms in mental health presenting to pediatric primary care providers.

OBJECTIVES

1. Identify the common presenting symptoms/complaints for behavioral/mental health seen in pediatric primary care that the advanced practicing clinician (APC) should be aware of.
   a. Understand the management of anxiety, depression, and attention deficit hyperactivity disorder (ADHD).
2. Identify mental health treatment and interventions that are practical, engaging to families, and effective for use by pediatric primary care providers.
3. Identify when to refer children to mental health services.
4. Identify signs for child abuse and neglect; the role of the mandated reporter.

ANXIETY

Introduction

Anxiety refers to excessive fears and worries that are more chronic, intense, and impairing compared with the normal fears and worries at different stages of development. The *DSM-5* includes seven anxiety disorders seen in children (American Psychiatric

Association [APA], 2013). Anxiety disorders in children include generalized anxiety disorders (GADs), social anxiety, separation anxiety (persisting after 2 years of age), selective mutism, obsessive-compulsive disorder, phobias (including school refusal), and panic disorder.

Etiology

The prevalence of anxiety disorders is 8% to 9% during childhood and adolescence. In addition, a family history of anxiety is often present. In pediatrics, children manifesting an anxiety disorder often present with physical symptoms.

Epidemiology/Risk Factors

Previous trauma or abuse may play a role in causing anxiety.

Symptoms

In pediatrics, children manifesting an anxiety disorder often present with physical symptoms, including excessive anxiety and worry. The anxiety, worry, or physical symptoms cause clinically significant distress or impairment in social, occupational, or other important areas of functioning (APA, 2013).

For the diagnosis for GAD in addition to the previously mentioned symptoms, a patient must also have disproportionate anxiety and worry occurring more days than not for at least 6 months about a number of events or activities (such as work or school performance), finds it difficult to control the worry, and is associated with one of the following symptoms: restlessness, easily fatigued, difficulty concentrating, muscle tension, and/or sleep disturbances (APA, 2013).

Focused Physical Exam Signs/Findings

Assessment for anxiety disorders in children and adolescents is performed through a face-to-face history as well as an interview with the child's parents. Detailed information should be obtained on the child's symptoms including frequency, duration, severity, and degree of distress or interference. It is important to ask about the child's specific thoughts and triggers underlying a particular anxious or avoidant behavior. In addition, when the history is obtained, it should include comprehensive questions pertaining to developmental history, medical history, and family psychiatric history.

A detailed social history includes questions about the family relationships, social relationships, school functioning, preferred recreational activities, substance abuse, and sexual history if age appropriate.

Differentials

Similar to depression, anxiety can have other mental health comorbidities such as ADHD. Rule out other potential causes of symptoms and identify comorbid conditions.

Don't Miss

- There is no test to diagnose anxiety.
- The pediatric APC should consider anxiety on the differential if a pediatric patient has symptoms such as not eating properly, quickly getting angry or irritable, being out of control during outbursts, or constantly worrying to encourage a visit.

Treatment

Behavioral therapy includes child therapy, family therapy, or a combination of both. Cognitive behavioral therapy (CBT) has the strongest evidence to support it as the recommended first-line treatment for all anxiety disorders in children and adolescents (with or without medications; Kozlowski, Lusk, & Melnyk, 2015). The school can also be included in the treatment plan. For very young children, involving parents in treatment is key.

1. Mild to moderate anxiety often responds to education, supportive care, and follow-up office visits.
2. Evidence-based treatments including CBT and/or a selective serotonin reuptake inhibitor (SSRI) are effective for moderate to severe anxiety disorders.

Prevention

While there is no way to prevent anxiety or depression, the American Academy of Child and Adolescent Psychiatry (AACAP) recommends that healthcare providers routinely screen children for behavioral and mental health concerns (https://www.aacap.org/).

Patient/Family Education

Patient and family education sheets can be found on AACAP.org website.

ATTENTION DEFICIT HYPERACTIVITY DISORDER

Introduction

ADHD is generally recognized as the most common neurobehavioral disorder of childhood. *ADD is no longer part of the nomenclature.* Instead, there are subtypes: ADHD, primarily inattentive type; ADHD, primarily hyperactive/impulsive type; and ADHD, combined type. AAP guidelines have now been expanded to cover ages 4 to 18 years. ADHD is a chronic condition that affects multiple domains of a child's functioning including academic performance, adaptive skills, peer relationships, and family dynamics.

Etiology/Epidemiology

The estimated prevalence of children with ADHD is around 8% in school-age children with boys more likely than girls to receive the diagnosis, some of which may be related to presentation. While the exact etiology of ADHD is not known, it is believed to involve catecholamine metabolism in the cerebral cortex. In addition, there is a genetic component to ADHD, which is supported by twin studies.

Symptoms

ADHD is characterized by two core symptoms: hyperactivity/impulsivity and inattention. Box 16.1 reviews the symptoms that give the diagnosis of ADHD. Other symptoms to look for include low frustration tolerance, emotional impulsivity, and executive functioning weaknesses including planning, working memory, and abstract reasoning.

Focused Physical Exam/Findings

Physical exam expected to be normal but should be done to rule out other conditions. This should include height, weight, head circumference, and vital signs (especially

BOX 16.1 PRESENTING SYMPTOMS CHARACTERISTIC OF ADHD

Hyperactive and impulsive: Symptoms are typically described as the inability to sit still or inhibit behavior. These are typically observed by 4 years of age with peak severity at 7–8 years of age. Hyperactive symptoms then begin to decline. However impulsive symptoms usually persist and can put adolescents at a greater likelihood of risk-taking behaviors (alcohol, drugs, unprotected sex).

Common observations: Fidgetiness difficulty remaining seated restlessness or hyperkinetic behavior (running/jumping) always on-the-go excessive talking difficulty waiting their turn and blurting out.
Frequent interruption difficulty with personal space.

Inattention: It is the impaired ability to focus attention.
Maintain attention and slow cognitive processing and response. Symptoms of inattention are usually lifelong.

Common observations: Poor attention to detail, careless mistakes, not listening, poor follow-through with tasks, difficulty organizing, task avoidance especially those that require sustained effort, loses objects, easily distracted by environmental stimuli, forgetfulness.

ADHD, attention deficit hyperactivity disorder.
Source: Data from Wolraich, M. L., Hagan, J. F., Allan, C., Chan, E., Davidson, D., Earls, M., . . . Zurhellen, W. (2019). Clinical practice guidelines in the treatment of ADHD. *Pediatrics, 144*(4). doi:10.1542/peds.2019-252

before and during treatment); assessment of dysmorphic features and neurocutaneous abnormalities; and a complete neurological examination, including assessment of vision and hearing.

Observation of behavior in the office setting can help with diagnosis but should be interpreted cautiously, as symptoms may not be apparent in the structured setting of the clinic visit or nervousness could be misinterpreted as symptoms of ADHD.

Medical history includes prenatal exposures, perinatal complications or infections, central nervous system infection, and head trauma/concussion. Developmental history includes especially early language development. Family history is important due to genetic component.

Lab Tests/Diagnostics

There are no specific lab tests for ADHD, but organic causes of learning difficulties such as iron deficiency anemia should be ruled out.

For the diagnosis of ADHD, a patient should have symptoms that are problematic in at least two settings: symptoms should be present before the age of 12 years, for at least 6 months, and impair function in academic, social, and/or extracurricular activities (APA, 2013). Furthermore, symptoms exceed expected developmental expectations for the age of the child, and symptoms cannot be explained by other mental health disorders (APA, 2013).

For children <17 years, the *DSM-5* diagnosis of ADHD requires ≥6 symptoms of hyperactivity and impulsivity or ≥6 symptoms of inattention. For adolescents ≥17 years and adults, ≥5 symptoms of hyperactivity and impulsivity or ≥5 symptoms of inattention are required for diagnosis. Conners Comprehensive Behavior Rating Scales and the ADHD Rating Scale IV have been validated in preschool-age children (≥4 years). The Vanderbilt rating scales are most commonly seen and are validated for 6 and older but probably can be used in younger children (Wissow et al., 2016).

Psychometric (neuropsychological or psychoeducational) testing is not necessary in the routine evaluation for ADHD but can be useful in excluding other disorders or confirming a diagnosis, particularly when multiple comorbidities present. Other neurodiagnostic testing (EEG, MRI) is not indicated.

Differentials

Developmental: autism, learning disability

Emotional/behavioral: anxiety, depression, conduct disorder, oppositional defiant disorder (ODD), posttraumatic stress disorder (PTSD)

Physical: seizures (absence in particular), sleep disorders (obstructive sleep apnea [OSA]), substance abuse

Don't Miss

1. Many conditions identified as differential diagnoses are also common comorbidities (i.e., learning disability, ODD, anxiety/depression, autism, sleep disorders), so their presence does not necessarily rule out ADHD and they need separate treatment/management.
2. Diagnosis is challenging in older school-age children/adolescents as overt hyperactivity declines, they have multiple teachers, and there is less parental observation. Self-reporting can be helpful.
3. To address parental concern regarding abuse potential of stimulants, they should be reassured that when prescribed appropriately, the risk is minimal, whereas untreated ADHD in adolescents increases risk of substance use (self-medication).
4. The final decision for pharmacological treatment is always left to family. Provider can educate and make recommendations, but they should not feel pressure from provider/school/extended family.
5. Be aware of cultural differences in recognizing and treating symptoms of ADHD.

ADHD Treatment

ADHD treatment (shown in Box 16.2) can be approached in a few ways; research has shown that the combination of therapy and pharmaceutical intervention tends to be most effective. The child's past medical history, age, symptom presentation, and family preferences all play important roles in the way management is approached.

As a very broad overview, these are the major nonpharmaceutical and pharmaceutical interventions that are typically recommended:

Nonpharmaceutical Interventions

- Cognitive behavioral therapy for the child
- Parent training for behavioral management
- Classroom accommodations (504 Plan, or IEP if child qualifies through school evaluation)
  - Examples of accommodations include extended time for testing/assignments, reduced homework demands, ability to keep study materials in class, and access to notes from the teacher.

BOX 16.2 AGE-BASED RECOMMENDATIONS FOR ADHD

Ages 4–6 years
- Parent Training Behavior Management
- Classroom accommodations
- Methylphenidate may be considered if other interventions are not successful
  - Guidelines for consideration of methylphenidate in this age group:
    - Symptoms persisting for at least 9 months
    - Dysfunction manifesting in both home and other settings
    - Has not responded adequately to Parent Training Behavior Management

Ages 6–12 years
- FDA-approved medications for ADHD with child/family agreement
- Behavioral interventions
- Educational interventions and individualized instructional supports (504 or IEP)

Ages 12–18 years
- FDA-approved medications for ADHD with child/family agreement
  - Assess for risk of substance abuse prior to initiating medication. If substance use identified, refer patient to subspecialist for support and guidance
- Training or behavioral interventions if available
- Educational interventions and individualized instructional supports (504 or IEP)

ADHD, attention deficit hyperactivity disorder; FDA, Food and Drug Administration.

Source: Data from Wolraich, M. L., Hagan, J. F., Allan, C., Chan, E., Davidson, D., Earls, M., . . . Zurhellen, W. (2019). Clinical practice guidelines in the treatment of ADHD. *Pediatrics, 144*(4). doi:10.1542/peds.2019-252

Pharmaceutical Interventions

- Nonstimulant medications—these tend to be more beneficial for children who are more hyperactive and are not as helpful for focus:
  - Guanfacine (Intuniv), atomoxetine (Strattera), clonidine (Kapvay)
- Stimulant medications (as shown in Box 16.3):
  - Methylphenidate and derivatives: Ritalin, Metadate CD, Concerta, Focalin/Focalin XR, Quillivant, Daytrana Patch
  - Amphetamine and derivatives: Adderall/Adderall XR, Vyvanse

Medication Considerations

Currently, there is no way to predict which medication will be most effective for a patient. Pharmacogenetic tools are not recommended due to lack of sufficient testing and reliability. The type of ADHD (hyperactive, inattentive, or combination) does not impact stimulant choice.

Before starting a stimulant medication, it is important to ensure there is not a significantly increased risk for cardiac problems in the child. To do this:

- Gather the patient's medical history.
- Gather family history for sudden death, cardiovascular symptoms, Wolff–Parkinson–White syndrome, hypertrophic cardiomyopathy, long QT syndrome.
- If any risk factors are present, an EKG should be done, and if EKG is abnormal, then a referral to a cardiologist should be made before starting medication.

Risk versus benefit of medication use should be considered and discussed with the family. Common side effects should be reviewed and are outlined in the following:

BOX 16.3 MEDICATIONS USED IN TREATMENT OF ADHD

Methylphenidate

    Short-acting (4–6 hr)—often used as initial treatment in children <6 years old
        Methylphenidate/Ritalin
        Focalin
        Methylin chewable or liquid

    Intermediate (6–8 hr)
        Ritalin LA
        Metadate CD

    Long-acting
        Focalin XR (8–10 hr)
        Concerta (10–12 hr)
        Quillivant XR (10–12 hr)
        Daytrana Patch (9–10 hr, or shorter depending how long patch is worn)

Amphetamine
    Short-acting (4–6 hr)
        Adderall
    Long-acting
        Adderall XR (8–10 hr)
        Vyvanse (10+ hr)

Nonstimulant Medications (all are long acting)
    Intuniv
    Kapvay
    Strattera

ADHD, attention deficit hyperactivity disorder.

Common Side Effects of Stimulants

- Decreased appetite
- Abdominal pain
- Headaches
- Sleep disturbance (most commonly difficulty falling asleep)
- Mood change/irritability
- Growth velocity changes are minimal—studies have shown diminished growth of 1 to 2 cm from predicted adult height
- Mild increase in heart rate and blood pressure, typically not clinically significant, but these measurements should be monitored
- Rare: hallucinations or other psychotic symptoms

Side Effects of Nonstimulants

- Guanfacine (Intuniv) and clonidine (Kapvay)
  - Common: decreased heart rate (HR) and blood pressure (BP), fatigue, dry mouth, dizziness, irritability, headache, abdominal pain
  - Medications should be tapered when discontinued to avoid rebound hypertension
- Atomoxetine (Strattera)
  - Common: increased HR and BP, fatigue, gastrointestinal upset, decreased appetite
  - The Food and Drug Administration (FDA) black-box warning for suicidal thoughts

- Growth delays in the first 1 to 2 years of treatment, with return to expected measurements after 2 to 3 years of treatment
- Rare: hepatitis

Medications

The stimulant medications are broken up into two major groups: methylphenidate (Ritalin) and amphetamine (Adderall). Within these two categories, there are multiple different options. In general, amphetamine agents are slightly more effective, but methylphenidates are better tolerated.

A combination of stimulants and nonstimulants can be used for 24-hour coverage while optimizing focus at school. Short-acting doses may be added to long-acting forms to provide adequate coverage for afternoon/evening (often called a booster dose).

What If a Child Cannot Swallow Pills?

The following medications come in a capsule that can be opened/sprinkled:

- Focalin XR
- Ritalin LA
- Metadate CD
- Adderall XR

The following medications are available in liquid/chewable/patch form:

- Quillivant XR (liquid)
- Methylin solution (liquid)
- Methylin chewable
- Daytrana Patch

Therapies that are *not* proven effective by research at this point, although anecdotal evidence exists:

- Omega 3/fish oil
- Diet modifications
- Cannabidiol (CBD) oil
- EEG biofeedback
- Mindfulness
- Supportive counseling
- Cognitive training
- External trigeminal nerve stimulation

Follow-Up

Close follow-up within 1 to 2 weeks is recommended after starting a new medication or after a dose change. Dose titration can be done every 1 to 2 weeks as needed. This could be by phone if you and family agree. Follow-up visit after medication initiation should be within 2 to 3 months. Once stable on a medication dose, follow-up every 3 to 6 months is reasonable depending on response and comorbidities.

Regardless of treatment choice (pharmacological and nonpharmacological), there should be ongoing monitoring of ADHD symptoms, adverse effects of medication, and impact on functioning.

CHILD MALTREATMENT

Child abuse and neglect takes on several forms. The main types of child abuse include physical, emotional, sexual abuse, and neglect. Injuries intentionally perpetrated by a caretaker that result in morbidity or mortality constituting physical abuse. Sexual abuse is defined as the involvement of a child in any activity meant to provide sexual gratification to an adult. Failure to provide a child with appropriate food, clothing, medical care, schooling, and a safe environment constitutes neglect.

Etiology

Nearly 700,000 children are abused in the United States each year. The youngest children were the most vulnerable; children less than 1 year of age had the highest rate of abuse and neglect with a rate of 24.2 per 1,000 children. About four out of five abusers were parents.

Epidemiology/Risk Factors

Despite the fact that child abuse and neglect occurs at all socioeconomic levels, it is more prevalent among certain populations or at-risk groups. Included in these at-risk groups are families with children with special healthcare needs (chronic illness, prematurity, etc.), families of children less than 1 year of age, children with caretakers who have themselves been abused or who have unrealistic parental expectations, or children of parents who are under significant stress or have a history of illicit drug abuse in the home and/or mental health issues.

Symptoms

Depends on the area/system of suspected abuse and neglect (see Differentials section).

Focused Physical Exam Signs/Findings

Physical exam depends on the area of suspected abuse and neglect, but red flags for abuse and neglect can include the following:

- Fractures in children less than 1 year of age
- Multiple fractures in different stages of healing
- Cuts and bruises in low trauma areas, such as the buttocks or back, are more suspect of abuse
- Injuries such as cuts or burns in patterns over the body

Red flags for possible child abuse and neglect include the following:

- When the history of present illness and the injury do not match up (for example, if a child rolls off of a couch and sustains a traumatic brain injury)

Most cases of suspected abuse are subsequently substantiated by child protective services.

Lab Tests/Diagnostics

Lab tests including a CBC with differential to show any hematologic abnormalities should be conducted. In addition, other organic causes of disease, including metabolic disorders and musculoskeletal and skin abnormalities, should be ruled out. Children less than 2 years old with musculoskeletal injuries (fractures) should have a skeletal survey to look for previous fractures or fracture in different stages of healing.

Differentials

The differential diagnosis depends on the type of injury, the age of the child, and the signs and symptoms. Differentials for child abuse and neglect by system include the following:

Hematologic Abnormalities

- Congenital dermal melanocytosis (Mongolian spots)
- Accidental bruises
- Hemangiomas
- Immune thrombocytopenic purpura (ITP)
- Henoch–Schönlein purpura (HSP)
- Petechiae or subconjunctival hemorrhage from vomiting or coughing
- Insect bites
- Bleeding disorder (congenital or acquired)
- Birth trauma
- Hemophilia
- Malignancy
- Erythema multiforme
- Alternative healing practices (i.e., coining, cupping)

Musculoskeletal–Related Abnormalities

- Accidental fractures
- Malignancy
- Osteogenesis imperfecta
- Rickets
- Osteomyelitis
- Bone fragility with chronic disease
- Scurvy
- Congenital syphilis
- Birth trauma
- Osteopenia

Skin/Burn–Related Injuries

- Accidental burns
- Impetigo
- Alternative healing practices (e.g., coining, cupping)
- Atopic dermatitis
- Inflammatory conditions of the skin
- Sunburn
- Contact dermatitis

Don't Miss

As the pediatric APC, remain nonjudgmental of the family/caretaker.

Document, document, document! Take pictures of suspected physical abuse for documentation.

History and PE being inconsistent and/or any delay in seeking medical treatment are key points for child abuse and neglect.

Treatment

The pediatric APC is a mandated reporter and should report any suspected child abuse and neglect. This means the first priority is creating a safe environment for the child, which begins with reporting suspected abuse to social services and/or law enforcement.

Prevention

Prevention of child abuse and neglect focuses on enhancing parental abilities and strengthening families who may be at increased risk of abuse and neglect.

- The National Association of Pediatric Nurse Practitioners issued a position statement supporting the development and implementation of maltreatment screening and ultimately supporting the concept that APCs should be involved in child abuse prevention.

Follow-Up/Patient/Family Education

Interventions that have been shown to decrease child abuse include the following:

- Parenting programs
- CBT
- Parent–child interaction therapy
- Child behavioral management programs
- Home visitation programs
- Peer support groups (Caneira & Myrick, 2015)

LOW MOOD/DEPRESSION

Etiology

Low mood (dysthymia) in adolescents (11 to 19 years old) is common. Estimates for depressive disorders suggest that 10 to 14% of adolescents have a mental health problem that impacts on function, with anxiety and depression being the leading conditions. Prevalence of a diagnosed depressive disorder is reported to lie between 1% and 6%. Unipolar major depression (major depressive disorder) is characterized by a history of one or more major depressive episodes in the absence of manic and hypomanic episodes. These differences are highlighted in Table 16.1. The severity of depression is often classified as mild, moderate, or severe. Mild to moderate depression is indicated by a score of less than 20 points on the self-report Patient Health Questionnaire (a nine-item survey [PHQ-9]; Spitzer, Williams, & Kroenke, 2019), whereas severe depression is greater than 20 points.

Epidemiology/Risk Factors

- Certain personality traits, such as low self-esteem and being too dependent, self-critical, or pessimistic
- Traumatic or stressful events, such as physical or sexual abuse
- Blood relatives with a history of depression, bipolar disorder, alcoholism, or suicide
- Being lesbian, gay, bisexual, or transgender
- History of other mental health disorders, such as anxiety disorder, eating disorders, or posttraumatic stress disorder
- Serious or chronic illness, including cancer, stroke, chronic pain, or heart disease

Table 16.1

Common Symptoms of Low Mood Versus Depression	
Low Mood	**Depressive Symptoms**
Sadness	Low mood lasting 2 weeks or longer
Feeling anxious or panicky	Not getting enjoyment out of life
Worry	Feeling hopeless
Tiredness	Appetite changes, or weight gain or loss
Low self-esteem	Trouble going to sleep or staying asleep, or sleeping too much
Frustration and anger	Fatigue or lack of energy
**A low mood tends to lift after	Feeling restless, irritable, or withdrawn
several days to weeks	Feeling worthless, hopeless, discouraged, or guilty
	Trouble concentrating, remembering things, doing daily tasks, or making decisions
	Thoughts of self-harm or suicide

Symptoms

See Table 16.1 for common symptoms of of low mood and depression.

Focused PE Signs/Findings

While children may not verbalize feeling depressed, they may exhibit irritability, temper tantrums, and mood lability and/or become easily frustrated, whereas adolescents may exhibit hypersomnia, decreased appetite, and weight loss.

Differentials

Unipolar major depression should be differentiated from low mood disorder. Depressed children and adolescents must be evaluated for suicide risk. In addition, depression in the pediatric patient is commonly a precursor to bipolar disorder. Other conditions on the differential can also be comorbid symptoms and include ADHD, anxiety, posttraumatic stress disorder, substance abuse disorder, and sleep disorders. The history should help to differentiate comorbid symptoms of depression from depression or low mood diagnosis.

Don't Miss

Indications for referral include uncertainty about the diagnosis of depression, discomfort managing depression in the pediatric patient, or, if the patient has suicidal ideation or homicidal behavior, the inability of the family to care for the child's safety, psychotic manifestations (i.e., delusions and/or hallucinations), recurrent and/or chronic depression, and/or acute comorbid disorders (i.e., conduct disorder, eating disorders, substance use disorders, bipolar depression; Cheung, Kozloff, & Sacks, 2013).

Treatment

Following screening for, and identification and assessment of, low mood or depression, APCs should provide general initial management (see Table 16.2). Standard treatment options for pediatric depression include psychotherapy, pharmacotherapy, or a combination of the two. For children with acute depression or moderate to severe depression, pharmacotherapy plus psychotherapy are initial treatment approaches, typically an

Table 16.2

Evidence-Based Interventions That Can Be Applied by a Primary Care APC	
Presenting problem area	Most common evidence-based practice interventions
Anxiety	Graded exposure, modeling
ADHD and oppositional problems	Tangible rewards, praise for child and parent, help with monitoring, time-out, effective commands and limit setting, response cost
Depression or low mood	Cognitive/coping methods, problem-solving strategies, activity scheduling, behavioral rehearsal, social skills building

ADHD, attention deficit hyperactivity disorder; APC, advanced practicing clinician.

Source: Wissow, L. S., Van Ginneken, N., Chandna, J., & Rahman, J. (2016). Integrating children's mental health into primary care. *Pediatric Clinics of North America, 63*(1), 97–113. doi:10.1016/j.pcl.2015.08.005

SSRI (i.e., fluoxetine) plus CBT. Once pharmacotherapy is initiated, treatment should be continued for the next 6 to 12 months before being discontinued. It is reasonable to treat with pharmacotherapy alone if other mental health services such as CBT are not available or patient declines this intervention. Furthermore, adolescents with mild depression can be managed with active support, and symptom monitoring may involve a referral to mental healthcare specialist. Pharmacotherapy may be associated with adverse events, including an increased risk of suicidal thoughts or behaviors (Cheung et al., 2013).

Prevention

There is no way to prevent depression; however, steps can be taken to help prevent depressive symptoms such as controlling stress and encouraging patients and families to get treatment at the earliest sign of a problem.

Follow-Up/Patient/Family Education

- Depression in children and adolescents can be safely and effectively treated. Psychological treatments and medication therapy can help with symptoms and help children and adolescents succeed in school and feel more confident.
- Although it is not clear that antidepressants cause suicide in children and adolescents, it is clear that depression can cause suicide.

SUMMARY

In summary, as pediatric APCs, it is critical to be appraised of the most common presenting problems to pediatric primary care in order to be effective at addressing the gap in mental health services. This is accomplished in several ways: (a) in being a gateway to specialty services and/or being part of a safety net; (b) in identifying and helping families who fall out of the specialized mental health system for one reason or another; and (c) by providing early intervention services and catching things before they get worse.

References

American Psychiatric Association. (2013). *Diagnostic and statistical manual of mental disorders* (5th ed.). Washington, DC: Author.

Caneira, L., & Myrick, K. (2015). Diagnosing child abuse: The role of the nurse practitioner. *Journal of Nurse Practitioners, 11*, 640–646. doi:10.1016/j.nurpra.2015.03.017

Cheung, A. H., Kozloff, N., & Sacks, D. (2013). Pediatric depression: An evidence-based update on treatment interventions. *Current Psychiatry Reports, 15*(8), 381. doi:10.1007/s11920-013-0381-4

Kozlowski, J., Lusk, P., & Melnyk, B. (2015). PNP management of anxiety in a rural primary care clinic with the EBP COPE program. *Journal of Pediatric Health Care, 29*, 274–282. doi:10.1016/j.pedhc.2015.01.009

Spitzer, R. L., Williams, J., & Kroenke, K. (2019). *PHQ: Patient health questionnaire (Modified from PHQ)* [Unpublished instrument]. Retrieved from https://www.evidencio.com/models/show/550

Wissow, L. S., Van Ginneken, N., Chandna, J., & Rahman, J. (2016). Integrating children's mental health into primary care. *Pediatric Clinics of North America, 63*(1), 97–113. doi:10.1016/j.pcl.2015.08.005

Wolraich, M. L., Hagan, J. F., Allan, C., Chan, E., Davidson, D., Earls, M., . . . Zurhellen, W. (2019). Clinical practice guidelines in the treatment of ADHD. *Pediatrics, 144*(4). doi:10.1542/peds.2019-252

17

Common Genetic Disorders Seen in Pediatric Primary Care

Leah Hecht and Sharon Lincoln

INTRODUCTION

The landscape of genetics and genetic testing is continuously evolving. The human body has about 20,000 different genes in each cell. Genes are located on chromosomes; each cell has 46 chromosomes grouped into 23 pairs. Each gene has a specific function. Aberrations in the genes or chromosomes can express themselves as various congenital abnormalities, which present as specific birth defects. The pediatric advanced practicing clinician (APC) is ever more involved with the ordering of genetic testing and discussing genetic testing results with families. Given the changes over time, the APC may not be familiar with available tests or their specific indications, which are included in this chapter.

The purpose of this chapter is to provide an overview of common abnormal findings that are seen in the pediatric primary care setting and to guide the approach to care around what may or may not warrant genetic testing and/or a referral to a genetics clinic.

OBJECTIVES

1. Identify common abnormal genetic findings often seen in pediatric primary care.
2. Guide the approach to care around what may or may not warrant genetic testing and/ or a referral to a genetics clinic.
3. Understand the most common types of genetic inheritance.
4. Understand the role genetics plays in the workup of the most common genetic disorders (including intellectual disabilities, autism, fragile X syndrome [FXS], and hereditary cancer syndromes).

CHROMOSOME ABNORMALITIES

Chromosome abnormalities in the baby may be inherited from the parent or may occur with no family history. These are the most common types of genetic inheritance (see Box 17.1).

BOX 17.1 THE FOUR DIFFERENT TYPES OF GENETIC INHERITANCE

1. Single gene is mutated (mutation can be dominant, recessive, or X linked).

2. Multiple genes are mutated.

3. Chromosomal changes—entire areas of the chromosome can be missing or misplaced.

4. Mitochondrial—the maternal genetic material in mitochondria can mutate as well.

BOX 17.2 MOST COMMON EXAMPLES OF SINGLE-GENE DEFECTS

Dominant

This means the abnormality occurs when only one of the genes from one parent is abnormal. If the parent has the disorder, the baby has a one in two chance of inheriting it. Examples include the following:

Achondroplasia: This is a bone development disorder that causes dwarfism.

Marfan syndrome: This is a connective tissue disorder that causes long limbs and heart defects.

Recessive

This means the abnormality only occurs when both parents have a copy of an abnormal gene. If both parents are carriers, a baby has a one in four chance of having the disorder. Examples include the following:

Cystic fibrosis: This is a disorder of the glands that causes excess mucus in the lungs. It also causes problems with how the pancreas works and with how food is absorbed.

Sickle cell disease: This condition causes abnormal red blood cells that do not carry oxygen normally.

Tay-Sachs disease: This is an inherited condition that causes the central nervous system to decline. The condition is fatal, usually by age 5.

X-linked

The disorder is determined by genes on the X chromosome. Males are mainly affected and have the disorder. Daughters of men with the disorder are carriers of the trait and have a one in two chance of passing it to their children. Sons of women who are carriers each have a one in two chance of having the disorder. Examples include the following:

Duchenne muscular dystrophy: This is a disease that causes muscle wasting.

Hemophilia: This is a bleeding disorder caused by low levels or lack of a blood protein that is needed for clotting.

A change in a single gene causes a defect or abnormality. Single-gene changes usually have a higher risk of being passed on to children. Single-gene changes can include those in Box 17.2.

DEVELOPMENTAL DELAYS/INTELLECTUAL DISABILITIES/AUTISM SPECTRUM DISORDER

Developmental issues are one of the most common referral reasons, and there are guidelines from multiple organizations, including the American Association of Pediatrics (AAP), which state that chromosomal microarray analysis is a first-tier test for any child with developmental delay, intellectual disability, and/or autism spectrum disorder (Committee on Bioethics, Committee on Genetics, American College of Medical Genetics, and Genomics Social, Ethical, and Legal Issues Committee, 2013). Fragile X testing is also considered a first-tier test for both genders (Oud, Lamers, Arts, & Ciliopathies, 2017).

Chromosomal microarray analysis is a test that looks primarily for deletions and duplications across the genome. Historically, microarrays were targeted and evaluated primarily only those chromosome regions known to be associated with a genetic condition. Arrays are now genome-wide, meaning they can detect deletions and duplications across the genome. Due to the differences in array technology, as well as the discovery of new syndromic deletions/duplications, if a patient had an array over 10 years ago, it may be worthwhile repeating.

In addition to detecting deletions and duplications, current microarrays are also able to detect areas of homozygosity (AOH). Usually, the sequence of gene and nongene regions of DNA on the chromosome differs slightly from one another. This is completely normal and is called heterozygosity. When the genes/chromosomes appear the same, however, it is called homozygosity. An area of homozygosity in and of itself is not an abnormal finding and can be seen when parents are related, are of the same ethnic origin, or are from the same small geographic region. AOH can be relevant if there is an autosomal recessive gene located in the area. This is because if a variant is present in one copy of the gene, it will automatically be present in both copies of the gene (because the sequence of the genes is the same on both copies of the chromosome due to the homozygosity).

There are three broad types of results for microarrays: normal/negative, abnormal/positive, and variant of uncertain significance. As with all genetic tests, a normal result does not rule out a genetic condition. Variants of uncertain significance (VUS) are relatively common and can cause quite a lot of undue concern for families. A VUS simply means there is not enough data in the literature or databases to know whether the finding is pathogenic or benign. Parental testing may be helpful in some situations, but even with those results, our interpretation of the variant often does not change.

Another important point for microarrays is the possibility of detecting incidental findings, such as adult-onset disorders or cancer predisposition syndromes. Incidental findings are not common (less than 1%) but have a very high impact on the patient and possibly the family.

Fragile X testing is also considered first-tier testing for individuals with developmental delay, intellectual disability, and/or autism spectrum disorder. FXS is most commonly caused by a triplet repeat expansion. Because the fragile X gene (FMR1) is located on the X chromosome, there are different implications for males and females with the full mutation.

Males with the full mutation will nearly always have FXS. The range for females is much broader and can range from apparently unaffected, social, or generalized anxiety, sensory integration issues, significant learning disabilities, and as affected as the males. Due to this significant range, females are often not tested or are tested significantly later than males, even in the setting of a family history of FXS. Although there is no specific treatment for FXS, there is a very good understanding of the neurodevelopmental profile, and earlier intervention targeting this profile may lead to better outcomes.

In addition to the full mutation, there are implications associated with the premutation. Approximately 20% of women with a premutation will experience fragile X-associated primary ovarian insufficiency (FXPOI). FXPOI is characterized by early menopause, defined as by or before the age of 40 years. Females with a premutation may have diminished ovarian reserves even if they do not have FXPOI, leading to fertility issues. In addition, both males and females with a premutation are at risk for fragile X-associated tremor/ataxia syndrome (FXTAS). Onset is typically not until the sixth decade of life and is characterized by tremors, ataxia, mood disorder, neuropathy, and cognitive decline.

There is a possibility of mosaicism in individuals with FXS. There are two types of mosaicism in FXS. Although individuals with mosaicism may have a milder presentation, this is not universal, and individuals with mosaicism can be as affected as those without mosaicism. As such, additional testing depending on other physical findings and/or severity of developmental delays may be warranted.

HEREDITARY CANCER SYNDROMES

It is relatively common to receive referrals for a known cancer history in the family. There are very few cancer predisposition syndromes that would be tested for in the pediatric setting. In general, if the condition has an adult onset, such as hereditary breast and ovarian cancer caused by BRCA1 and BRCA2 and Lynch syndrome, it is not recommended to test the child until they are of legal age (Oud et al., 2017). If there can be a pediatric onset, such as with familial adenomatous polyposis or MEN1/MEN2, genetic testing may be indicated depending on the age of the child.

It is important to keep in mind that if a family member other than a sibling or parent has a genetic diagnosis of a cancer predisposition syndrome, a first-degree relative of the patient should be tested first. For example, if the maternal aunt has a BRCA1 mutation, the patient's mother should be tested before testing the child. This applies for both adult-onset and pediatric-onset disorders.

If there are questions as to whether a referral is appropriate, we would encourage reaching out to the local genetics' clinic or a cancer genetic counselor.

HYPERMOBILITY

Hypermobility and joint laxity are becoming very common referral reasons to genetics clinics. In the past, any individual with hypermobility was lumped under the diagnosis of hypermobile Ehlers–Danlos syndrome (EDS). Within the past couple of years, there have been updated diagnostic criteria for hypermobile EDS. The new criteria require additional findings, including but not limited to abnormal skin findings, positive family history, chronic joint pain, and exclusion of other connective tissue disorder etiologies (Committee on Bioethics et al., 2013).

An important part of the diagnostic process is an echocardiogram and ophthalmology evaluation looking specifically for findings seen in connective tissue disorders. If a referral to genetics is going to be made, we would encourage these evaluations be performed prior to the genetics visit. It is important to note that genetics are involved in the diagnostic process of hypermobility and connective tissue disorders, but not in the management. Management includes joint protection, physical therapy, and pain management. Contact sports are strongly discouraged given the risk for injury.

MULTIPLE CONGENITAL ANOMALIES

Congenital anomalies are common. Many individual anomalies have an incidence of at least 1/1000, and the overall risk for each pregnancy is 3% to 4%. It is difficult to recommend a single genetic test when an infant has one or multiple congenital anomalies, and it is important to realize that a congenital anomaly (even a severe one) can be isolated and not part of a larger genetic syndrome. In general, many genetic practices will recommend a chromosomal microarray analysis as a baseline test, unless there is high suspicion for one specific condition.

Noninvasive prenatal screening (NIPS) via cell-free fetal DNA is becoming more and more common. This can be a way that a diagnosis of a syndrome with multiple congenital anomalies is diagnosed.

NEWBORN SCREENING

The process of newborn screening (NBS) is an incredibly complex yet simple tool used around the world to identify rare diseases in the neonatal period, with the aim of preventing or slowing the progression of what otherwise would often be devastating conditions.

There has been a continuously increasing number of conditions included within NBS tests. There are currently more than 30 disorders screened for on NBS in the United States; however, the exact number of tests on each screening varies from state to state. Many states have active pilot screening programs in place for potential candidate tests to be added.

The pediatric APC may potentially be the first to discuss the many possible indications of an abnormal screening result to the family. When the office is notified of an abnormal NBS result, they will also receive an ACT sheet, outlining basic information pertaining to the flagged result along with a list of local referral centers.

We hope to provide some guidance around the pediatric APC's approach to a positive result within the increasingly lengthy NBS panels.

Key Points

1. NBS is not a diagnostic test.
2. An abnormal NBS result requires referral to a genetic or metabolic specialist for confirmatory diagnostic testing, which may find the following:
   a. Neonate is a carrier for a condition.
   b. Neonate has mild to severe form of a condition.
   c. Screening was a false-positive result.
   d. Screening found to be secondary to primary maternal condition, requiring mother undergo further diagnostic testing.
3. A normal repeat NBS result does not negate the need to at least speak with the genetics specialist to determine if any next steps are needed.
4. The differential diagnoses for abnormal NBS results are increasingly complex as testing is expanded and molecular analysis is more often included. This complexity may often require more detailed genetic analysis to confirm a diagnosis, or it may be that the diagnosis remains unclear, despite further testing. The latter group of individuals will require ongoing follow-up with the specialist due to this uncertainty.
5. Ultimately, it is important to communicate both with the caretaker/parent of your patient and with specialist teams and refer the child to a geneticist to assure that the family receives appropriate and timely education and intervention.

SHORT AND TALL STATURE

As with congenital anomalies, genetic testing recommendations for stature anomalies can be difficult. There are many reasons a child may have short or tall stature, one of the most common being parental height. Another cause for short stature can be nutrition.

Disproportionate short stature may be more likely to have a genetic component than proportionate short stature, which may be more likely due to an underlying endocrinologic or nutritional issue.

Tall stature alone is not an indication to refer to genetics. As with short stature, it is important to keep in mind parental height. However, if there are other findings, such as congenital anomalies or connective tissue disorder symptoms, it may be reasonable to refer to genetics.

RESOURCES AND IMPORTANT CONSIDERATIONS

Additional resources for APCs practicing in pediatrics include the following:

1. *GeneReviews* has detailed reviews about genetic and metabolic disorders that include the natural history of the disorder, medical management guidelines, and information about risks to family members.
2. Unique is a support organization based in the United Kingdom for rare chromosome disorders.
   i. It has pamphlets on many different disorders, which include literature reviews, information from its own dataset, and parent/family testimonies. These pamphlets are family-friendly, and although Unique is based in the United Kingdom, many of its members are from the United States.

There are several situations where genetic testing may be indicated and pursued in the pediatric primary care setting. Pediatric APCs are uniquely situated to provide first-tier testing to their patients. This is particularly the case in settings where the wait time for a genetics appointment is 6 months or more.

Important considerations when ordering genetic testing include:

- As the pediatric APC, making a chart of the family history can help show risks for certain problems.
- Many insurance companies require prior authorization for genetic testing. Some companies are starting to require genetic counseling prior to ordering testing, which limits the ability for pediatric primary care offices to order testing.
- Genetic tests can be quite expensive, and even if testing is covered, patients may still have out-of-pocket costs due to deductibles, copays, or coinsurance. It is important to have this discussion prior to ordering any testing.
- If genetic testing is ordered, it is essential that the ordering provider be able to interpret and provide information about the results.
- There are companies now providing telemedicine consults for genetics, and this may be an option to consider for your patients in instances where wait times for appointments are extremely long.
- Genetic testing continues to advance. Whole exome sequencing is becoming a more common first-tier test in many situations, although, due to the complexities of this testing, it has not made its way into the primary care setting yet.
- As there continues to be a move toward personalized and precision medicine, genetics will play a larger and larger role in the pediatric primary care setting.

References

Committee on Bioethics, Committee on Genetics, American College of Medical Genetics, and Genomics Social, Ethical, and Legal Issues Committee. (2013). Ethical and policy issues in genetic testing and screening of children. *Pediatrics, 131*(3), 620–622. doi:10.1542/peds.2012-3680

Oud, M., Lamers, I. J., Arts, H. H., & Ciliopathies, G. (2017). Genetics in pediatric medicine. *Journal of Pediatric Genetics, 6*(1), 18–29. doi:10.1055/s-0036-1593841

III

Point-of-Care Testing

18

Point-of-Care Testing in Pediatric Primary Care

Kristine M. Ruggiero

INTRODUCTION

Point-of-care tests (POCTs) (shown in Table 18.1) are being used more often in pediatric practices to facilitate clinical decision-making, including regarding the screening and monitoring of a variety of pediatric conditions. POCT is testing that occurs at the time of the patient encounter, and results are known before the end of the encounter. There are many conditions for which POCTs can be used; however, time, accuracy, and cost are some of the considerations practitioners must consider when using POCTs.

Some of the more beneficial and commonly used POCTs and procedures of pediatric primary care will be reviewed in this chapter. POCTs can help practitioners identify, diagnose, monitor, and treat conditions such as diabetes mellitus, sexually transmitted infections (STIs), pharyngitis, and respiratory tract infections.

Table 18.1

Common Point-of-Care Tests Used in Pediatric Primary Care				
Diagnosis	**Screening for**	**Method**	**Background for Test**	**Sensitivity and Specificity of Test**
Bacterial pharyngitis (strep throat)	GAS	RSAT	A throat culture or strep test is performed by using a throat swab to detect the presence of GAS bacteria (most common reason for strep throat). This bacterium can cause strep throat, scarlet fever, and rheumatic fever.	**Rapid** tests for **strep** throat have a high specificity (98–99%), meaning there are very few false positives. They have a rather low sensitivity, around (90–95%), meaning there are more false negatives. The sensitivity is higher in pediatrics than adults.
Mononucleosis	EBV	Rapid heterophile antibody test, aka the Monospot, tests for heterophile antibodies that are produced by the immune system in response to the EBV infection	Viral, often self-limiting infection, presenting with swollen lymph nodes, sore throat, and fever.	Literature shows decreased sensitivity in patients <13 years of age. Also, many patients do not produce heterophile antibodies; therefore a negative heterophile does not rule out infectious mono and should be followed up with EBV-specific serologies if clinically suspected.
Trichomonas	Motile protozoan parasite called *Trichomonas vaginalis*	OSOM Trichomonas Test	Aka Trich is a nonviral STI affecting the vagina and/or urethra causing symptomatic vaginitis; very common and curable; often underdiagnosed.	95% agreement compared with combined testing method of microscopy and culture.
Flu	Influenza A and B	PCR test (the cobas® Liat® Influenza A/B assay) for the diagnosis of influenza detects viral RNA A NP swab is used to collect a respiratory secretion sample from patients with suspected influenza.	Various types of POCTs result. Rapid, accurate screening can help reduce the unnecessary use of antibiotics that may result from incorrectly diagnosing a patient with a bacterial infection based on symptoms alone.	

(continued)

Table 18.1

Common Point-of-Care Tests Used in Pediatric Primary Care (continued)				
Diagnosis	Screening for	Method	Background for Test	Sensitivity and Specificity of Test
DM (type I or type II)	Elevated blood sugar.	Single use lancet is used to elicit a small drop of capillary blood usually from a finger tip (0.3–1 μL). This small drop of blood is then added to a single use reagent strip and read by a glucometer.	Test is appropriate for patients that present with symptoms of hyper- or hypoglycemia and also can be used as a monitoring for blood glucose control in diabetics.	Sensitivity and specificity varies between various brands of testing kit. However, most brands have been found to be accurate when compared to laboratory measurements.

DM, diabetes mellitus; EBV, Epstein–Barr virus; GAS, group A *Streptococcus*; NP, nasopharyngeal; PCR, polymerase chain reaction; POC, point-of-care; POCTs, point-of-care tests; RSAT, rapid streptococcal antigen test; STI, sexually transmitted infection.

*Sensitivity is the ability to correctly detect people who have the disease. Specificity is the ability to correctly identify people who do not have the disease.

Index

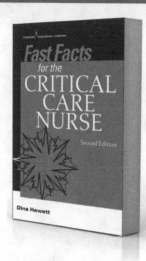
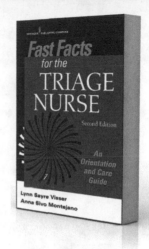
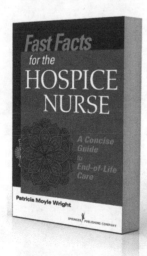
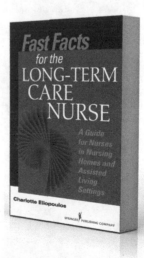

Printed in the United States
by Baker & Taylor Publisher Services